INVASION
– of the –
BODY

INVASION
– of the –
BODY

Revolutions in Surgery

NICHOLAS L. TILNEY

HARVARD UNIVERSITY PRESS

Cambridge, Massachusetts

London, England

2011

Santa Fe Springs City Library
11700 Telegraph Road
Santa Fe Springs, CA 90670

Copyright © 2011 by Nicholas L. Tilney

All rights reserved

Printed in the United States of America

Many of the designations used by manufacturers and sellers to distinguish their products are claimed as trademarks. Where those designations appear in this book and Harvard University Press was aware of a trademark claim, then the designations have been printed in initial capital letters.

Library of Congress Cataloging-in-Publication Data
Tilney, Nicholas L.
    Invasion of the body : revolutions in surgery / Nicholas L. Tilney.
        p. ; cm.
    Includes bibliographical references and index.
    ISBN 978-0-674-06228-3 (alk. paper)
    1. Surgery–History. 2. Surgery–History–20th Century. 3. Surgery–History–21st Century. I. Title
    [DNLM: 1. General Surgery–history. 2. History, 20th Century. 3. History, 21st Century. WO 11.1]
    RD19.T56 2011
    617–dc23   2011013287

To Michael J. Zinner, Surgeon-in-Chief of the
Brigham and Women's Hospital and Moseley
Professor at Harvard Medical School

CONTENTS

Introduction   1

1. Three Operations   7
2. The Teaching Hospital   35
3. Evolution of a Profession   52
4. Steps Forward and Steps Backward   75
5. War and Peace   97
6. The Promise of Surgical Research   128
7. Operations on the Heart   153
8. The Mechanical Heart   186
9. The Transfer of Organs   213
10. Making a Surgeon, Then and Now   240
11. Shifting Foundations   267
12. Unsolved Challenges   295

Notes   325

Acknowledgments   345

Index   347

INVASION
— *of the* —
BODY

The chirurgic art! Is it your fashion to put the masters of the science of medicine on a level with men who do carpentry on broken limbs, and sew up wounds like tailors, and carve away excrescences as a butcher trims meat? A manual art, such as any artificer might learn and which has been practiced by simple barbers.

–George Eliot

As art surgery is incomparable in the beauty of its medium, in the supreme mastery required for its perfect accomplishment, and in the issues of life, suffering and death which it so powerfully controls.

–Sir Berkley Moynihan

The concept that one citizen will lay himself horizontal and permit another to plunge a knife into him, take blood, give blood, rearrange internal structures at will, determine ultimate function, indeed, sometimes life itself–that responsibility is awesome both in the true, and in the currently debased, meaning of that word.

–Alexander Walt

Introduction

All of us grew up hearing that knives are dangerous. The accidental cuts and punctures we inevitably sustained as children intensified our ingrained fears of pain, bleeding, and infection. Even the word *knife* carried the potential of danger, mutilation, or death. The media buttressed this instinctive response with endless reports of the implement as a weapon, noting that crimes involving knives account for about one-fifth of the almost million aggravated assaults in the country every year. Despite such formative influences, however, some young doctors enthusiastically choose careers that allow the legal application of a razor-sharp scalpel to the body of a patient, an instrument of considerably more salutary connotation than a knife. Indeed, as the enduring symbol of surgery and of surgeons, the scalpel implies the gentle and precise dissection of tissues for the reconstruction of defects and deficiencies or the control of disease. In expert hands it can perform wonders. If used badly, catastrophe may result.

While most people do not consider surgery an agreeable subject of contemplation, it is of potential importance to all of us. An astonishing 85,000 elective operations are carried out in hospitals and clinics *each weekday* throughout the United States.[1] Emergency cases, particularly at night and on weekends, add to the total. This means statistically that every citizen will undergo over nine surgical procedures during his or her lifetime, a number of some consequence. Obviously, the knowledge, experience, and expertise of those who perform such operations are crucial in correcting or treating relevant problems as they arise.

When I was in high school, my older brother, a surgeon, invited me to watch him remove a football-sized cyst of the ovary. I immediately realized that the green drapes exposing only a portion of the lower abdomen of the patient neutralized much of any emotional response I might have had in witnessing the invasion of a body for the first time. Nevertheless, seeing the actual incision was too much. Heeding my brother's warning to "fall backward, away from the table" if I felt faint, I quickly left the room. It didn't take me long to regain my equilibrium and return. By the time he had closed the incision, I had become a convert. Still, I was nervous and tentative years later when, as a surgical house officer at the Peter Bent Brigham Hospital in Boston, I was instructed by the staff surgeon I was assisting to make an incision. I drew the blade gingerly across the skin. A scratch appeared. Exhorted to press harder, I incised too deeply. Blood from the underlying yellow fat and red abdominal muscles flooded the field. Sweating despite his coaching, I continued through the layers and finally entered the abdominal cavity.

I arrived at the Brigham, as it is known, in 1964, completed much of my training there, and joined its faculty nine years later. Renowned as an academic and educational center, this original teaching arm of Harvard Medical School received its first patient in 1913. It merged with two neighboring institutions in 1980 to form the Brigham and Women's Hospital, an internationally recognized force in patient care, specialty training, and research. It subsequently partnered with the Massachusetts General Hospital (MGH), the third oldest general hospital in the United States and Boston's first major medical institution, opening in 1811. Their partnership, despite previous decades of sometimes intense competition, has created an even more influential medical presence.

The 120 university-affiliated hospitals like the Brigham represent a potent force in health care in the United States. They are responsible not only for about 20 percent of patients in the country, but for upholding optimal medical practice, advancing the treatment of disease, producing biologic and technical innovations, applying scientific knowledge, and training future doctors. Innervated by the earlier introduction of anesthesia, asepsis, and the subsequent formulation of educational and professional standards, surgery in the twentieth century experienced a trajectory of growth and maturation that may never be repeated. These three seminal revolutions—anesthesia, asepsis, and the establishment of medical standards—were critical to the maturation of the modern field and its adjunctive disciplines. I describe the discovery and introduction of antibiotics, insulin, and modern pharmaceuticals as the fourth revolution, and discuss the unresolved current turmoil in medical education and reforms in health care as the fifth. As a result of these transformations and other emerging dynamics, modern surgery little resembles its counterpart of even a few decades ago. I portray high points and trends in surgical history with a broad brush for those perhaps unfamiliar with them, and depict some of the pioneers responsible for the advances. Because a more encyclopedic exposition would exceed both the stamina of the writer and the patience of the audience, I intersperse throughout the text various significant developments that have arisen in the department of surgery of a single teaching hospital of one major medical school as examples of and background for parallel progress in comparable academic institutions. Examples from my personal experience illustrate the types of challenges that surgeons everywhere may encounter during their careers.

Despite a deluge of information from an array of media sources, the subject of surgery, its indications, its contributions, and its related scientific achievements are outside of most people's knowledge until a medical crisis affects their lives. Many seem to take what happens for granted, even when they allow surgeons to remove their tumors, replace their joints, transplant their organs, and correct their heart disease. Indeed, in my own clinical experience, it has struck me forcefully how little the public and even the patients themselves want to know about what intrusive steps a relative stranger may take with their bodies, their well-being, and occasionally their lives.

My curiosity about this apparent general disinterest crystallized several years ago when I accompanied my wife, Mary, to a center for diseases of the eye. She had developed a cataract that interfered with her vision and had gone there electively for its removal and the implantation of an artificial corrective lens. Neither of us felt unduly nervous about the procedure or its outcome. We were well aware of the reputation of the surgeon and the statistically low risks. But it was still her eye! Patients, accompanied by relatives or friends, had already filled the waiting room by the time we arrived. On schedule, they disappeared one by one through a door into the operating room complex. Each emerged an hour later, wearing dark glasses and carrying a small pot of violets, presumably a reward for or remembrance of their experience. Looking around, they collected their companions and left for home. After the nurse called my wife, I began to look at the large television set at one side of the room on which the operations were shown live.

A cataract is an opacity of the lens that prevents clear vision. Normally transparent, the lens is elliptical in shape, about one-half inch in diameter and about one-quarter inch thick. It lies toward the front of the eye surrounded by clear gelatinous fluid that protects it. Images from the outside pass through the structure to stimulate the light-sensitive retinal cells at the back of the organ that mediate sight via impulses to the brain. When a cataract forms, the lens thickens, hardens, and loses its clarity. Although often a consequence of aging, the condition may occur as a result of injury, radiation, diabetes, or the use of steroids. It can also run in families; two of Mary's siblings developed the disorder at a relatively young age.

Intrepid practitioners in ancient times treated the cataracts of those desperate enough to allow them by pushing the clouded lens backward out of the line of vision with a probe or thin blade they inserted through the surface of the eye. They termed the procedure "couching" or "reclining." Eighteenth-century French surgeons introduced a method of cataract removal that remained routine until recent years. They made a half-inch incision through the transparent covering at the front of the eyeball. Via this aperture, they dissected the lens free from its surrounding fibers and removed it with a hook. After the procedure, thick magnifying glasses allowed some vision. Without anesthesia, the forbearance of those experiencing such treatment can only evoke awe. Even patients of a generation ago recall lying flat in bed for days after the operation, their heads held immobile with sandbags. Improvements since have been nothing short of extraordinary.

Mary's surgeon performs over forty cataract procedures two days a week on lightly anesthetized patients, supporting his hands on a stand of an operating microscope and manipulating the miniature instruments precisely. Fascinated, I watched the screen as he made an incision through the tough outside tissue of the eyeball about the size of the tip of a ball-point pen. He then pushed the tiny knife blade deeper into the eye to puncture the membranous covering of the opaque lens lying beneath, inserted a minute high-frequency probe into its substance to liquefy the abnormal tissue, and removed the remains with a micro-suction device. Under magnification, he slipped a new plastic lens already chosen to produce perfect vision into position. No sutures were necessary. His skill in executing each step flawlessly seemed, even for a surgeon such as me, almost miraculous. It did not escape my attention, however, that few of those sitting in the waiting room were watching. They coped with boredom and anxiety by chatting, reading magazines, or staring out the window. Some appeared bemused, even disgusted, as they occasionally glanced at the events on the screen.

An individual facing an elective operation may reflect on its rationale, intricacies, and risks, but an emergency situation requires the patient to accept unquestioningly what the surgeon deems necessary. My own memories of eye surgery, for instance, were very different from Mary's. It was late in the afternoon during a squash match during the early 1970s, before the use of safety goggles was common. My opponent, a surgical colleague, inadvertently hit me in the eye with his racquet while trying to retrieve a ball. I remember a hard blow. Although there wasn't much pain and I still had some vision, we both immediately realized that I had been severely injured. We hurried to the Brigham emergency room where he called the staff ophthalmologists (who also happened to be playing squash). They confirmed that my eyeball was badly torn. For four hours that night, they struggled to repair the long rent, intermittently sending messages of gloom to Mary and my daughters, who were waiting nearby. I recall nothing of the ultimately successful procedure but do remember weeks of wearing a black patch and enduring an intense and painful sensitivity to light in my other eye. I also recall vividly the removal of the sutures. The procedure was carried out under the bright magnification of a microscope, and I felt as if the instruments were boring into the center of my brain, deep into my very being. It was only then that I began to grasp that the accident could have ended my career, and that my colleagues, with their specialized skills, had saved my vision.

Although we may occasionally find detailed particulars of operations on cable television or the Internet, the usual descriptions of surgery come via popular dramas that draw the viewer's attention to dramatic human interactions and intense moments in which life, disability, or death are characterized in naked form. The better programs relate the actor-patient to his or her illness and accurately describe the background, development, and overall aims of the treatment. Most, however, concentrate more superficially on those working directly in the operating room, infrequently consider the less immediate concerns of the families, and do not dwell on the unseen presence of the third-party payers standing in the shadows behind, relentlessly urging more rapid turnover and shortcuts to reduce the costs. It is difficult for these media sketches to portray, except in cursory fashion, those involved in the surgical act or its sometimes far-reaching complexities and consequences for the individual lying on the table.

The story of surgery is incomplete if seen merely as the chronicle of surgeons and their craft. Four distinct but inexorably linked forces compose the broader picture. One is the professional who spends five or six years of general surgical residency after medical school, extended by additional years in specialty and laboratory training before entering practice. If she pursues a career in a university-affiliated institution, teaching and research are added to clinical responsibilities. The patient is the second and most important individual, presenting a variety of expectations, anxieties, and concerns with which caregivers must deal. Language barriers, class, cultural differences, and divergent value systems may compound effective communication with the doctor, an important reason for misinterpretations, misconceptions, and misunderstandings about a given condition and its treatment strategies. A third entity is the hospital or clinic in which the operation takes place. The resources of these complex centers include a bedazzling array of specialty physicians, nurses, and physician's assistants; laboratories and their technicians; social and food services; general administration and lawyers; public relations; educational facilities; and psychological and spiritual counseling. The expense of modern medical care has made health insurance and cost containment an omnipresent fourth part of the whole. These forces are the players in the story ahead.

— *one* —

Three Operations

Welcome to a representative surgical suite of my teaching hospital. Let us look at three procedures, each performed approximately a half-century apart from the others. These snapshots of surgery over the last one hundred years illuminate the respective differences in the surgeons and their skills, the facilities, the instruments, and those seeking help. The professional staff introduced here are real people. With the exception of Mrs. Turner and a few historical figures, I have changed the names of the patients, although their conditions and operations are as described. Their experiences represent events that occurred routinely in similar hospitals during the periods discussed.

Mary Agnes Turner was the first patient admitted to the newly completed Peter Bent Brigham Hospital in Boston on January 22, 1913. She was 45 years old. Following the birth of her first child, the veins in her legs, once fine blue traces beneath the skin, became progressively swollen and unsightly. They grew larger during each subsequent pregnancy. Then, as she became older and gained weight, the distended vessels became quite painful. Since her mother and two of her sisters suffered the same symptoms, her condition had genetic roots. It may have been exacerbated by the sustained time she spent on her feet as a servant and later caring for her family and her home. Indeed, as an upstairs maid in one of the great houses downtown, she toiled for long hours. As a result of these influences, her varicose veins had become so bothersome that she sought help.

She lived with her husband, employed as a laborer, and their five children on the top floor of a triple-decker frame house in a working-class neighborhood in the Roxbury section of the city. Her neighbors all lived in similar wooden buildings, one family to a floor. A nearby school, grocery store, Catholic church, and a couple of bars made up their world. Each day Mr. Turner took the electric trolley to work, where he was employed building new streets and houses. Although the family rarely ventured the three miles into Boston proper, they occasionally spent summer weekends picnicking and wading on beaches along the Charles River or those lining Boston Harbor.

The Peter Bent Brigham Hospital, a long, low structure housing 110 beds and sitting directly across the street from the newly constructed, marble-clad buildings of Harvard Medical School, was within walking distance of Mrs. Turner's house. The choice to seek help there was obvious despite the distrust of hospitals that she and her contemporaries had held for generations—that one only entered such institutions to die, particularly if one was poor. The affluent who lived comfortably downtown on Beacon Hill and in the Back Bay would never have considered patronizing such a place. They preferred to undergo their surgery at home or in private clinics. They also expected their surgeons to visit their houses to monitor their postoperative recovery. Only on rare occasions did they enter the nearby MGH. Because Mrs. Turner could not have afforded any type of private treatment, the newly completed Brigham, a charitable institution dedicated to "the care of sick persons in indigent circumstances in the county of Suffolk," was her only option. Whether she appreciated it or not, the location of the hospital had been chosen both to be convenient for persons of her modest means who lived in the spreading western suburbs and to provide teaching material for the medical students and residents in training.

Her doctor, David Cheever, was one of the two general surgeons in the new department. A Bostonian who had attended Harvard College and its medical school, he was reserved and scholarly. Men in his family had been surgeons ever since an ancestor had treated the wounded in the Revolutionary War. Mrs. Turner knew the patrician type well from her years as a domestic and accepted his advice without question. Cheever arranged to admit his patient to the thirty-bed open female ward three days before an operation to remove her varicose veins. This period of rest gave Mrs. Turner time to get acquainted with the nurses and staff and allowed the intern to conduct an unhurried and complete medical history and general physical examination. The house officer also ordered a blood count and urinalysis, virtually the only laboratory tests then available, to determine if she was anemic, infected, or spilling protein in her urine, a sign of kidney disease.

On the day of her operation, Adolf Watska, the general factotum of the recently appointed surgeon-in-chief, Harvey Cushing, wheeled Mrs. Turner into surgery. The gentleness of the huge orderly as he lifted patients from the litter to the operating table became legendary. Everyone except Watska wore cotton face masks, a recent innovation that did not fully enter surgical routine until after World War I. Before their use, conscientious surgeons had insisted on minimal talking during the procedure, believing that droplets from the mouths and noses of the team were often a primary source of wound infection. Curiously, Cushing allowed his giant assistant to go without a mask after he assured his employer that he never breathed or spoke in the operating room.

Being the first admission to the new hospital, Mary Agnes Turner was wheeled into the largest of the five operating rooms. It was stark, high ceilinged, and smelled of the antiseptic solution that Watska had mopped onto the wooden floor. Large windows on the outside wall, open in the summer to catch any breeze, provided natural illumination. Electric bulbs, an improvement from the ubiquitous gas lamps of only a few years before, hung above the operating table to supplement the daylight. Although some visitors and students stood on stools directly behind the surgical team during subsequent operations, most viewed them from seats in a glass-fronted balcony built high on the wall opposite the windows. Furnishings were limited to a cast-iron operating table covered with a thin mattress, an instrument table, a few iron and wood stools, and a wooden rack to store laundry and equipment. A rudimentary suction device was available to remove blood and other fluids from the surgical field. Cotton gowns, towels, and drapes were washed after each use until disposable paper products became available in the 1980s. The nurse was directed to collect the blood-soaked sponges at the completion of each case, wash and sterilize them, and refold them for later operations. Despite the continuing antipathy of some surgeons to using rubber gloves, she carefully saved those worn during surgery, cleaned them by hand, then powdered, sorted, repackaged, and sterilized them for future use. I performed these same tasks as a student volunteer at the MGH in the late 1950s, for disposable sterile gloves only became universally available in the next decade.

The surgeons, wearing rubber aprons and boots to protect against fluid spill, scrubbed their hands at a large porcelain sink just outside the operating room door. Conrad Jacobson, a new resident assigned to the case, washed both of Mrs. Turner's legs with soap and alcohol to kill bacteria. Having donned masks, gowns, and gloves, he and Cheever wrapped her feet in sterile towels and draped the rest of her body with sterile sheets. Jacobson had traced the course of her distended varicose veins with ink the night before as she stood upright. Easily seen when standing, they emptied and collapsed when she lay flat. If left unmarked, they would have been difficult to locate.

The nurse moved her instrument table into position, having laid out a scalpel, a few clamps, a needle holder, needles, gauze sponges, and spools of cotton, silk, and dissolvable catgut thread. The needles were reusable; one of Watska's tasks was to sharpen them on a whetstone between cases. The scalpel, an integral part of every operation, has a long history.[1] Flint knives, used to open the skull to relieve headaches, epilepsy, and melancholy, have been found among artifacts of 8,000 years ago. The ancient Romans used surgical tools of bronze and iron. Those of fifteenth-century surgeons were often works of art–single units consisting of a blade and an elaborately carved handle. By the eighteenth century in Europe, creation of such implements had become a specialized profession, part of the manufacture of cutlery. Instrument makers also flourished during the American Civil War; production was stimulated by the need for long, sharp knives for amputations. The design of the modern scalpel dates from the beginning of the twentieth century, when Mr. King Gillette perfected a safety razor with a detachable and disposable blade. Although the safety razor had gained popularity among many surgeons by 1910, its square shape was difficult to use. Disposable blades that would snap on and off a common scalpel handle, a design now used universally, first appeared in 1915 and was refined in 1936. Scalpels currently come in several sizes and shapes that vary from large curved blades for opening the chest or abdomen, smaller blades for fine work, and pointed stilettos to pierce an abscess.

Impressively sharp, the blades may be easily changed during a long case as they become dull.

Mrs. Turner, at first anxious and wide awake, lost consciousness as Walter Boothby, a specialist in anesthesia, dripped ether onto the gauze mask that he held over her face. This experience was inevitably unpleasant for the patient because sedatives were still unavailable. Jacobson had to restrain her firmly on the table until she had passed through the transient excitatory phase of involuntary muscular movement common during the initial administration of the agent. She long remembered the intense feeling of suffocation before unconsciousness ensued, an unforgettable sensation that those of us who were put to sleep with ether as children recall with enduring clarity. Although Cushing had introduced the blood pressure cuff to the United States from Italy some years earlier and insisted on its use during all operations, other monitoring methods to determine the depth of anesthesia or the respiratory state of the patient did not exist. If not deep enough, patients would struggle. If too deep, their lips or fingers would turn blue from lack of oxygen. Only Boothby could see Mrs. Turner's face and ensure that she was breathing satisfactorily and that her color was normal.

Stripping of varicose veins was a relatively new operation when the Brigham opened in 1913. For millennia physicians had followed the traditional custom of opening veins and draining blood to remove harmful humors from the body, restore equilibrium, and assuage the symptoms of disease. They had never understood the functional role of these vessels in particular and of the vascular system in general until William Harvey, an English physician working in Padua in the seventeenth century, demonstrated that the heart pumps the blood continuously throughout the body. He substantiated this novel observation in a patient, a young nobleman who had survived severe open fractures of the ribs on the left side of his chest.[2] The site had become infected, leaving a large and permanent cavity. Harvey inserted his fingers into the defect, felt the beating heart covered only with a layer of "fungous flesh," and noted that it contracted in precise synchrony with the pulse at the wrist. He also made the unique discovery that the moving organ elicited no sensation when touched. He went on to prove in living animals that the rhythmically contracting left side of the heart pushes a stream of oxygen-rich red blood through the arteries to all organs and tissues. Veins return the oxygen-depleted blue blood to the right side of the heart. Propelled from there through the lungs, the blood regains oxygen before re-entering the left side of the heart to begin another circuit. About the same time Harvey made these discoveries, an Italian microscopist, Marcello Malpighi, described the tiny capillaries that connect the arterial and venous systems throughout every bodily structure.

Harvey's demonstration of the circulation of the blood, so intrinsic to life itself, subjected him to prolonged and vituperative attack by physicians throughout Europe, who were outraged that the radical nature of the new teachings contradicted the concepts then in vogue. Some believed the arteries contained air from the lungs that mixed with venous blood and crossed the heart via small perforations in its muscular wall. Others felt that arterial and venous blood were manufactured in the liver and ebbed and flowed as separate entities to and from the tissues with each heartbeat. Still others felt that the movement of the lungs agitated the blood mechanically but denied that air entered the circulation. Like many advances in science, Harvey's careful observations transcended existing but erroneous dogma and superstition. He made them, after all, during the period that Galileo was under ecclesiastical condemnation for his revelations about the universe.

Varicose veins are obvious both to the afflicted and to those around them. For centuries healers and natural philosophers could not explain why they developed. Realizing that the condition occurred most frequently in women and was characterized by dilated and tortuous venous channels snaking along calf and thigh, the physician-teachers of ancient Greece blamed their development on stagnant blood pooling in the legs during child bearing, or remarkably, on "standing too much before kings."[3] Seventeenth- and eighteenth-century practitioners believed that menstrual blood collected in the legs during pregnancy. The condition was so common that nineteenth-century medical texts barely mentioned it; the authors only addressed the complications. A few surgeons in Victorian London treated extreme cases by tying off the major varicosed channel in the upper thigh. This ill-considered maneuver often made the situation worse, as the swollen vein and its branches became even more distended from blood that then lacked any direct path back to the general circulation. Skin ulcers developed, and abscesses formed. Infected veins ruptured, and patients sometimes died. Commenting on an 1864 report of eight deaths following such interventions, one of the foremost surgeons of the day, Sir Astley Cooper, declared publicly that anyone performing such a procedure deserved to have the ligature applied around his own neck!

The origins of the varicosities remained a mystery until 1916, when John Homans, the other general surgeon in the four-person Brigham department, clarified the pattern of blood flow through the veins of the lower extremity by demonstrating the importance of the separate but interconnecting superficial and deep venous systems.[4] Like Cheever, Homans came from a distinguished medical family in Boston, was of independent means, and spent his entire career at the hospital. Unlike his more circumspect and formal colleague, however, he was outspoken and iconoclastic, possessing both a rollicking wit and a contagious laugh. He influenced generations of students and residents in the care of the ill. Surgeons treasured his 1931 *Textbook of Surgery* in all of its six editions.

The main superficial venous trunk and its smaller tributaries run beneath the skin from the inside of the ankle to the groin. At the groin, this channel empties into the deep vein that carries blood from the muscle and bone of foot, calf, and thigh. These sizable, thumb-sized deep vessels, one from each leg, join together in the pelvis to form the inferior vena cava, the major conduit that transports blood from the entire lower body back to the heart. A series of one-way valves divides both superficial and deep leg veins into segments to prevent undue static pressure on the entire channel while the individual is standing. In addition to every contraction of the heart pushing the circulation forward, walking and other muscular activity of the calf muscles milk the venous blood upward, causing the valves to open as the blood column ascends. When the heart dilates or the muscles relax, they snap together to prevent backflow. In contrast to the deep vessels, which are supported by surrounding structures, the superficial veins lying in soft fat may lose their elasticity and widen. As a result, the edges of the valve leaflets cannot meet. Blood leaks backward.

The added weight of the fluid column in one dilated portion of vein places more pressure on the segment below, causing it to expand and its valve to become incompetent in turn. The entire affected vein and its tributaries enlarge progressively over time to form unsightly and bothersome varicosities. If large and symptomatic, these functionless vessels can be removed with impunity, as all venous blood flows through the deep system.

In celebration of the first operation performed at the Brigham, Cheever had invited the newly appointed surgeon-in-chief into his operating room. Forty-four years old and already internationally recognized as the founder of the new specialty of neurosurgery, Harvey Cushing made a "ceremonial" skin incision, using the newly introduced razor-blade scalpel. He had recently arrived from Johns Hopkins in Baltimore, the recruitment of star talent between universities and academic hospitals being as familiar then as it is now. His symbolic action suggests something about the ritualistic aspects of surgery, although it is unlikely that a chief would risk a similar gesture in a new hospital today. With Jacobson's help, Cheever then made a series of small incisions down the leg over the marked vessels, clamping bleeders in the overlying skin and globules of fat and tying them off with catgut from a spool he held in his hand. Using techniques introduced only a few years before, he stripped segments of the large, whitish, thick-walled varicosities from beneath the skin by running a cable down their lengths, securing the end of the veins around a button on the head of the cable, and pulling out the diseased structures forcefully. He slid a metal ring on a handle along the outside of smaller, thinner, and more fragile vessels to rupture their connections before removal, controlling bleeding with pressure. Once he had extracted as many of the enlarged veins as possible, he and Jacobson closed the overlying fat with catgut and the skin with silk on straight milliners' needles threaded individually by the nurse. It was a tedious process, although little different from that carried out today on large, dilated varicosities.

After the team had wrapped Mrs. Turner's legs in bulky pressure dressings to prevent swelling, nurses observed the awakening patient for a time in an adjacent room before returning her to the ward. Sustained vomiting marred her early recovery, for no drugs then existed to control this inevitable sequel of ether anesthesia. Postoperative management of patients who underwent this surgery remained relatively unchanged until well into the 1970s. Care was designed to prevent bleeding and promote clotting of the small, torn venous branches. The intern instructed Mrs. Turner to remain on bed rest for several days with her legs raised on pillows before allowing her to sit in a chair with her feet on a stool. He forbade standing to prevent blood pooling in the healing tissues but required her to walk intermittently so that her leg muscles could push the blood upward in the deep veins. Her incisions did not become infected, enabling her to escape a common surgical complication. This was perhaps a benefit of being admitted to the new hospital before others shared their bacteria. After having made friends with some of the other patients gradually filling the ward during her ten-day postoperative stay, Mrs. Turner was discharged by Cheever and sent home. The hospitalization was undoubtedly one of the highlights of her life, long remembered, oft recounted, and with any terror and discomfort forgotten.

Although records from the period are no longer available, we may safely assume that the hospitalization cost the Turners little or nothing. They did not have to pay the daily room rate, which was set at $15–$18, "comparable to the 1910 charge of $17.50 per day that the MGH had raised from $16.52 in 1909."[5] Competition between the institutions had begun.

If a granddaughter of Mary Agnes Turner had visited the neighborhood in the mid-1960s, a half-century after that first operation at the new hospital, she would have seen that the landscape was little changed. Block after block of triple-decker houses remained as before. The Brigham had grown to accommodate about three hundred beds, most notably by the addition of a three-story wing for "private" patients to help sustain its finances. A few modest extensions had also been added to house new laboratories. While Boston Brahmins from Beacon Hill and Back Bay patronized the MGH, conveniently located nearby, those seeking care from the western side of the expanding city (and increasingly from across the country and around the world) were gravitating to the Brigham as the teaching hospital most closely associated with Harvard Medical School. The founder, Peter Bent Brigham, surely could not have anticipated that his charitable initiative would become a world-renowned center of research and treatment within fifty years of its inception. Of course, affluent patients wanted their amenities, hence the new private wing. The presence of a paying clientele was essential. The medical school could not contribute, and Mr. Brigham's original $5 million endowment could no longer underwrite the expenses of wards, laboratories, and academic departments in the economy of the 1960s. The indigent, however, continued to occupy half of the hospital's beds.

An operation on which I assisted in 1965 during the second year of my residency illustrates some of the advances in surgery that had accrued in the five decades following the opening of the institution. The patient, Joseph Costello, a stocky, muscular man with a large abdomen, was 68 years old when he arrived for a workup. The owner of a construction company in a nearby town and still fully involved in its management, he was hard driving and hard drinking. A heavy smoker throughout much of his life, he had experienced two heart attacks. When he complained of a feeling of fullness and discomfort in his stomach and a persistent "heartbeat" below his ribs, his wife insisted that he visit his local doctor. This is a common medical sequence: a man seeks consultation only after his wife demands it. The physician noted a chronic cough and high blood pressure. Although he could feel nothing unusual on palpating the thick abdominal wall, calcifications on an X-ray suggested that a portion of the largest artery in the body, the aorta, was abnormally widened. Because of the potential for this weakened area to rupture, an often-fatal catastrophe, he advised operative intervention and referred the patient to the surgeon at the Brigham interested in the new field of vascular reconstruction. He also advised him that repair of the condition was just coming into general acceptance. Relatively few such operations had been carried out, and the risks were substantial.

Arteriosclerosis, a generalized process involving predominantly the arteries of the heart, neck, abdominal aorta, and the legs, produces hardening, degeneration, inflammation, and roughening of the arterial walls. No one knows why other vessels such as the aorta in the chest or those that supply the upper extremities and abdominal organs are usually spared. Running in families and usually occurring among people in their sixties and beyond, particularly those with a history of smoking or high levels of fats in their blood, it presents in one of two forms or occasionally in combination. In a common type, the affected arterial wall, normally pliant, smooth-walled, and elastic like a supple garden hose, thickens and stiffens as calcium deposits build up on its inside layers and surfaces. Clots may suddenly form in a critically narrowed segment of vessel, stopping blood flow and causing death of the tissues it supplies. This sudden event is most commonly manifest when a coronary artery is blocked and the patient suffers a heart attack, when sudden closure of a vessel to or in the brain causes a stroke, or when the foot or toes become gangrenous after obstruction of the main artery in thigh or calf. The other form of arteriosclerosis involves the same process, but instead of progressive narrowing, the involved portion of vessel widens progressively to form a balloonlike but often calcified sac. The majority of aneurysms involve the four- to six-inch segment of aorta in the upper abdomen that lies between its branches to the kidneys and its division in the pelvis into the two arteries supplying the legs. Occasionally, aneurysms may form in the artery behind the knee. It is not clear why some diseased vessels narrow and others expand except that the proteins responsible for normal structural strength and elasticity selectively diminish during aneurysm formation.

Richard Warren was the surgeon interested in carrying out vascular repair. Another example of the enduring family legacies of the Boston medical community, he was the last of seven generations of surgeons. One ancestor served in the Revolutionary War. Another, John Collins Warren, performed the first successful operation under anesthesia at the MGH in 1846. A third, J. Collins Warren, a professor of surgery at Harvard Medical School, became heavily involved in the gestation and birth of the Peter Bent Brigham Hospital. After graduating from Harvard College, Richard Warren studied classics at the University of Cambridge, an experience that enabled him to translate Latin poetry for pleasure throughout his life. An adventurous man who sailed his boat between Boston and his house on the Irish coast, he was the first surgeon in the United States to remove successfully a pulmonary embolus, a blood clot that had migrated from the leg veins to the lung. Editor of a major surgical text and a surgical journal, he was instrumental in forming an affiliation between the Veterans Administration and Boston teaching hospitals after World War II, a unique and valuable relationship both for those damaged in combat and for the house officers who cared for them. This innovative connection between a government medical facility and a university hospital was subsequently repeated throughout the country and remains an integral part of health care for many patients.

Richard Warren returned to the Brigham after World War II, having served in Europe in the army. He was intrigued by the possibilities of surgical intervention for involved arteries of patients with arteriosclerosis. Because he realized that substituting normal blood vessels from cadavers for the abnormal ones was relatively ineffectual despite ongoing investigations by some of his colleagues, he and a few other pioneers in the United States and Europe began to replace the diseased section of the aorta with tube grafts made of synthetic cloth. Introduced in the 1950s, materials such as nylon, Orlon, Dacron, and Teflon gradually entered general use, although no one at the time knew how long the body might tolerate them. One of my tasks as a resident in the early days of vascular surgery was to make grafts for arteries by sewing together pieces of an old nylon spinnaker from Warren's boat. Sometimes we added legs like a pair of trousers to sew to the arteries leading to the lower extremities.

Mr. Costello was assigned to a room on one of the new private floors. Its relative seclusion, large windows, and air conditioning contrasted with the older open public wards and semiprivate, curtained cubicles throughout the rest of the hospital. His workup was far more extensive than Mrs. Turner's had been. Laboratory technicians still carried out blood counts and some chemical determinations by hand but assessed the function of other organs, such as liver and kidneys, on recently introduced automatic analyzers. Most of the results were normal in his case, although smoking had reduced his lung capacity substantially. An electrocardiogram identified old injuries to the heart.

I visited him after he was settled in bed to take a history and perform a physical examination. We spent about an hour together. Our teachers in medical school had drilled the structure of the workup into our heads. We went through it compulsively on each admission so as not to forget anything. The questions came in sequence: the chief complaint and present illness, past medical history, queries about each part of the body, and a family and social history. The physical began at the top of the head and progressed to the feet. Not only did this structured approach allow us to define the primary disease, it provided information about other conditions and risk factors, recognized and unrecognized. At the beginning of our interview, Mr. Costello was abrupt, evasive, hostile, and apparently angry. As we continued, it became apparent that he was frightened of the operation and unhappy about his relationship with his wife. He spoke of his difficulties with drinking, concerns about the future of his company, and anxiety about one of his sons. Beneath the bluster lay a fragile and insecure man.

Once I had gained the basic information, even though I was unable to feel anything significant in his abdomen, the next step was to study the suspected aortic aneurysm by injecting radio-opaque dye into the artery and taking an X-ray. The use of arteriograms had come into use a decade or more after World War II. Previously, one could only conjecture the general site and severity of the vascular disease by physical examination or by noting suspicious flecks of calcium on a standard film. Before radiologists became interested in the subject in the 1970s, surgeons and residents carried out the procedures. To visualize the state of Mr. Costello's abdominal aorta and the arteries of his legs, we brought him to the X-ray room and positioned him on his stomach over a long film cassette.

The aorta is the largest artery in the body. It arches downward from its origin at the left side of the heart to descend along the backbone through the chest and abdomen. Normally about two inches wide in the chest of a male and somewhat smaller in females, its abdominal portion is about an inch in diameter. Large branches from the arch supply the head and arms; smaller branches nourish the lungs. Upon emerging through the diaphragm, the muscular partition that divides the chest from the abdominal cavity, the vessel gives off branches to the liver, stomach, intestines, and kidneys. Finally, at the level of the umbilicus, the aorta divides into two large branches that supply the pelvic organs and the legs. We were interested particularly in the section of vessel from the diaphragm to the pelvis.

This was the first arteriogram I had ever performed. I was caught up in my own nervousness, my hands trembling and my brow sweaty.

Apparently accepting that he was in a teaching hospital, Mr. Costello was stoic and seemingly failed to notice the whispered instructions of the senior resident who stood nearby, coaching me through the procedure. With trepidation I inserted a stout six-inch needle slowly through his back muscles, hugging the bony vertebral column. Most of the needle disappeared during what seemed an eternity. Finally, I felt a "pop" as its tip penetrated the side of the thick-walled vessel and bright red arterial blood boiled out of its base. I still remember the sense of overwhelming relief. I attached a large glass syringe to the needle, then injected the viscous dye by pushing as hard as I could on the plunger, calling to the technician to "shoot" the X-ray at what I thought was the correct moment. The patient's immediate sensation of a hot flush through his legs confirmed the correct distribution of the dye. Once developed, the single, long X-ray plate showed the arterial tree from the upper abdomen to the calves. Although the film was of relatively poor quality, we could see the dye-filled normal aorta entering the abdomen from the chest, then suddenly ballooning into a large sac. Its width was that of a fist.

How different this all was from the technical diagnostic advances that followed within a few years. These days the patient lies sedated on his back in a darkened room beneath a sophisticated X-ray machine. The interventional radiologist inserts a large-bore needle into the artery at the groin under local anesthesia, then slides a long, flexible catheter through the needle into the bloodstream. Watching the position of the tube on a fluoroscopic screen, he advances it up the aorta to a point just above the diaphragm. Dye is injected rapidly via a computerized automatic pressure device. At the same time, multiple films are taken in sequence, several each second. The images define any abnormalities well. Even less invasive methods have become available for specific conditions. These not only provide more exact definition of the vascular tree but are considerably easier to carry out. Technicians administer dye intravenously to the patient, who lies in a full-body scanner. The resulting three-dimensional computerized pictures resemble the illustrations in an anatomy text, improving substantially the precision of diagnosis and enhancing patient safety and comfort. They are even in color, with the red arteries and blue veins contrasting strikingly with the yellow background tissues.

Despite substantial improvements in surgical technique, the mortality rate for elective repair of aortic aneurysms both in the 1960s and at present remains at 5 to 10 percent. Generalized arteriosclerosis places the affected patients at risk from heart attacks or strokes during the postoperative period.[6] If uncorrected, however, over 80 percent of individuals with aneurysms larger than two or three inches in diameter die from rupture within five years. This catastrophe is usually heralded by an acute onset of abdominal or back pain. The peritoneum, the membranous envelope encompassing the abdominal organs and adhering to the front of the aorta, may contain the leak in its early stages. However, this membrane is thin and often tears, allowing sudden free flow of blood into the abdominal cavity. Death occurs within a few heartbeats. The death of Charles de Gaulle, famed general of World War II and later president of France, was one of the more dramatic examples of such a catastrophe. While working at his desk in 1969, he suddenly experienced severe pain and collapsed minutes later.

Even if emergency repair is carried out effectively and rapidly, half of the patients with a ruptured aneurysm do not survive in the days following the surgery because of the development of "multiple organ failure." This feared condition may ensue even if the surgeon controls the bleeding and replaces the diseased arterial segment successfully. The kidneys may cease to function because of sustained low blood pressure and shock from the acute hemorrhage, despite aggressive replacement with multiple transfusions. Although such patients may be supported with dialysis, they not infrequently develop coincident failure of the liver, bleeding from the stomach and intestines, lung dysfunction, and other relatively irreversible conditions.[7] It is like a house of cards falling down despite heroic efforts by all involved.

I still remember with distress the attempt I made to save one such unfortunate individual, a 75-year-old man named John Kelly. Although his peritoneum still transiently contained the blood that had burst from the arterial sac, it was obvious that the aneurysm was huge, beginning high in the abdomen, almost out of reach beneath the rib cage. The residents and I managed to place a clamp on the neck, the short length of normal, uninvolved vessel emerging beneath the diaphragm and leading into the dilated portion. We positioned the instrument blindly in a welling pool of blood. Despite control of the inflow of the circulation, brisk back-bleeding from the arteries of the pelvis and legs continued to obscure the field as we opened the overlying membrane to get to the rupture itself. It was with difficulty that we finally managed to gain full control, so we could let the anesthesiologist replace the lost volume. Although we still felt that we might be able to save the patient, we noted that his urine volume had markedly diminished, a grave sign. In addition, the neck of the aneurysm, usually of relatively normal quality, was so diseased that it wouldn't hold stitches. Over and over we sewed the cloth graft to the fraying arterial remnant. Over and over the sutures pulled out. He bled to death, his vessel disintegrating in my hands. We had been at it for eight hours.

In stark contrast, Mr. Costello's operation was elective and calm. He was sedated, then taken to the same operating room into which Adolf Watska had wheeled Mrs. Turner five decades before, one of the seven available. By 1965, however, the walls were tiled and the floor covered with glistening linoleum. All furniture and equipment were of stainless steel. Shiny reflecting lights on adjustable arms hung above the table, directing intense and focused illumination onto the operative site. The large window was still present, but the surgeon no longer had to rely on daylight to see the field—an important advance. The anesthesia machine automatically delivered appropriate mixtures of oxygen and anesthetic agent to the patient. Oscilloscopes monitored heart rate and blood pressure continually. A device that provided electric current for cutting or cautery stood ready. A table overflowed with specialized instruments.

As the junior resident and most inexperienced member of the team, I was responsible for readying several pints of blood from the blood bank the night before and to ensure that all X-rays were hung properly in the room at the start of the operation. I placed a catheter into Mr. Costello's bladder to measure urine volumes at intervals throughout the operation and passed a tube through his nose into his stomach to release swallowed air and remove any liquid that would accumulate thereafter. I then inserted two large intravenous lines into arm veins for the administration of salt solutions and transfusions during and after the procedure, and an additional line into the artery at his wrist to measure blood pressure directly and to sample arterial blood for oxygen content.

The procedure and its preamble progressed in an orderly and practiced fashion. The anesthesiologist, now a member of a separate department, no longer faced the obstacle of a patient struggling under ether. He put Mr. Costello to sleep with intravenous drugs, then paralyzed him with a muscle relaxant to allow insertion of a breathing tube through his mouth into his windpipe. Once in place, he attached the tube to the anesthesia respirator. He administered antibiotics as an added precaution; if the synthetic graft material were to become infected, the suture line could weaken and give way. After I had scrubbed the abdomen and groins, we draped off the rest of his body. The gowns and sheets were still made of cloth, although the gloves and sponges were disposable. Two suction devices were available to clear the field of blood.

The surgeon and the senior resident used an electric knife to open the abdomen from breastbone to pubis. This automatically coagulated small bleeding vessels, although they had to tie off the larger ones. My unenviable job was to hold open the thick abdominal wall with one retractor and to pull the liver and the intestines out of the way with another so as to bring the aneurysm into view. The intestines in particular can be compressed into a relatively small space with cloth pads, allowing full view of the area of dissection. With the anesthesiologist adding small doses of relaxant as necessary to prevent the patient from straining and tensing his abdominal wall, the operators explored the viscera for other abnormalities, then gingerly freed the huge, pulsating structure from the surrounding tissues and tied off individual vessels on its back wall. They also sacrificed the single branch on its surface that ran to the large bowel. Other channels would supply enough blood to this organ. The aneurysm was an impressive sight, about five inches across and six inches long, expanding and contracting with each heartbeat. Although my role was only to assure full view of the area, I was seized with anxiety. Despite carrying out scores of such operations during my later career, I never lost the fear that the massive artery might rupture in my hands. The remark of Sir William Osler, the foremost physician of the previous century and one of the founding professors of the new Johns Hopkins Medical School, that "there is no disease more conducive to clinical humility than aneurysm of the aorta," still reverberates in my ears.

Warren isolated and clamped the neck of the aneurysmal sac and the uninvolved vessels with noncrushing instruments. This maneuver was safe because smaller channels could carry enough blood around the site to nourish the lower extremities for the duration of the operation. He then removed the entire structure, a formidable and lengthy undertaking, and bridged the large defect with a synthetic woven tube graft of appropriate diameter and length. He used silk sutures that the nurse threaded individually on half-round needles. Smooth, pliable, nonreactive synthetic substitutes attached directly to sharp disposable needles had not yet come into general use. In retrospect, silk had limitations. Not only could bacteria survive in the interstices of the braided material, but the patient's white blood cells could attack it as a foreign body. The weakened sutures holding the graft to the artery might occasionally fracture years later, allowing blood to leak from the ever-unhealed junction. The result is a "false aneurysm," which could slowly enlarge and even rupture. These require repair or graft replacement, an operation of considerable risk and difficulty because dense scar tissue from the original surgery makes the subsequent dissection a taxing experience.

When Warren released the clamps, the suture holes left by the stout needles needed to pierce the calcified arterial wall bled substantially before tiny clots formed to seal the areas. Overlooked small vessels, disrupted during the dissection, also made their presence known. Despite our best efforts of control, we still needed four units of blood to restore the loss, not an unusual amount. The senior resident and I then replaced the bowel and closed the abdominal wall in layers. The procedure took nearly five hours. Mr. Costello remained stable throughout. With the small recovery room already filled with patients on respirators, we brought him directly to the surgical floor, where nurses monitored his vital signs frequently and checked if his urine output was satisfactory; the concept of intensive care was still rudimentary at the time. Recovering without incident despite his substantial risk factors, he was discharged after ten days of gradually increasing diet and activity. He lived comfortably for another four years before dying suddenly of a heart attack.

Health insurance took care of most of his hospital expenses. No one in the present hospital administration could tell me the cost of this 1960s operation, however. Data accrued before the advent of computers apparently cannot be retrieved. I should also note that the rate of a private room at the Brigham and most other hospitals at that time had just risen to a hundred dollars a day, a source of incredulity to the staff and consternation to the patients.

Few of us involved with Mr. Costello and other patients in the 1960s could have imagined that changing patterns of disease and the accelerating progression of new concepts and innovations would increasingly challenge traditional approaches, diagnostic tools, and operative techniques. The evolution came before many of us realized it. Shirley Laverne sought treatment for morbid obesity, an emerging and rather unexpected health problem, at the Brigham and Women's Hospital in 2007. Mrs. Laverne was 37 years old. She lived in a suburb south of Boston with her ten-year-old daughter and her husband, an accountant. Ample food was a consistent feature of her childhood. Although her father had remained slim—due no doubt to his physical activity as a stonemason—her mother and sisters were heavy. Mrs. Laverne had always been overweight and still remembered the ridicule she endured from her school classmates. The sedentary life she spent as a telephone operator in the years before her marriage compounded the problem. Gaining additional weight since the birth of her child, she had tried a variety of diets without long-term success. Now weighing nearly 350 pounds, she could no longer care for her house and family. Depressed and embarrassed, she rarely ventured outside. Related physical problems emerged. To move was an effort. The damp skin between the folds of fat of her breasts, abdomen, and groins were chronically inflamed and infected. Her hips and knees ached when she walked. A nonhealing skin ulcer developed on one of her ankles. Her primary care physician told her that her blood sugar was elevated and that she had become diabetic. Her very existence had become a burden.

She slept in a chair during much of the day because her loud snoring and shortness of breath woke her at night, and periods of breath-holding lasting many seconds frightened her husband. Increasingly concerned, she returned to her doctor. He realized that her breathing difficulties (sleep apnea) were a result of her massive obesity and referred her to David

Lautz, a young staff surgeon at the Brigham, about the possibility of a gastric bypass operation. After completing five years of surgical training, Lautz had taken an extra fellowship year in bariatric surgery, as this new specialty of treating the obese is known, and had become expert in caring for those with the condition.

Morbid obesity, defined in part as body weight at least twice normal or a hundred pounds or more in excess, has become virtually epidemic in some developed countries. Nearly 100 million people in the United States, one-third of the population, are seriously overweight; 5–10 million are morbidly obese.[8] The resulting medical and economic costs total nearly $100 billion per year nationwide. Morbid obesity affects school children, adolescents and young adults, the middle aged, and the elderly.[9] Reasons given for the ubiquity of the disorder range from lack of exercise and overuse of the automobile, to hours of television watching each day, to the unending promotion and availability of relatively inexpensive, highly caloric junk foods in schools and fast-food establishments. It has become a major public health issue both in regard to immediate quality of life and the development of long-term complications. Life expectancy may be shortened as much as seven years. Indeed, the situation has become so important that the governments and industries of France and Britain, for instance, are taking active steps to change the dietary habits of their children. Because of public complaints, companies in the United States are also beginning to alter the type of food available in schools. First Lady Michelle Obama's recent "Play 60" campaign, which encourages children to be active for at least sixty minutes each day, has brought particular attention to the problem.

Mrs. Laverne met Lautz for the first time during an introductory visit to the bariatric clinic. Later attending a general information session conducted by specialty nurses, she and the others in the audience learned details of the condition; indications for and alternatives to surgery; the consultations needed before any procedure could be considered; the types, risks, and benefits of the surgical options, and the necessity of prolonged follow-up. They also found that stringent and demanding treatment protocols were well worked out and discovered that about 200,000 such procedures are performed in the United States each year. Although this seems a large number, obesity surgery is performed on less than 1 percent of those who would be eligible. Finally, each met with an administrator in a separate office to go through the nuances and intricacies of insurance coverage.

Following these initial visits, Mrs. Laverne returned to the clinic for a protracted and careful evaluation. After she filled out a computerized form detailing her medical history, a physician's assistant interviewed her closely about patterns of weight gain, attempts at dieting, and the presence of related physical abnormalities. The assistant then carried out a full physical examination and ordered a series of laboratory screening tests. Because of the demands of their other duties and the vagaries of current work-hour regulations, no residents were involved in the workup, a striking departure from earlier practices. Finally, Lautz arrived for further discussion and to answer additional questions. Mrs. Laverne emphasized that her life was miserable and that she needed whatever aid he could propose. She later expressed her satisfaction with the information given, the completeness of the initial appraisal, and the attention her surgeon had given her.

Considering Mrs. Laverne an appropriate candidate, the team asked her to undergo psychiatric clearance and extensive interviews with a dietitian. The weight of her chest wall and breasts made breathing difficult, so she submitted to a sleep study to assess the extent of her sleep apnea. A cardiologic evaluation was organized as well; she had once been treated with an appetite inhibitor that had suddenly been removed from the market in 1997 because of unexpected and deleterious effects on heart valves. A radiologist checked for the presence of existing gallstones, as more may develop during the period of rapid weight loss after surgery. Reports from each of these consultants were then sent to Lautz for his final evaluation and to the insurer for authorization for payment.

Although some of the other attendees of the clinic were adolescents, Mrs. Laverne is typical of persons with morbid obesity seeking surgical help. Often weighing well over 300 pounds, they develop high blood pressure, elevated levels of cholesterol, and diabetes. Because of their sedentary lifestyle, they may form blood clots in their leg veins with subsequent skin breakdown. The frequency of hip and knee replacement in these difficult and at-risk patients is rising appreciably. The prospect of anesthesia is intimidating; their thick necks make placement of a breathing tube for controlled ventilation difficult. Their diminished capacity to breathe may even require the use of a respirator after the operation, sometimes for prolonged periods. They also learn that they must commit themselves to a strict diet and continuing exercise for the rest of their lives. The surgical procedure, gastric bypass, although the most common operation currently performed in the United States, is not a panacea.

The team explained the bypass operation in detail to Mrs. Laverne, using pictures to illustrate the various steps. The object is to create a gastric pouch, a remnant of the stomach so small that the individual will become full after eating only small amounts of food; the pouch contains four to eight ounces as compared to a normal stomach that can hold one to one-and-a-half quarts. In most instances, the surgeon enters the abdominal cavity either through a traditional open incision or using the minimally invasive technique of laparoscopy. He staples across a small portion of upper stomach and detaches it from the rest of the organ. He then connects a limb of small intestine to the gastric remnant to carry food through the intestinal tract, and finally rejoins the remaining bowel anatomically to drain secretions from the large, nonfunctioning segment of stomach, pancreas, and liver.[10] Two years after the operation, patients generally have lost 60 to 70 percent of their excess weight.

The instructors also described an alternate approach that involves creation of the pouch by positioning an adjustable plastic noose around the upper stomach, like placing an elastic band around the end of a balloon. The surgeon tightens the noose to isolate the segment from the remainder of the stomach, and joins the intestinal segment to it as before. While this procedure is the simplest to perform and does not involve division of the stomach, it is less effective than the surgically divided pouch, for readjustment of the tension of the band not infrequently becomes necessary. However, the Food and Drug Administration (FDA) recently approved this technique for patients who are only moderately obese and can afford to lose weight at a relatively slow pace. Mrs. Laverne was not presented with a third option in which the patient swallows a balloon that is then filled with fluid to occupy the stomach. The balloon is retained over a period of months. Used more commonly in Europe, this noninvasive technique has not gained popularity in the United States.[11]

Mrs. Laverne and her group learned about the ease and convenience of tissue stapling compared to the individual placement and tying of dozens of sutures. The walls of the stomach and the intestine comprise three layers. The outside layer is smooth and glistening, allowing free and normal movement of the organs within the abdominal cavity; the thick, muscular middle layer contracts and dilates to churn the food and push it along; the inside layer contains specialized cells that digest and absorb nutrients into the bloodstream. Since the end of the nineteenth century, surgeons treating cancer and peptic ulcer disease have sewn together divided portions of stomach or bowel in two steps, inverting the approximated full-thickness walls with stitches of absorbable material and then buttressing the outside layer with multiple silk sutures to prevent leakage and reduce the formation of adhesions to adjacent structures. During the past two decades, the stapling has increasingly replaced hand suturing. With a standard abdominal incision, large staplers are used. With a laparoscopic approach, tiny stapling instruments on long handles are introduced into the cavity via a half-inch port. Although surgeons occasionally used earlier stapler prototypes in the late 1960s, improving technology has enhanced the general utility of this approach. With a device that combines cutting and stapling, for instance, the operator can divide, seal, or join portions of stomach or intestine in considerably less time than by sewing. Overall, these instruments have effectively enhanced the more traditional operative methods.[12]

The nurses informed Mrs. Laverne and the others about the operative approaches. Patients who undergo the traditional open procedure, a diminishing minority, experience considerable pain in the long abdominal incision, particularly with moving or coughing. They stay in hospital as long as a week, or until they can eat a full diet and care for themselves. They cannot resume activities such as lifting or driving for six weeks thereafter. Wound infections may develop in the layer of fat, sometimes many inches thick, between skin and abdominal musculature. Hernias may develop in the large incisions at a rate as high as 20 percent and are often difficult to repair. As a result, bariatric surgeons have increasingly shifted to the use of laparoscopes for gastric bypass, expending much effort to master the new techniques. It was easy for Mrs. Laverne, 200 pounds overweight, to choose this newer strategy. She would go home in two days, experience little pain, and return relatively quickly to her normal activities with little risk of hernia formation.

Although operative mortality is low (about 0.2 percent in most current series), complications may develop with either method (a total incidence of about 7 percent with the laparoscopic approach, 14 percent with the open operation). If a patient develops bleeding or leaks when sutures pull out or staple guns misfire with laparoscopy, the surgeon must open the abdomen and correct the problem. There may also be occasional long-term side effects. Although infrequent, late bowel obstructions may occur. The new anatomical rearrangement may inhibit the normal uptake of essential minerals such as calcium, which may eventually lead to bone disease. In considering whether to pursue the operation, each individual must balance improved quality of life and sustained health with the risks of significant acute surgical complications and delayed metabolic disturbances.

The minimally invasive technique of laparoscopy has become increasingly dominant. In fact, it has changed the entire field of general surgery and the education of those performing it.[13] The abdominal wall is an obvious obstacle to adequate viewing of the anatomy and manipulation of the structures within. For optimal exposure, a substantial incision must be made. In contrast, when the surgeon inserts a telescope and small ports or rigid tubes through skin and muscle, the integrity of the abdominal wall is maintained. He or she may then carry out the necessary surgical maneuvers using an intense light source and specialized instruments. With limited disruption of anatomical structures, a new era has emerged in the continuing effort to reduce postoperative pain and accelerate recovery.

Like many advances in medicine and science, the idea of peering through a port at the patient's insides to make a diagnosis or to carry out a simple procedure was not new. Physicians in ancient Greece inserted short pipes into the anus to diagnose hemorrhoids and fistulae. Not until the beginning of the nineteenth century, however, did European investigators begin to visualize the inside of hollow structures with external orifices such as bladder, rectum, or stomach, using a rigid straight cylinder illuminated by the reflected light of a candle. By midcentury they had added lenses to the tube to concentrate the source of light, now a flame of gazogene, a combination of turpentine and alcohol. Prismatic lenses for angled viewing followed. A platinum loop and then a miniature electric bulb eventually provided brighter light to see through the telescope. In 1910 a Swedish surgeon first examined the intestines and other viscera via a tube he inserted through the abdominal wall. Several clinical groups then began to manipulate internal structures, placing a telescope to see into the abdominal cavity through one port and inserting long instruments through another. With one hand to hold the eyepiece and the other to move and apply the instruments, they could biopsy the liver. The introduction in the 1950s of a flexible image transmission camera system positioned by an assistant and shown on a television screen allowed the surgeon to use both his hands. Gynecologists had embraced such improved techniques for operations on the female pelvis for decades, but not until 1986 did a French surgeon successfully remove a gallbladder through a laparoscope.

While enthusiasm for this novel method slowly grew among a few French, German, and American surgeons, particularly those in private practice, the majority accepted it more slowly. One reason was a prolonged learning curve. Older professionals trained before the advent of the new methods found the approach particularly difficult and perhaps threatening to their long-established and painfully acquired open operative skills. In contrast, younger individuals, raised in an age of computers and video games that improve hand-eye coordination, have embraced the emerging technology. Indeed, public demand for smaller and less painful incisions, shorter hospitalizations, and quicker return to normalcy thereafter encouraged wider use of the technology. At the same time instrument designers provided progressively more sophisticated equipment to enhance precision and safety. For some cases, innovators have reduced the usual four or five ports to a single scope placed through the umbilicus for adequate visualization, retraction, and manipulation. No scar is apparent. In operations in which a hand must be inserted to stabilize or retract particular tissue, or when an organ like a kidney, spleen, or portion of colon must be removed, an additional small incision is made. Only two inches long, these are relatively inconsequential. Overall, this minimally invasive approach is currently used in 30 to 40 percent of abdominal operations. It has also spilled over into increasing numbers of thoracic procedures (thoracoscopy). Some have even used the technique to remove the thyroid gland via the armpit to obviate an obvious neck incision.

Laparoscopy is such a departure from traditional operative approaches that training is lengthy. For several years teaching programs have offered courses in the subject, attended in large numbers both by surgical residents and qualified surgeons. In addition to hours of instruction and individual coaching, all must complete ten laparoscopic procedures on patients under direct supervision before they can be credentialed. But despite stringent standards, such operations still pose occasional risks; as with any surgery, there is the ever-present possibility (less than 5 percent) of a heart attack or pulmonary embolus. For example, even after extensive experience with gallbladder removal, the most common procedure performed with the method, the incidence of injuries to important adjacent structures, although low (0.3 to 0.5 percent), remains constant. Reunited portions of intestine may leak. Inadequately controlled vessels may bleed. The method is neither easy nor foolproof.

As Lautz knew well, most trainees begin in a laparoscopic surgery laboratory. Once they have mastered maneuvering the long-handled instrument outside the "body," they learn to shift the perception of their movements from a normal three-dimensional view to two dimensions by looking constantly at a TV monitor attached to the inserted telescope. This takes much practice, for now they can only see the screen, not the actual structure they are handling. Many learn on animals such as pigs. Alternatively, they use a cardboard box or a plastic or rubber mannequin that startlingly resembles a patient. In the box model, the instructors staple a piece of plastic sheeting inside the cover to represent the peritoneal membrane lining the abdominal cavity. The student first learns how to insert the instruments through the membrane and to cut, clip, or staple a sponge placed inside to simulate an organ or tissue. The mannequin, in contrast, is a sophisticated, realistic, and expensive virtual training tool. Small holes in its abdominal wall accommodate the ports. Realistic organs lie in the mock cavity. The efficacy of these teaching aids has been striking.

Mrs. Laverne arrived at the hospital at five o'clock the morning of her operation, having arisen hours before, to face a complex and potentially life-threatening procedure. The large entrance hall was empty except for a few figures sleepily buying coffee in the adjacent cafeteria. Accompanied by her husband, she checked with the admissions officer, who arranged for an orderly to push her in a large wheelchair to the preoperative area, a floor beneath the street. This huge space is a collecting point for patients entering the forty operating rooms, so different from the cramped quarters of the original institution. After she had changed behind curtains and said goodbye to her husband, two nurses helped her onto an extra-wide bariatric bed. The anesthesia team quickly greeted her, placed an intravenous line in her arm, and gave her sedation.

Once in the operating room—a pristine aggregate of gleaming tile, stainless steel lights, and sophisticated monitoring equipment—the team moved Mrs. Laverne to the "Hercules," a special operating table of substantial width and strength to accommodate morbidly obese patients. They had to do this carefully using a roller, as she could do little to help position herself. To diminish the possibility that a clot might form and migrate to her lungs, a nurse placed flexible pneumatic boots on her legs. Air from a delivery pump sequentially compressed and deflated segments of the boots to milk venous blood upward toward her heart and prevent pooling and clotting in her legs. The anesthesiologist administered small doses of a blood thinner as a further precaution. After she lost consciousness within seconds of receiving a powerful hypnotic, he paralyzed her muscles with another drug and slid a breathing tube into her windpipe with some difficulty because of the size and shortness of her neck. As in Mr. Costello's case, he connected this to an automatic respiratory unit. Via a line placed in the artery at her wrist, he determined blood levels of oxygen and carbon dioxide at frequent intervals to ensure adequate ventilation. The resident placed a catheter in her bladder, inserted a tube into her stomach, and arranged intravenous lines. He then scrubbed her skin and draped the field with sterile, disposable paper drapes. Much of the equipment had been disposable for several years, including the gowns, gloves, knife blades, and even some of the laparoscopic instruments themselves.

Lautz pushed a sharp instrument into her peritoneal cavity with care, so as not to injure the underlying bowel. He introduced a finger-sized tube around it and filled her abdomen with air to elevate the abdominal wall from the organs beneath. He then inserted a telescope with a wide-angle camera at its end and positioned two smaller tubes in the left side and two in the right side of her upper abdomen to carry the appropriate instruments. Visualizing the magnified field on the large television monitor on the wall, the assistant used graspers on long handles to retract the liver and large bowel away from the small bowel and stomach. With the operative site in perfect view, the surgeon could dissect and isolate precisely structures to be cut or vessels to be tied. He stapled closed and divided a portion of the small intestine. He used a similar but larger device to isolate the top portion of the stomach as a gastric pouch, reinforcing the staple lines with silk sutures he tied with the instrument tips. With yet another stapling device, he restored intestinal continuity by attaching one end of a divided portion of small bowel to the stomach and the other to a loop of normal bowel. After testing the integrity of the suture lines with fluid and air instilled through the stomach tube, the team sewed shut the small defects in the abdominal wall and skin, and returned Mrs. Laverne to the recovery room. Blood loss was minimal.

The postoperative course was smooth. On a follow-up visit to the bariatric clinic three years later, she told the team that she was a new woman. And indeed she was. Her diabetes had disappeared, blood pressure had decreased toward normal, and levels of blood sugar, cholesterol, and other serum fats had declined. She weighed 140 pounds and was actively involved with her child and with community activities. She underwent two additional operations to remove excess aprons of skin from her abdomen, a result of her extensive weight loss. She enjoys her life, remains grateful for her surgery, and is still impressed that she sees Lautz during every visit. Her insurance company, once they had admitted the medical necessity of the procedure and the hospitalization, paid the $45,000 bill.

two

The Teaching Hospital

Mrs. Turner walked down the hill from her house to the hospital on the day of her admission. Few people were on the street. A trolley clattered by. Only an occasional motorcar passed as she crossed the road near the recently opened nursing school and toiled up the steep driveway past the entrance lodge toward the Doric columns that embellished the front of the main building. Pulling open the large glass door, she entered the white, wood-paneled central rotunda. Overhead balconies with cast-iron railings led to doctors' offices. Behind a semicircular mahogany reception desk stood an imposing figure available to answer questions and direct patients to their destination. Mrs. Carr, as one of the older surgeons remembered, was "tall and stately, with a regal hairdo, a commanding voice, and an impressive bosom."[1] After appropriate greetings, she called the admitting nurse to meet Mrs. Turner for a brief interview and accompany her to the ward.

Although the halls were relatively empty when the first patient entered the new building, the scene changed over the ensuing weeks and months as the beds filled. Each day at 1:00 PM, visitors gathered in the rotunda to obtain information about their family or friends. Mrs. Carr made sure that the four senior house officers were present for interviews and questions. With the beginning of visiting hours at 2:00 PM sharp, she opened the doors and allowed the multitude to stream down "The Pike," the long walkway that connected the various wards and clinics interspersed along its length. Its south side, open to the air, was draped with wisteria vines. Pleasant in the summer, driving sleet or snow often filled it in the winter. Indeed, as they occasionally struggled through drifts to visit the wards, the staff confirmed despairingly that the architect of the Brigham, who had won a prize for his design, had never spent a winter in New England.[2] The outside wall was not closed in until the 1960s. In addition, many considered some of the buildings of the new complex to be outdated by the time they were built.

Mrs. Turner and the growing number of in-patients soon discovered that although efficiency was lacking, much about the arrangement was pleasant. Lawns, fruit trees, and a tennis court separated the four circular, thirty-bed open wards. When the weather was fine, the nurses opened skylights in the high ceilings and pushed the beds outside through wide doorways. Private patients on the second floor occupied individual cubicles divided by wooden partitions, with a curtain in front for privacy. Adjacent porches were available for sunning. One curious deficiency in the new hospital, as newly admitted patients discovered when they tried to hang up their clothes, was a lack of storage space. This seeming omission was in fact a purposeful provision in the architect's plans. He was apparently concerned that healthy female nurses would, upon occasion, be subject to sexual temptation. To eliminate opportunities, he omitted spacious closets from the plans.[3]

Two large brothers crammed into the narrow front seat of the 1913 electric ambulance to transport Mrs. Turner and other patients home upon discharge. Taking turns driving, they struck a large brass bell mounted on the left door with a hammer to call attention to their progress and to warn loiterers to get out of the way. The hard rubber tires on the wooden-spoked wheels provided a rough ride. When the steepness of the hill exceeded the capacity of the inefficient batteries, as it did on this trip, one of the brothers got out and pushed. They controlled the speed on the downward journey by throwing over the side a timber attached to the frame with a chain, regulating the resultant drag pressure with a brake lever. The hospital superintendent retired this remarkable vehicle in 1939, ostensibly because its battery charger became obsolete when the hospital converted its electrical power supply from DC to AC.

Established in 1782, Harvard Medical School had already occupied several sites in Boston. All were three miles distant from the main campus and its graduate schools across the Charles River in Cambridge.[4] After the school celebrated its one hundredth anniversary with a move to yet another downtown location, professors and students alike realized that the new facilities lacked both adequate laboratory space and spare land for expansion. Even the curriculum was a source of controversy among some of the less scientifically oriented faculty, who reproached their more serious colleagues for insisting that the students spend time learning chemistry and physiology.

The school had been a proprietary concern administered by a few self-interested individuals from the Boston medical establishment until Charles William Eliot, a mathematician and scientist at Massachusetts Institute of Technology, became president of Harvard University in 1869. Like virtually all comparable institutions of that period, the medical school was essentially a money-making diploma mill for students whose literacy was often in doubt.[5] In fact, Eliot noted pessimistically, "The ignorance and general incompetency of the average graduate of American Medical Schools at the time when he receives the degree which turns him loose upon the community, is something horrible to contemplate."[6] Newer hospitals in Boston, such as Boston City Hospital (1864) and Children's Hospital (1869), like the MGH, insisted on autonomy for both their administration and their staff appointments, and the school was completely dependent upon their choices for its own clinical faculty. Cronyism was rife. Eliot instituted a series of far-reaching educational and financial reforms to raise the standards of this weak section of the university, anticipating the coming revolution in medical education. He demanded strict entrance requirements, a relative novelty. He arranged a stringent course structure to be presented over a three-year period, and insisted that the students take written examinations. Although a conservative faction from the MGH, led by a forceful surgeon, and other faculty opposed Eliot, his innovations were enforced, and academic performance improved dramatically.

In 1900 Eliot and his advisors learned that a twenty-three-acre tract of land west of the city center, named *Longwood* after Napoleon Bonaparte's site of exile on St. Helena, might be for sale. They hoped that the area could accommodate an expanded medical school and university hospital under its control, based on similar developments under way at Johns Hopkins University in Baltimore. The location of the site was desirable. It was close to a growing population center, accessible, and distant from the MGH on the other side of the city.[7] Although for the first time in its history Harvard assigned unrestricted funds for the proposed venture, the prospects of an underfinanced multimillion-dollar project remained frightening. Even Eliot became nervous. Despite the substantial endowment of the university, considerably more money was needed to buy, build, and equip the intended complex. It was an ideal moment to raise such funds, however. The nation was prospering in an age of large enterprises initiated and guided by men of great wealth and vision. Encouraged by interested and enthusiastic philanthropists and entrepreneurs, several benefactors in Boston and New York supplied financial aid. The land was bought and the buildings designed. Construction of the new medical school buildings around their own quadrangle began in 1903, using Italian marble acquired at a bargain price from the New York Public Library, which had discarded the stone because it was the wrong color. The new complex was completed in 1906.

The prospect of an adjacent university hospital for Harvard Medical School was becoming increasingly attractive to many of the faculty and other supporters of the project. Almost by happenstance, those involved became aware that a Boston merchant, Peter Bent Brigham, had left a will a quarter-century before directing that the proceeds of his trust should be used to build a charitable hospital for the deserving poor. Brigham was born in 1807 on a farm in Bakersfield, Vermont, to which his parents had moved ten years earlier from Massachusetts. They were reasonably well off and well educated. The family possessed a library and subscribed to the Boston newspapers. But after Peter's father, Uriah Brigham, died in 1818, the family became impoverished. The boy spent his childhood in reduced circumstances with his widowed mother and eight predominantly older siblings. Hoping to improve his expectations, he started for Boston by horseback at age 17, carrying his few belongings and fourteen dollars in a saddlebag. He planned to sell the horse and bag upon his arrival and send the money to his mother. The animal became lame on the way, forcing him to trade it to a minister for his old mare plus six dollars. The newly acquired mare soon foundered. Brigham had to continue his journey by working on a canal boat, finally arriving in the city on foot and virtually penniless.

He began his career by selling oysters and fish from a wheelbarrow. As oysters were plentiful and a popular food among the public at the time, he was able to open an oyster bar in a nearby hotel and eventually buy and operate a successful restaurant. He invested shrewdly throughout his life-time, making much money in local real estate and as a director of a nearby railroad. Now a millionaire, he lived in a fine house in the center of Boston. A bachelor of regular habits and abstemious of tobacco and alcohol, he was a model of Victorian probity. His growing reputation for integrity and civic responsibility caused city officials to seek out his opinions on munici-pal improvements. Perhaps in response to his disadvantaged childhood and regretted lack of education, his interest in aiding the underprivileged included strong opinions against slavery. Indeed, his executors later found among his belongings two cancelled wills, dated 1862, which left the bulk of his estate for furthering the emancipation of slaves.[8] His final will, the contents of which later enraged his hopeful relatives, was probated upon his death in 1877. It stipulated that much of his property be kept in trust for twenty-five years and then be used to found a hospital for the indigent of Boston. He left additional funds to improve the educational system of his birthplace in Bakersfield. Further contributions from a sister and other cooperative members of his family allowed acquisition of land for a new school. The Brigham Academy still stands.

Peter Bent Brigham's philanthropy inspired others in his family to make similar accommodations. Shortly after Brigham went into the restaurant business, Brigham's nephew also left Vermont to begin work at his uncle's establishment. An upright and community-spirited man like his uncle, he too accrued resources to open his own hotel and to involve himself in local real estate. He ultimately set aside funds for a hospital for those with arthritic disorders. The Robert Breck Brigham Hospital opened in 1914. Three-quarters of a century later, these two neighboring institu-tions merged with a third to form the Brigham and Women's Hospital.

With the potential carrot of the Brigham trust dangling before them, members of the Harvard Corporation opened discussions with the execu-tors of the estate in 1907 about creating a teaching institution for the new medical school.[9] The executors agreed to a relationship but insisted on full independence. With the arrangement becoming public, disquiet arose in the corridors of the Boston State House about the prospect of an institution to care for the poor and provide a venue for the teaching of students and residents. The concerns centered particularly around the unwelcome prospect that money designated for the benefit of the impoverished sick of the city might enrich Harvard's coffers, a possibility anathema to the politicians. A young alderman, James Michael Curley, who later became one of Boston's most famous (or infamous) mayors and then governor of Massachusetts, led an ultimately unsuccessful charge against the scheme.

The controversy surrounding Harvard and its desire for a teaching hospital was not unique. Hospitals in the United States since the Civil War had cooperated relatively marginally in the education of future physicians. They consistently limited close involvement with trainees, feeling that their primary responsibility was to their patients.[10] Despite persistent overtures by both medical instructors and their students for more visibility on the hospital wards, teaching remained rudimentary into the first decade of the twentieth century. The relationship between the MGH and Harvard Medical School is a good early example of this divide. Hospital practitioners at the MGH considered themselves independent of the admittedly rudimentary educational administration. The new Johns Hopkins Hospital in Baltimore provided the only example of a university hospital dedicated both to clinical care, particularly of the poor, and to the teaching of residents and students.

The formation of Johns Hopkins Medical School in 1889 and its affiliation with Johns Hopkins Hospital four years later were critical events in the history of modern medicine, the first in America to capitalize on the advances ongoing in Europe. The university president, Daniel Coit Gilman, appointed four distinguished academic professors identified following national searches to define and orchestrate the reforms. These prescient individuals revamped the curriculum and training of young doctors, related the basic sciences to clinical questions, and emphasized research as part of the four-year course of study. Entrance requirements became more stringent than for any other school in the country. For the first time, a college degree was required. Basing their concepts on the structured courses of study of the French and German systems of higher education, the Hopkins professors led well-defined departments. The

German model was particularly appealing, with its highly organized, research-oriented hospitals and universities, productive scientists, traditions of scholarship, and devotion to postgraduate training. In contrast, the few other American university-affiliated institutions continued to adhere to the British system, in which students gained knowledge by trailing a handful of faculty members who ran small clinical services for poor patients and spent several months each year in private practice.

A variety of stimuli encouraged a closer relationship between universities and their evolving hospitals. The success of the novel venture in Baltimore was obvious. The scientific treatment of disease was coming into sharper focus, and both students and faculty demanded clinical improvements. Important partnerships and mergers formed in cities in the United States, first at the University of Michigan Medical School, which owned and operated its own hospital, then between Columbia University's School of Medicine and the Presbyterian Hospital in New York, and Washington University and Barnes Hospital in St. Louis. With similar relationships forming elsewhere, American medical education became increasingly influential. However, despite subsequent decades of comprehensive improvements in patient care, more inclusive methods of instruction, and progressive productivity in research, some aberrant differences in roles and mission between hospital and school still exist. Harvard, for instance, still has no university hospital per se but is served by several affiliated but autonomous institutions, each with its own board of trustees, administration, and faculties.[11] Indeed, some hitherto firm connections between medical schools and teaching hospitals seem increasingly threatened by ongoing financial and social dynamics.

Construction of the Peter Bent Brigham Hospital in 1911 occurred several years after initial considerations about a proposed teaching hospital for Harvard Medical School. A distinct departure from long-established Boston medical traditions, the hospital appeared as an interloper to at least some of the existing local institutions. This attitude was particularly true at the MGH. Heavily endowed through the sustained efforts of generations of trustees and interested citizens, it had provided care to those around it for a century. As a result, it considered itself and its works independent of the medical school. The Brigham, steeped in the Johns Hopkins philosophy and staffed with doctors trained at Johns Hopkins, quickly assumed a prominent role in the evolution of modern medical care, education, and research. It soon became apparent that even though the new establishment was of modest size and bed capacity, it emerged fully mature and able to attract a select full-time academic faculty of physicians and surgeons of national stature, free from the parochialism of the local professional and social elite, who were equipped to refine and extend scientific investigation and residency training.

The changes that Peter Bent Brigham's legacy instituted were not easy to implement in a city so sure of its rank as the "Athens of America." Boston had become a place of consequence during Brigham's lifetime. By the time of his death it contained 250,000 inhabitants, with over half a million living in the surrounding metropolitan area. Commerce thrived. In the years before the Civil War, speculators had amassed great wealth through trade with China. Following the conflict, the manufacture of textiles and shoes in the mills on the banks of the nearby rivers gradually became dominant, as did coastal trading, sugar refineries, and foundries.[12] Powerful banking interests, controlled by a relative few at the top rungs of society with business connections abroad, provided capital for the construction of transcontinental railroads.

Enriched by these activities, the Boston Brahmins built fine houses on Beacon Hill and on the new streets that stretched along land reclaimed from the surrounding tidal flats. Members of this entrenched and powerful group were not infrequently related to each other by marriage. Their social and financial worth encouraged them to act as stewards of the culture, education, and civil betterment of the city. Their Puritan traditions imbued them with a highly developed social conscience. Many felt it was their duty to act as "God's trustees" for the immigrant working class, whom they perceived as helpless, impoverished, and downtrodden. The formation of hospitals as charitable foundations also allowed them to promulgate their Christian values and engender a sense of stability among those entering the doors. Indeed, social responsibility was an overriding sentiment among the Brahmins who assumed leadership roles at the MGH, Boston City Hospital, and Children's Hospital.[13]

As protective of their wealth and privilege as they were of their social position, they viewed newly wealthy entrepreneurs as a threatening and unwelcome force. A specific example of this thinly veiled antipathy was their refusal to assign Brigham a pew in church suitable to his influence and standing in the community. This and other snubs may have sharpened Brigham's already well-developed social conscience. Brahmin insularity may also have stemmed from the growing presence of "foreign" institutions such as the Catholic Church and the increasing success and power of outsiders, particularly the Irish, in local politics. By 1870 35 percent of the population had been born abroad, primarily in Ireland.[14] Many worked as laborers in the seaport; others filled the mills and factories. Fourteen thousand female domestics served the rich. They huddled in tenements and boarding establishments in undesirable parts of the city, enduring overcrowded conditions and inadequate sanitation. Although her lot in life had improved from that of her mother and grandmother, Mrs. Turner provides a later example of this social milieu.

The need for health care was large. As in many cities in the United States at the time, communicable diseases were rife, with the common conditions of childhood, in particular, causing many deaths. Although Boston had escaped the cholera epidemics that periodically ravaged New York, tuberculosis remained the primary cause of mortality. Pneumonia and diphtheria were endemic. Accidents constantly threatened the workers in the burgeoning industries. Those jostled off the narrow brick pavements into streets crowded with horse-drawn streetcars and carriages often sustained injury. They had nowhere to go for care but the hospitals, despite their enduring reputation as places of last resort.

Physicians and surgeons in Boston came from the Brahmin class. Inevitably male and usually educated at Harvard, they often undertook additional training in their profession at famous centers in Scotland, France, and Germany. The gulf between these exalted beings and those in the lower social strata needing help was as deep as the medical aristocracy's contempt for outside doctors who had learned their trade by apprenticing with often inadequately educated local practitioners. The few hours they spent each week with the underclass that crowded the hospitals provided them the opportunity to deal with a spectrum of disease states. With extensive clinical material at their disposal, they could practice treatments, perfect techniques, and instruct medical students and interns. The reward for these activities was not pecuniary but ensured both faculty status at Harvard Medical School and proper social and professional connections that increased their reputation among their private patients. These wealthier individuals, in turn, received their medical care in convenient and comfortable settings in which they could escape the all-pervasive infections and meager conditions in the public hospitals.

The education of doctors and their approaches to disease at the turn of the twentieth century were relatively recent departures from enduring historical precedent. For centuries, healers in the West had combined mystical practices and supernatural beliefs with traditional treatments based on teachings of early Greek physicians that were later translated and embellished by Arab sages. Even with investigations in anatomy, physiology, and natural law by Renaissance scholars, most aspects of medicine remained rudimentary, with the majority of physicians mired in ignorance, superstition, and folk customs. Only a few retained practical skills and considered the fabric of the body, the care of wounds, and the nature of contagion. After the Reformation, Protestant culture added a moral meaning to disease, preaching that sin and wickedness predisposed one to illness, which was an expression of God's displeasure. In the absence of satisfactory explanations for physical conditions, these doctrines flourished, later finding their most obvious expression in Puritan America.

Despite ongoing beliefs in witchcraft, sorcery, and astrology, the scientific discoveries of the seventeenth century were a watershed. Experimental thinking shifted increasingly from philosophical interpretations of natural events to those based on objective observations. Novel findings in mathematics and physical science by European thinkers were often at odds with religious dogma. Innovations in agriculture, navigation, industry, engineering, and biology set the stage for advances that followed. New classes of manufacturers, workers, and consumers emerging during the Industrial Revolution in eighteenth-century England demanded opportunities to gain cultural and scientific knowledge. Interest in natural phenomena exploded, encouraged by the voyages of exploration and accounts of the flora and fauna of far-off lands. In response, universities in the nineteenth century promoted science and technology.

Inevitably, a significant proportion of the population did not benefit from the advantages of the new industrialism. An increasing birth rate, migration of those from the countryside desperately seeking jobs in the smoke-belching factories, and entry of cheap Irish labor into the British workforce created unprecedented urban crowding and draconian living conditions. Health and hygiene received low priority. With unqualified midwives officiating, childbirth was dangerous. Two-thirds of children born in London died before they reached the age of five from malnutrition, ill treatment, or infectious disease. Smallpox sprung up periodically while other epidemics ravaged populations in Britain and the Continent. Across the ocean, the situation was similar. In Massachusetts, Cotton Mather, the eminent Puritan preacher and author of the first medical textbook in the colonies, *The Angel of Bethesda*, lost his wife and three of his fifteen children in less than two weeks during the measles epidemic of 1713. Diphtheria was particularly virulent among indigenous peoples. Cholera and typhoid fever were uniformly dreaded. Lice spread typhus. Mosquito-borne yellow fever assailed Philadelphia in 1793. Even as late as 1878, half the population of Memphis died from that disease.

Hospitals also changed over the centuries. Despite only rudimentary understanding of medicine and science, medieval hospitals in Europe had been sanctuaries for the poor, providing reasonable, kindly, and charitable care. Expanding numbers of such benevolent institutions during the eighteenth century stimulated clinical and educational interests with demonstrations of anatomical dissection, instruction in diagnosis of disease, and training in surgery. By the nineteenth century, however, admission to a hospital became virtually a death threat, with conditions deteriorating to little better than those of the streets. As we have seen with Mrs. Turner, this fear persisted into the early twentieth century. Overcrowding and lack of sanitation could lead to often fatal infections, and open wards promoted the spread of disease. Surgical patients lay between those dying of pneumonia or with the pox. Drunkenness, fighting, filth, and despair prevailed.[15] But in the midst of such chaos, Florence Nightingale and her followers brought some order and improved standards of patient care. Despite her nursing reforms, however, institutional conditions remained primitive for decades thereafter.[16]

It is no wonder that the profession of medicine was not well respected. In Roman times, practitioners in this poorly regarded field were primarily foreigners, slaves, or freemen. Throughout the Middle Ages, those in religious orders took responsibility for care of the sick, providing more spiritual than practical help; unguents and salves, concocted from herbs in the monastery gardens, were only occasionally effective. The relatively few physicians in eighteenth-century England balanced precariously on the lowest rung of the gentry, striving to provide their services to those above them. Later, some of the more powerful in the profession gained reputations for being corrupt. Treating persons of rank became more important than developing skill, and greed and ignorance transcended empathy and knowledge.[17]

The majority of early medical practitioners in the United States faced substantial challenges in their unregulated profession. Despite the presence of a few enclaves of professional privilege in cities on the Eastern seaboard, most doctors led a difficult existence serving subsistence populations. Unqualified individuals practiced indiscriminately. Most made a poor living, which they supplemented by owning farms or by producing and dispensing uncontrolled patent medicines. Suspicious of any elitist propensities, many Americans felt that the vocation of medicine should be open to all and, like the law, be part of basic education.[18] Even as late as the time of Brigham's death, some pedants proclaimed the field to be the most despised of the professions. Indeed, the anti-intellectual and antischolastic culture of the Republic discouraged professional superiority, an attitude that encouraged local women to conduct domestic medicine and lay healing in their homes. Quackery abounded. The original universities in America, like the universities of Oxford and Cambridge, emphasized the classics and theology in preparation for the ministry. Medical education was particularly chaotic, lacking standards of quality and structure. But as the frontiers of the country expanded, the need for doctors increased. Training opportunities at early hospitals such as Pennsylvania Hospital in Philadelphia (1751), New York Hospital (Kings College, 1775), and the MGH were limited in number, so informal apprenticeships to local practitioners became the norm.

For-profit "proprietary" medical schools, often without serious credentials and regulations, proliferated. They were supported by highly individualistic physicians who decried as unnecessary and meddlesome the formation of the American Medical Association in 1846 to bring order and organization to the system. Many sold diplomas through the mail; students never even had to attend. In 1850 fifty-two such fly-by-night organizations existed. By 1900, 160 more had opened, including forty-two in Missouri; thirty-nine in Illinois (fourteen in Chicago alone); twenty-seven in Indiana; eighteen in Tennessee; eighteen in Cincinnati, Ohio; eleven in Louisville, Kentucky; and forty-three in New York.[19] Homeopathy, an unorthodox alternative method of treatment, vied for power with established practices. Competition, feuds, and antipathy among professionals were common. An extreme but amusing example of such fraternal strife and sectarianism occurred in 1856 at the Eclectic Medical Institute of Cincinnati, where a schism opened between the faculty and its supporters regarding finances and the introduction of new medicines. One faction locked the other out of the school building, declaring a state of war and displaying weapons. The feud was finally settled when the opposition brought in a six-pound cannon.[20]

After the Civil War, academic leaders considered means to organize professional training to the level already existing in other graduate fields such as engineering, law, and divinity. The presidents of private institutions such as Yale, Columbia, Chicago, and Washington University, and state universities such as Minnesota and Wisconsin began to take more control of their marginally affiliated medical schools or to establish a relationship with an already existing school. Their efforts raised standards of admission and enhanced the quality of instruction. President Eliot's substantial reforms at Harvard were followed soon thereafter by the more effective innovations at Johns Hopkins in Baltimore and improvements at the Universities of Michigan and Pennsylvania. New, relevant courses in science were added, and students worked in well-equipped laboratories under the direct supervision of full-time faculty members. These early forays initiated an important revolution in medical care.

Adequate financing of medical education was a long-standing problem. In 1891, for instance, total endowment for all medical schools in the
United States was $5 million. In contrast, funding for schools of theology
had risen to $18 million.[21] But the atmosphere was changing. The 1910
report *Medical Education in the United States and Canada* by the educator and
reformer Abraham Flexner was so influential that it permanently altered
the landscape of medical education. Energized by the findings, the trustees
of John D. Rockefeller's vast foundation, the General Board of Education,
increased funding for the schooling of doctors to $61 million by 1928.
The Carnegie Corporation contributed substantially. Private philanthropists and local and regional governments added revenue. Support for the
effort finally became secure.

Professional payment has been a contentious subject of debate throughout the history of academic departments in the United States, beginning
with the founding of the Pennsylvania Hospital in 1752. Then as now, the
majority of practitioners concerned themselves primarily with their private
patients, carrying out clinical teaching on an ad hoc basis. With encouragement and funding from the Rockefeller Foundation in the 1890s, those
at the new Johns Hopkins Hospital initiated a plan: under contract with
the university, the faculty would receive a salary from patient interactions paid directly to the institution itself. This departure from the long-
established system of fee for service was not without controversy. For
years following its introduction, the debate raged at Hopkins. Would the
professors neglect their academic responsibilities, spending too much time
with their private patients? Administrators worried that high surgical fees
in particular would be directed away from the coffers of the institution.
Flexner's report expressed concern that the private wards in academic
hospitals would detract from teaching by becoming "high priced sanitaria
for the well-to-do private patients of the prominent clinicians connected
with the hospital and medical school."[22] The additional proposal of placing those "prominent clinicians" on salary was and still is heavily debated.
The full-time plan generated considerable heat, first at Hopkins and then
at other teaching hospitals that accepted it. While some academic professors embraced the overtures (and money) of the Rockefellers, those with
large private practices did not. Indeed, the chair of medicine at Hopkins,

having first welcomed the idea, reconsidered and resigned his position rather than accept the proposed salary. The dissenting faculty placed his successor under such pressure that he fell ill. Shortly after the turn of the twentieth century, members of the foundation offered Harvard a similar arrangement to convert its existing laissez-faire program to the full-time system. Opposition rose so high that the university politely turned down their proposal.

The Brigham trustees had formulated strict salary arrangements for the staff, but Cushing continued to hold mixed opinions about the impact of the full-time faculty system on clinical departments. He did feel that such an arrangement would be more effective for a teaching hospital, and that the private practice plans of the MGH and most other teaching hospitals of the time introduced conflicts of interest among lucrative clinical work, research, and education. He arranged for a proportion of professional fees to be returned to the department to fund its educational and investigative activities. This modified full-time program spread throughout other institutions. Ultimately, at the Brigham clinicians received a base salary but were allowed some private practice using a few beds that the hospital had set aside for the purpose. Although Cushing was the only one of the original faculty who benefited, those in the department since have subsequently adhered to this plan.

With these gradual changes commercial American medical schools offering a degree for a fee eventually disappeared. The profession became more cohesive as advances in scientific knowledge complemented standardized training.[23] The plethora of patent medicines, so prevalent in earlier decades, came under state regulation. The numbers of charlatans and quacks declined with increasing professional specialization. Infant mortality diminished, and overall life expectancy lengthened as public health measures began to control the spread of infectious diseases. Anesthesia and surgery improved. The American faith in simplicity and common sense began to yield to a celebration of science and technology. Finally, the prestige of a medical career increased; it was becoming desirable to be a doctor.

With the United States an increasingly formidable industrial presence, its expanding and increasingly well-funded educational enterprises began to rival those of Europe and Great Britain. Hospitals progressed from places dreaded by those lacking alternative recourse to institutions that based comprehensive care on biological discoveries. Patients actually survived their operations. With the Johns Hopkins model of medical education and patient care providing a fresh force in American medicine and with reform in the air, the time was propitious for the creation of an academic medical complex in Boston different from the long-established and autonomous MGH. The Peter Bent Brigham Hospital and its faculty refined the new system substantially, blending an organized program of residency training under dedicated clinician-teachers with comprehensive patient care through clinical observation, relevant scientific knowledge, and progressively more accurate laboratory determinations. The Baltimore and Boston institutions produced continuing advances in diagnosis and treatment, education, and investigation in concert with others throughout the country that gradually began to follow their lead.

Despite the excitement engendered by these changes, however, we must remember that medical knowledge was still relatively underdeveloped as the twentieth century dawned. Efforts by practitioners were often limited to the relief of symptoms; many illnesses still ran their natural course little influenced by the tools, techniques, and medications that we now take for granted. Indeed, no less an international authority than Sir William Osler had suggested only a few years before that doctors could cure only four or five conditions, and that often the most they could do for a patient was to alleviate suffering and ensure proper nursing care. Many practitioners of the day took umbrage with those remarks, although Osler was only confirming, rather more subtly, Voltaire's tongue-in-cheek opinion of two centuries earlier that nature alone is responsible for cure while the purpose of medicine is only to amuse its adherents. These sentiments were entertainingly echoed in the 1870s by the Harvard anatomist and clinician Oliver Wendell Holmes, who declared: "I firmly believe that if the whole materia medica, as now used, could be sunk to the bottom of the sea, it would be all the better for mankind and all the worse for the fishes."[24]

Even with acceptance of the germ theory of disease and identification of specific microorganisms, control of infections remained inadequate.

Diabetics often died; insulin would not be discovered until after World War I. Although digitalis was available to improve the function of a failing heart, antibiotics, antihypertensives, antidepressants, anti-inflammatories, and other pharmaceuticals so ubiquitous in our lives today still lay in the future. Blood transfusions were exceptional. Anesthesia and asepsis were used routinely, but surgical intervention remained limited to relatively simple procedures. Even these procedures had a long evolution.

three

Evolution of a Profession

Giles Mullins was a middle-aged butcher who worked during the 1840s at London's Smithfield meat market in the shadow of the seven-century-old St. Bartholomew's Hospital. He had become increasingly incapacitated by intense spasms in his lower abdomen, intermittent stoppage of his urinary stream, fever, and bloody urine. In recent months his life had become unbearable.

Although the incidence of bladder stone has inexplicably declined in the modern world, it was all too common throughout much of human history. The condition occurred so frequently in sixteenth-century France, for instance, that the kings kept court experts in the surgical removal of the concretions. Practicing throughout all levels of society, these and other lithotomists formed specialty schools dedicated to the subject. Samuel Pepys, the English diarist, survived a successful operation in 1658 and kept the tennis-ball-sized memento near him for the rest of his life as a reminder of his mortality. Napoleon Bonaparte suffered for years with stones and spent much time during the Battle of Borodino in the Russian Campaign of 1812 dismounted from his horse and leaning against a tree trying to empty his bladder. The clouded judgment that led an ill and debilitated Napoleon III to declare war on Germany in 1870 was apparently related to the disease. Three years later the emperor died following unsuccessful surgical removal. Those in America were no less spared. Benjamin Franklin suffered agonies during the last eight years of his life, chose to defer operative intervention, and succumbed at age 84 in sustained misery.[1]

In despair, realizing that he was probably under a death warrant regardless of treatment and unable to afford to call the surgeon to his house, Mullins entered St. Bartholomew's for help. He could not realize what he would have to endure, as operations at that time were inevitably brutal exercises of final desperation. With a variety of nostrums doing little to dull the pain, surgeons worked as rapidly as they could on the screaming and struggling patients. The best lithotomists could enter the bladder and take out the stone within a minute; the worst took considerably longer. Indeed, it was a dictum that "Long and murderous operations where the surgeon labors for an hour in extracting the stone [lead] to the inevitable destruction of the patient."[2] The most experienced operators could amputate a leg, another common undertaking, in a few seconds. Baron Dominique Larrey, surgeon general of the French armies during the Napoleonic Wars and a pioneer in military medicine, allegedly removed 200 legs in twenty-four hours in the field during one of the major battles.[3] According to a perhaps apocryphal story, a mid-nineteenth-century London surgeon, well known for his speed in leg amputation, included both testes of his patient and two fingers of his assistant with a single sweep of the knife and flash of the saw.[4]

The operating theaters were torture chambers. Onlookers crowded around the table to view the relatively small numbers of procedures performed. Some were built as actual amphitheaters. In the Royal Infirmary of Edinburgh in 1750, for instance, 200 spectators sat on the high tiers of seats gaping down at the scene below. Once the floor had been cleaned of blood, the chamber could be used as a lecture hall, autopsy room, or chapel.[5] The young Charles Darwin was so appalled at the blood, screams, and violence he experienced while viewing surgery in 1825 that he gave up any thoughts of entering medicine.[6] "I attended on two occasions the operating theater in the hospital at Edinburgh, and saw two very bad operations, one on a child, but I rushed away before they were completed. Nor did I ever attend again, for hardly any inducement would have been strong enough to make me do so; this being long before the blessed days of chloroform. The two cases fairly haunted me for many a long year."

Extraction of bladder stones lived up to its horrific reputation. Celsus, a nonphysician medical writer of ancient Rome, portrayed in detail an enduring technique for "cutting on the gripe," incising through the prostate gland directly into the bladder. The patient lay face-up on a table, ankles and wrists tied together, knees spread, and head and body restrained by burly attendants. This "lithotomy position," still used for rectal procedures and in gynecologic and urologic surgery, allows full access to the perineum, the area between the external genitalia and the anus. The operator inserted a finger in the rectum, felt the bladder, and pushed the stone forward toward the skin. Quickly opening the intervening tissues, he removed the hard object with his fingers, a hook, or as methods of performing the procedure changed, with scoops or instruments.[7] Surgeons used this approach for centuries before an itinerant French practitioner, Frère Jacques de Beaulieu (the Frère Jacques of nursery-rhyme fame) designed and popularized a less-disruptive incision made through the intervening tissues to the side of the midline and away from the prostate and the urethra, the tubular passage between the bladder and the outside. With the stone extracted and urine escaping freely from the defect, the intense bladder spasms the patient had experienced for so long disappeared. If he or she survived without infection, the fistulous tract would close. The introduction of anesthesia within a few years of Mullins's ordeal allowed more convenient entrance into the bladder through the lower abdominal wall.

An alternate strategy first attempted by the ancient Egyptians and undergoing many modifications thereafter involved a crushing device that the surgeon inserted through the penis directly into the bladder. He could then locate the stone by feel, grasp it, and break it into pieces that he then could pull out with the instrument.[8] Occasionally he could fragment the material into bits small enough for the patient to void. This method has been further refined in modern times with a thin fiber-optic light source that allows full visualization of the bladder contents through a scope for precise instrument placement. Even more sophisticated are the current methods of disintegrating the concretion via high-frequency shock waves transmitted from outside the body.

Despite the short duration of Mullins's operation, the actual experience must have been beyond agony. Although the removal of a stone the size of a hen's egg relieved his urinary symptoms, he predictably began to sicken within a few days from the almost inevitable sepsis that the unwashed hands of the surgeon and the inadequately cleaned, encrusted instruments had introduced into the incision. During his final week of misery, his attending doctors tortured him further with blistering, enemas, laxatives of senna and rhubarb, and administration of opium and aromatic spices.[9] Toward the end of an aggressive session of copious bloodletting, he died. His wretched experience was all too common throughout centuries of surgical intervention.

A harrowing description of an actual case was the subject of a lawsuit in 1828 brought by a surgeon who sued for libel Thomas Whatley, the editor of the fledgling British medical journal, *Lancet*. Whatley had published an eyewitness account of the operation.[10] The surgeon was apparently unable to find the bladder through his increasingly large incision. His assistants described the events:

> Various forceps employed: a scoop, sounds, and staves introduced at the opening. "I really can't conceive the difficulty–Hush! Hush! Don't you hear the stone? Have you a long finger? Give me another instrument. Now I have it! Good God! I can hear the stone when I passed the sound from the opening, but the forceps don't touch it–O dear! O dear." Such were the hurried exclamations of the operator. Every now and then there was a cry of, "Hush!" Which was succeeded by the stillness of death, only broken by the horrible squash, squash of the forceps in the perineum. "Oh, let it go–pray let it keep in," was the constant cry of the poor man.

The operation took fifty-five minutes. The patient died twenty-nine hours later.

In past centuries, custom often took precedence over surgeons' direct experience or clinical trials. For example, in preparation for his operation, Mullins had been purged and bled. Long considered a panacea for all illness, the letting of blood was not infrequently carried out before surgery to weaken the patient and make him or her less conscious of pain. More value was assigned to such surgical traditions than objective evidence, a shortcoming that endures in some instances to this day. While the origins are obscure, the ancient practice of bloodletting is documented

in Egyptian papyrus scrolls. The Greeks, Romans, and subsequent healers throughout the ages carried it out in both the healthy and the ill. At
least some of its beginnings may be attributed to Hippocrates, the Greek
Father of Medicine, who taught in the fifth century BC that imbalance of
the four humors of the body and their respective associated personality
traits—black and yellow bile, blood, and phlegm; melancholic, choleric,
sanguine, and phlegmatic—were the cause of all disease. Remedies, particularly bleeding, were designed to correct this imbalance. Galen, a prolific
medical popularizer of the second century AD, extolled the practice of
selectively removing "tainted" blood from afflicted sites to restore equilibrium. A surgeon to the Roman gladiators, he also described operations for
varicose veins, the repair of cleft lips, and the closure of loops of intestine
penetrated by sword or spear.[11] He encouraged enthusiastically bloodletting before these ordeals.

One of the few invasive procedures that early surgeons could perform
easily, the purposeful removal of blood persisted long after William
Harvey's demonstration in 1628 that blood circulated continuously
throughout the body. Indeed, the entire concept that bleeding restored
humoral balance was based on false premises.[12] By 1750, nearly three-
quarters of patients in at least some large British hospitals were bled
routinely, many on a daily basis. Practitioners in America were no
less eager. During the yellow fever epidemic in Philadelphia in 1793,
Benjamin Rush, arguably the foremost clinician of his time, let blood from
sick patients so assiduously that he undoubtedly shortened many lives.
His almost fanatical zeal presumably influenced those treating George
Washington's sore throat six years later; their unrelenting bleeding
ensured his demise.

The tradition died slowly despite mounting evidence against its benefits. Sir William Osler advocated the treatment in the seventh (1907)
edition of his highly popular and enduring textbook, *The Principles and
Practice of Medicine*, the last he wrote entirely by himself. He admitted,
however, that in many cases, "a hypodermic of morphine [was] more
effective."[13] A section of the 1948 sixteenth edition still discussed bleeding to treat a wide variety of conditions that included pneumonia, emphy-
sema, stroke, pleurisy, peritonitis, delirium, and mumps, although this

advice disappeared in subsequent editions. Even during the early years of my residency in the 1960s, physicians still bled patients to improve the symptoms of cardiac failure. The diseased hearts of these individuals do not function well enough to propel blood at a normal rate throughout the body. As a result, fluid leaves the circulation and collects in the tissues, especially the lungs. Breathing becomes increasingly difficult. Lacking effective medications to increase urine output, we removed a liter or more of blood, believing we might reduce excess body fluid and improve shortness of breath. Although such maneuvers worked transiently, the fluid inevitably returned.

A quite different approach involved the application of leeches to the chest of patients with pneumonia to decrease congestion, drain blood from fresh surgical dissections, or diminish swelling in inflamed or engorged areas. In 1833, for instance, over 41 million leeches were imported into France for medical purposes.[14] Even now, reconstructive surgeons occasionally use the worms to reduce swelling and promote healing of tissue flaps they have transferred from one bodily site to another, joining the incredibly small vessels under a microscope. Despite their lack of aesthetic appeal, the leeches are remarkably effective.

The first two revolutions of the modern field, anesthesia and the principles of antisepsis and asepsis, were not fully accepted until the late nineteenth century. Until then, having an operation was the final brutal recourse of hopeless individuals with advanced disease like Giles Mullins. It was little better for the operators themselves, who had to disregard the incalculable suffering they were producing with their fingers, the knife, and the red-hot iron. Success was equated with survival.

Although practitioners of the ancient world carried out a variety of relatively sophisticated surgical maneuvers with forceps, probes, saws, and long-bladed knives, application of their techniques remained static as learning shifted from Sumeria and Egypt to other Mediterranean countries, Asia Minor, and westward into Europe. The manuscripts that resided in the great libraries of the Middle Ages and provided the bulk of medical and scientific knowledge were predominantly Latin translations of the writings of Arab and Christian savants. The information these individuals produced was less than objective. They combined their own, often erroneous, interpretations of and commentaries on the tenets of Greek and Roman physician-teachers with contemporary beliefs and mixed syllogistic precepts, theoretical dialectic, and theological dogma. Despite surgery having been an important part of the repertoire of the Greek physicians, Arab pedagogues disapproved of the craft, believing that to touch the human body, particularly blood, with the hands was unclean and unholy. Cloistered Christian scholars solidified this belief in an edict issued by the Council of Tours in 1163, *Ecclesia Abhorret a Sanguine*. This and subsequent ecclesiastical doctrines separated those who actually tried to relieve or correct the physical problems of patients by operative intervention from physicians, who remained aloof from such practical matters.

The philosophical differentiation between physicians and surgeons has been an enduring one. In seventeenth-century Paris, for instance, physician-teachers, who the educational academies of the time considered qualified to instruct on any subject, lectured in Latin to aspiring students. However, they imparted little useful knowledge. Never lowering themselves to examine the patient, these lofty figures diagnosed from on high with pretense and pedantry, prescribing usually ineffective medicaments and relegating bleeding and purging to the surgeons, far beneath them on the social scale. Their fatuous Olympian attitude, which Molière portrayed in his plays, and Thomas Cruikshank and Honoré Daumier later characterized in their satirical drawings, continues to amuse. Unhappily, similar impressions of the disinterest and arrogance of some medical professionals may still exist in the minds of more than a few patients.

The early surgeons took a different route. Throughout the Middle Ages the individuals who performed operations were usually relatively untrained itinerant barbers, sheep gelders, bath keepers, and even occasional executioners. Although disdained by the self-important physicians, they set fractures, drained abscesses, opened fistulas, and excised superficial ulcers. They occasionally dealt with depressed cranial fractures, as had ancient practitioners before them, by boring a series of holes through the skull to produce an opening large enough to remove the penetrating shards of bone; these remnants became popular as charms. They sutured lacerations and, as we have seen, even couched cataracts with a probe. Even though early surgeons lacked adequate anesthesia or knowledge of the importance of sterile practice, these relatively minor procedures not infrequently benefited the patients.

The successful treatment of the fistula-in-ano of Louis XIV of France did much to raise the profile of surgery. This was a common condition in centuries past, particularly among the nobility who spent much time on horseback wearing heavy suits of armor. Perspiring freely when the weather was hot and remaining damp and cold in the winter, the knights often developed painful abscesses near the anus. Not infrequently, these burrowed inward through the fat of the buttock and eventually formed a tract between the skin near the anus and the rectal wall. The result was a chronically infected, intermittently discharging, inflamed, and tender connection between the two sites. Treatment was relegated to the usual purging, bleeding, or application of leeches. Often in desperation in the age before anesthesia, some surgeons passed a string or wire through the tract, tying it ever tighter to cut through the intervening tissues during weeks of torture. Others thrust a red-hot iron into the site, hoping in vain that the cooked area would heal.

In severe distress from the condition, the Sun King consulted his surgeon, Charles François Félix. Because Félix had never operated upon an anal fistula, he gathered together a group of patients with similar problems from the charity hospitals of Paris to practice and perfect his skills. Early in the morning of November 18, 1686, he entered the king's bedchamber.[15] Several people were present, including Mme. de Maintenon, the minister of war, a priest, three surgeons, and four apothecaries to hold His Majesty still. Using a knife with an especially narrow blade, Félix made two incisions, then used scissors to open the connection between rectum and skin widely with eight snips. Although he had to perform three additional procedures in the ensuing weeks to keep the tract open, this radical approach allowed the open wound to fill in and heal gradually. By January, the king was cured. The technique is used to this day.

Louis not only endured the ordeal and the prolonged convalescence, but was so pleased with the result that he elevated Félix to the nobility, gave him a large estate, and insisted on paying a huge fee. In a further gesture of appreciation, he improved significantly the status of surgeons and their education in the universities by endowing five academic chairs. Despite the royal gratitude and support, the alleged intellectual and educational superiority of the socially elite physicians to the surgical journeymen persisted. The Paris Faculty of Medicine continued to force surgeons to take an oath swearing to the superiority of physicians and their medical treatment over the adherents of an allegedly less acceptable discipline. This rule was not abolished until 1750. Indeed, modern surgeons are still occasionally made aware of this enduring concept.

Understanding the location and relationships of the structures of the body took centuries. Comprehension of their function took even longer. The Greeks initiated the earliest anatomical research, usually at public dissections of the bodies of criminals. Ultimately, however, this practice fell out of favor, and animal subjects replaced humans. Indeed, Galen, with his vast and usually inaccurate writings on anatomy, never dissected a human body. It was an activity ultimately forbidden by law. The practicalities of science slumbered in medieval times, with their schematic and usually inaccurate renderings of anatomy, theological concepts about the sanctity of the body, conjecture about its ultimate ascent to Heaven, and uncritical attention to the doctrines of higher authority. Knowledge introduced during the Renaissance plus the loosening and eventual removal of a papal ban on human dissection enhanced the new emphasis on assimilating accurate information from direct observation. The several causes for this gradual rebirth included Johannes Gutenberg's introduction of the printing press around 1440 and the formation and growth of universities throughout Europe.

During the late fifteenth century, Leonardo da Vinci introduced the subject of functional anatomy, based directly on his detailed human dissections and recorded in his 750 sketches and unique cross-sectional renderings of the musculature and underlying organs. Andreas Vesalius elevated the subject further with his 1643 text, *On the Fabric of the Human Body*. He and a few equally renowned colleagues and disciples described a variety of disease states by carrying out autopsies and reintroducing ancient surgical techniques that had been lost during the Middle Ages. Their discoveries discomforted many of their more doctrinaire peers. At least one of the free thinkers who continued to place fact before dogma, Michael Servetus, was burned as a heretic for reporting that blood mixes with air in the lungs before it re-enters the heart.[16] The surgical anatomists also moved from the dissecting room to the side of the patient. Dealing with the distress of those unfortunate individuals undergoing operations without anesthesia, they were able to carry out a variety of procedures that included removal of bladder stones, ligation of bleeding vessels, amputation of the leg, and excision of superficial tumors, despite little real appreciation of disease processes and the almost invariable development of infection in an age before there was any inkling of the existence of bacteria.

With both scientific discoveries and public curiosity about the natural world increasing during the eighteenth and early nineteenth centuries, surgeons formed competing schools of anatomy, particularly in London, where no medical school yet existed. Advertising for students, who paid a fee to attend, the lecturers taught their craft through anatomical demonstrations. In contrast, such institutions had been long established in cities in continental Europe, Scotland, and Ireland. The Munros in Edinburgh and the surgeon-scientists William and John Hunter in London popularized this type of instruction. Similar practices spread across the Atlantic to America.

A constant influx of fresh subjects for dissection was necessary for the sessions. Although King Henry VIII had formed the Company of Barber Surgeons under royal charter in 1540 and allowed chosen anatomy schools the right to dissect the bodies of four, then six, hanged criminals each year, this official supply of cadavers could not meet the burgeoning demand. As a result, a lucrative underworld trade of bodysnatching began that flourished well into the twentieth century.[17] The "resurrectionists," as they were dubbed, supplied the needs of the anatomy schools by procuring the newly dead illegally from graves or directly from the hangman's gibbet. Outraged and offended, the public cried out against these practices. Families hired guards to watch over freshly dug gravesites. Battles for possession of the body at the site of execution became routine. Even more nefarious irregularities surfaced when fresh corpses arrived secretly at the schools for dissection. The most infamous of the procurers, William Burke and William Hare of Edinburgh, sold the bodies of victims they had murdered to the eminent surgical teacher Robert Knox. Hare gave evidence against his partner and escaped execution. Knox's career was ruined. Burke was eventually hanged and dissected in 1829, but achieved relative immortality with the introduction of the word burke—murdering to order—into the English language.

The clandestine trade in bodies for anatomical dissection also thrived in the United States. Many subjects came from populations lacking social or political influence, particularly the denizens of almshouses and other urban poor. The majority were African Americans, although in Boston they were predominantly Irish paupers. Although some medical schools expected their students to remove bodies from graves, professional resurrectionists, kept informed by caretakers of graveyards, undertakers, and even doctors, routinely exhumed bodies of the recently deceased from their coffins.[18]

Even though public antipathy was strong and social mores condemned such defilement of the dead, little could be done to lessen such practices. The Doctor's Riot in April 1788 was one violent exception. This occurred behind New York Hospital after some boys spotted a student dissecting an arm. A gathering mob rampaged through the building, destroying anatomical preparations and carrying off several bodies for reburial. The following day, still angry and unassuaged, they stormed the jail that housed several surgeons and their students. The guards opened fire on the throng, killing seven and wounding several more. Protests occurred periodically in other cities.[19] In general, local officials did not become involved until well-publicized indignities provoked action. In Philadelphia in 1882, for instance, the newspapers reported that an organized group of grave-diggers were systematically looting the main African-American burial ground in the city.[20] The headlines trumpeted "Graveyard Ghouls Arrested with a Cartload of Corpses," and "Thousands of Bodies Taken for Dissection." Occasional "mistakes" gained additional publicity. One in particular involved a former congressman of Ohio and son of President William Henry Harrison, who was found hanging in a dissecting room in the Medical College of Ohio in 1878. Resurrectionists had stolen his body from the family mausoleum at a highly reputable cemetery in Cincinnati.[21] As a result of these and other examples, and despite ineffectual attempts at regulation by individual states, concerned national, political, and medical leaders eventually collaborated in the 1930s to pass strict anatomy laws controlling such practices, and instituted anatomy boards to identify and distribute unclaimed bodies.

It is all too obvious that the majority of surgical treatments from ancient times to the latter half of the nineteenth century, as cruel as they were, represented the only realistic options to relieve suffering. For good reason, the majority of individuals like Giles Mullins rarely sought help unless the disorder from which they suffered was completely intolerable, totally incapacitating, or acutely life threatening. Other patients were denied surgical intervention as too dangerous. Indeed, an operation was a relatively infrequent event; only forty-three were performed at the MGH between 1821 and 1823.[22] The procedures were not only distressing to all but often failed.

One representative catastrophe feared by patients and their doctors alike was obstruction of the intestine, with its predictable downhill course of worsening abdominal cramps and distension, intractable vomiting, dehydration, and death. The condition may arise from a twist in the bowel, adhesions, or the presence of a tumor. A loop of intestine may enter the sac of a hernia at the groin or umbilicus. If the bowel cannot promptly be pushed back into the abdomen, it may become fixed in place (incarcerated). If the trapped segment distends with gas and fluid, its blood supply may become compromised; this results in strangulation, tissue destruction, and perforation.

Physicians throughout the ages contended with the problem in a variety of ways. If no external hernia was visible and the obstruction was a result of some abnormality within the abdominal cavity, some practitioners suspended the patient upside down for prolonged periods, hoping that the drag on the intestines would cause the affected portion of bowel to open. Others gave copious water enemas. Still others made the unfortunate individuals swallow as much as three pounds of mercury or lead shot, thinking that the weight of the metal would relieve the blockage.[23] Later, a few used the newly introduced electric shocks, placing one electrode in the rectum, the other on the abdominal wall.[24] Bleeding, leeches, cold baths, and ice packs were always in vogue. Occasional surgeons were more proactive if the site of obstruction was the result of an obvious hernia, and they could puncture the trapped bowel with a needle or open it with a knife. They occasionally relieved the problem by dividing the constricting tissue with blade or cautery. Returning a portion of strangulated bowel to the abdomen, however, meant certain rupture and the spread of its bacteria-laden contents throughout the peritoneal cavity. Death after days of suffering seemed merciful.

With surgery becoming more successful by the turn of the twentieth century, operative control of intestinal obstruction improved. Hernias could be repaired. The abdomen could be opened and constricting adhesive bands divided. Twisted bowel could be straightened. Tumors could be excised and the ends of the bowel rejoined. When a tumor of the large bowel or rectum was too large for immediate and definitive treatment, a diverting colostomy could be formed, with an artificial anus on the abdominal wall to allow free egress of bowel contents. If a segment of bowel was dead, it could be removed and the healthy ends approximated. Despite these advances, the well-known London surgeon Sir Frederick Treves noted in 1899, "It is less dangerous to leap from the Clifton Suspension Bridge than to suffer from acute intestinal obstruction and decline operation."[25] These sentiments remain true to this day.

As an example of how serious the condition was before effective operative relief, let us consider the events surrounding the death of Caroline of Ansbach, queen consort of King George II of England.[26] Her early ample proportions grew to obesity by middle age through good food and bearing seven children. During her sixth pregnancy she developed an umbilical hernia that slowly enlarged in size. In early November 1737 Caroline experienced progressive cramping, abdominal pain, and vomiting. With actual physical examination of the Royal Person transcending existing protocol, her physicians administered a variety of medicaments and stimulants. They repeatedly bled her.

Finally granted permission to examine her two days later, her surgeon discovered a swollen and tender loop of bowel firmly stuck in the hernia sac. No one favored opening the constricting ring of surrounding tissue, thinking the procedure would be too risky. Several attempts to drain the contents of the distended bowel were unproductive. The segment finally burst and copious fluid gushed out. Eleven days following her initial symptoms, after prolonged and unbearable suffering, the queen died at age 54 with the most distinguished medical experts in the land standing helplessly by.

Yet a few examples indicated that surgical intervention in the eighteenth and nineteenth centuries under particular circumstances could yield positive results. Two operations performed by innovative country practitioners in remote areas in the United States belied gloomy public and professional attitudes about the effectiveness of surgery. Ephraim McDowell carried out the first on a table in his living room in Danville, Kentucky, late in 1807, the successful removal of a huge ovarian cyst. Although working by himself in a rural environment, he was well educated for his time, having spent three years reading medicine with an Edinburgh graduate practicing in Virginia and two additional years in Edinburgh with Sir John Bell, a celebrated surgeon in what was then the most famous medical school in the world. In his lectures, Bell had discussed the possibilities of surgical treatment of these huge cysts but had never attempted the feat.[27]

The patient, Jane Crawford, rode sixty miles through the Kentucky mountains to McDowell's house and its adjacent apothecary shop, balancing her hugely distended abdomen on the pommel of the saddle. He had already informed her that surgery was the only solution. Knowing its formidable risks, she agreed. Medicated with opium and alcohol, she was said to have kept her mind off the pain of the twenty-five-minute procedure by repeating the Psalms. Unable to deliver the huge cyst through the modest abdominal incision, he opened its wall and drained out fifteen pounds of gelatinous contents. He then tied off the vascular stalk, removed the empty cyst, which itself weighed seven pounds, and sewed the abdomen shut. She recovered nicely. Eight of the thirteen patients in McDowell's eventual series survived the procedure and returned to normal life, an enviable record at the time. Several factors probably contributed. The peritoneum, the glistening membrane lining the abdominal walls and the viscera inside, can withstand a single insult but not continuing contamination. In Mrs. Crawford's case, the surgery was performed rapidly in a clean environment. Neither infection nor bleeding occurred.

The second surgical advance involved the closure of a vesico-vaginal fistula, a connection between bladder and vagina that may occur when tissues tear during a complicated obstetrical delivery. Described throughout history and still common in underdeveloped countries, this tragic condition ostracizes afflicted women from their families and communities, relegating them to a life of misery, with leaking urine soaking their clothes and inflaming the skin of their thighs.[28] Surgeons over the centuries had attempted to close the defects using linen or silk sutures. The inevitably infected fistulae always reopened. There were only a handful of successes.

Marion Sims solved the problem. He was born in a village in South Carolina in 1813. After completing his education in that state, he spent several months observing surgeons in Philadelphia. His father, a lawyer, reinforced the prevailing public disdain toward the practice of medicine by noting, "if I had known [of your career choice] I certainly would not have sent you to college!"[29] Opening his office in a town in rural Alabama, Sims was soon faced with several slaves with this fearful condition. Possibly because of pelvic distortion from childhood rickets, they had experienced tissue disruption during traumatic deliveries that left them incapacitated, wretched, and near suicide. The young surgeon had previously corrected uterine displacement by asking the patient to kneel with her back arched and her forehead and arms on the table. Manipulation of the uterus then became easy. He adopted this knee-chest position to close the first two fistulae with fine silk, incorporating lead shot over the stitch for added support. Both attempts were unsuccessful. Realizing that the permeable silk promoted infection, he substituted fine silver wire from a jeweler to close the defect and inserted a urinary catheter to keep the bladder from filling and stressing the suture line. These relatively simple innovations provided him with the first of many successes. Indeed, the new approach was a revelation. Moving to Europe during the Civil War because of his support for the Confederate cause, he convinced surgeons there to use the inert wire. Again, there were many successes. Eventually he migrated to New York, having made a critical improvement in surgical technique.

Adherence to established traditions and preservation of the status quo rather than assessing the worth of proposed innovations by direct trial has been a constant theme throughout medicine, science, and progress in general. Convincing colleagues that new ideas may improve the norm is inevitably difficult. The obvious advances that McDowell and Sims had instituted remained objects of suspicion to many of their peers. Indeed, even after a number of surgeons in Europe and America had followed McDowell's lead and successfully removed ovarian cysts, members of the French Imperial Academy of Medicine still refused to vote to accept the procedure before enduring months of debate and demands for continued assessment. In our own time, startlingly original departures, such as Mrs. Laverne's minimally invasive laparoscopic gastric bypass operation, are not accepted easily. But increasing numbers of believers have persevered and supported innovation. Spencer Wells, for instance, a well-known London surgeon, reported that he had removed a thousand ovarian cysts between 1858 and 1880. The mortality of his final one hundred patients was a respectable 11 percent, although competitors on either side of the Atlantic questioned his statistics for some time thereafter.[30] Satisfactory closure of vesico-vaginal fistulae using Sims's method also became routine. Other types of surgery became more common. Some surgeons removed cancers of the breast plus adjacent lymph nodes. A few carried out amputations through hip and shoulder with survival of the patients. Surgery was slowly coming of age.

Within a few years after Mullins's death from bladder stone removal, the revolution of anesthesia, followed by a second revolution of antisepsis and asepsis, transformed long-established surgical traditions.

The introduction of anesthesia changed surgical operations from unbearable ordeals of terror and despair to calm and elective events. Throughout the centuries surgeons had administered a variety of ineffective medicaments to temper the agony. These included mandrake root, henbane, opium, hemp, alcohol, and tobacco enemas. Some tried hypnosis. A practice in the Royal Navy was to beat a drum loudly near a victim's ears to keep his mind off the pain. The strong arms of the assistants were inevitably more effective. A description by the highly popular English diarist, playwright, and novelist Fanny Burney of the removal of her own breast is a disturbing recollection of what happened before the first revolution in modern surgery. Baron Larrey carried out the procedure in her apartment in Paris in 1811 while the completely awake patient glimpsed portions of the procedure through a thin cloth covering her face.[31] "I refused to be held; but when I saw the glitter of polished steel–I closed my eyes. When the dreadful steel was plunged into the breast–cutting through veins–arteries–flesh–I began a scream that lasted intermittently during the whole time of the incision. I almost marvel that it rings not in my ears still! So excruciating was the agony. I felt the Knife rackling against the breast bone–scraping it." Months later and still with nightmare-laden nights, she had difficulty putting her experience into words in a long letter to her sister.

The use of inhaled gases transformed this appalling picture. Humphry Davy, a young chemist working in "pneumatic medicine" near London in 1800, became interested in the effects of nitrous oxide, a gas that Joseph Priestley, who isolated oxygen, had discovered over twenty-five years before. Davy noted that those who breathed the fumes exhibited sensations of pleasure, particularly laughter, and seemed impervious to pain. Christening it "laughing gas" and trying it himself, he found that it relieved his toothache. His colleagues, however, thought it merely an amusing diversion and did not take seriously his suggestion of a potential use in surgery. In 1815 Michael Faraday, one of Davy's assistants who later worked out the theory of electricity, found that if individuals inhaled another substance, ether, they experienced effects similar to those of nitrous oxide. Although recognized a century previously as a sleep inducer, the gas had never been thought of as an agent for dulling pain. Both nitrous oxide and ether became popular recreational drugs for "frolics" among undergraduates in London and among medical and dental students in America.

Three more decades passed before some in the medical profession, particularly in the United States, seriously considered that the agents might be advantageous during operations. A country doctor from Jefferson, Georgia, produced the first clue. Indulging with his friends in an "ether frolic," Crawford Long realized that those who breathed the gas and fell down felt no pain, despite sometimes sustaining cuts or bruises. In 1842 Long administered the substance to a friend, James Venables, before removing a growth in his neck. Again, there was no pain. Unfortunately, Long, a modest man, did not publish the results of this and probably other cases for seven years. In 1844 a dentist from Hartford, Horace Wells, heard a lecture on the effects of inhaling nitrous oxide. Intrigued, Wells convinced a colleague to pull one of his molar teeth under its influence. Wells remembered nothing of the procedure. Despite several further successes, however, a public demonstration failed because the patient suddenly awoke screaming. An ex-partner of Wells, William Morton, moved to Boston, where a chemistry professor, also impressed by what he had seen at the fashionable "ether frolics," advised him to switch from nitrous oxide to ether in his dental practice. Morton used the latter agent on a dog, his assistant, on himself, and on a patient so successfully that he convinced the surgeon at the MGH, John Collins Warren, to allow him to give a demonstration of its effectiveness before a large crowd of medical onlookers.

It was October 16, 1846. Faculty and students filled the operating suite, a small amphitheater still preserved as the "Ether Dome" and used as a lecture hall. With an inhaler device he had constructed specially, Morton anesthetized the patient, Edward Abbott. To the astonishment and relief of the audience, Warren isolated and calmly tied off a large vascular anomaly in Abbott's neck without causing pain. The operation took thirty minutes. Abbott awoke, amazed and gratified. The news spread quickly. Unhurried and precise operative dissection of tissues in asleep and relaxed patients replaced forever rough and rapid intervention in frightened and struggling victims. The successful use of ether by British surgeons and the effectiveness of chloroform in childbirth cemented the new concept further into general use. Queen Victoria, who received it during her eighth delivery, approved. "We are," she allegedly proclaimed, "going to have this baby and we are going to have chloroform."

Even so great a contribution as general anesthesia, however, was controversial. Despite its ability to remove the pain of childbirth, it incited a raging battle between those fully convinced (notably the women who had benefited during delivery), and those opposed. The supporters quoted Genesis, noting that "the Lord caused a deep sleep to fall upon Adam." The doubters noted that "in sorrow thou shalt bring forth children," as well as arguing, remarkably, that a mother's sufferings during birth were responsible for her love of the child. Even more vituperative were discussions concerning credit for its discovery. Lack of recognition and acclaim caused Wells, a man of volatile temperament and burning ambition, to become increasingly depressed. He committed suicide by ether overdose three years later.[32] Morton attempted to hide the identity of ether by patenting it under the name "Letheon." Soon discovered, he gave up his practice and spent a great sum of money to protect what he considered to be his legal rights. For a time he became impoverished until a sympathetic colleague rescued him.

Despite the mercy of anesthesia, operations remained potentially deadly. The cause was infection. The scourge of puerperal fever in many hospitals, the often-fatal infection of the uterus that disseminates throughout the body after childbirth, stimulated the first formal efforts to control sepsis. Only a few had even considered the possibility that a surgeon or other attendant could prevent the spread of contamination among patients by simple measures of hygiene. Oliver Wendell Holmes was one of the lone voices insisting in 1843 that practitioners should not tend women in labor immediately after they had conducted postmortem examinations on those who had died of infection, a hitherto routine practice.

About the same time in Europe, Ignaz Philipp Semmelweis, appalled by the soaring obstetrical death rate in his renowned Viennese hospital, the Allgemeines Krankenhaus, noticed that puerperal fever occurred infrequently in wards attended by midwives, who adhered to strict rules of personal cleanliness. In contrast, the complication was epidemic in the wards immediately adjacent to the dissection room, from which the doctors and medical students emerged to examine the patients. Indeed, the mortality rate of the new mothers was 1–2 percent when midwives were in charge, but 18 percent among those treated by doctors and students.[33] Semmelweis's insistence on washing the hands with soap and warm chlorine water between patient examinations and the use of a nailbrush to remove particulate matter from beneath the fingernails caused the mortality rate to fall precipitously. These simple but radical departures from established protocols provoked such hostility among their respective colleagues, however, that Holmes was ostracized and Semmelweis driven to insanity and death. Their contributions took years to become routine.

In 1865 a surgeon in Glasgow, Joseph Lister, initiated a further critical improvement. Until that time, operating room behavior, traditions, and culture were inviolate. Instruments were rarely cleaned between cases. Surgeons officiated in frock coats encrusted with pus and blood, with ligatures hanging from a buttonhole for use during the procedure. Under such conditions, operative sites almost invariably became septic and thus almost always fatal. In some hospitals eight out of ten patients died after an operation. Hospital gangrene, an invasive infection leading to tissue destruction and death, was rife. Many surgeons removed the most obviously affected areas with the red-hot cautery, an agonizing and relatively unsuccessful strategy.

By chance, Lister noted that a portion of the Clyde River receiving effluent from an adjacent chemical plant ran clear while the surrounding water remained cloudy and polluted. Phenol, flowing with the factory waste, was identified as the responsible agent. Based on this observation and from the corroborative evidence of gypsies who had used the material to cleanse wounds for generations, he began to operate in a continuous antiseptic spray of phenol-containing "carbolic acid" that enveloped surgeon, patient, and the operative field. He initially used the technique when treating compound fractures, a usually fatal misfortune because bacteria entered the tissues and spread throughout the body via the bone ends protruding from the skin. Amputation was frequently the only recourse. With his spray filling the air, his routine bathing of the wound and surrounding skin with the carbolic solution, and his insistence on clean instruments, Lister's successes were unprecedented. Between 1864 and 1866, for instance, he and his colleagues carried out thirty-five leg amputations for compound fracture. Sixteen patients died, a 46 percent mortality rate all too common at the time. In contrast, following the introduction of routine antisepsis, they performed forty amputations between 1877 and 1880. Six patients died, a mortality rate of 15 percent.[34] The lesson was clear.

The Scottish surgeon's radical divergence from established custom undeniably decreased the incidence of postoperative infection. However, like the reaction to Holmes and Semmelweis before him, many of his peers accepted the new advance only after years of opprobrium. For instance, Lister presented his results in lectures and demonstrations in several cities throughout the United States during the country's centenary celebrations in 1876. Many surgeons heard him but remained unconvinced.[35] No less a figure than Samuel Gross of Philadelphia, the most prominent surgeon in America at the time, publicly dismissed Lister's contribution, noting that few of the "enlightened or experienced surgeons on this side of the Atlantic" had faith in his innovations, and that care in dressing the wound was all that was necessary. He went on to predict that "the honor, the dignity and the glory of American surgery will be safe" without such radical changes.[36] It is also interesting that in Thomas Eakins's huge 1875 portrait, *The Gross Clinic*, we see the master teaching and operating with his team while wearing a suit, flowing bow tie, pearl buttons, and watch chain. The Scot's carefully considered concepts were obviously lacking.

Antisepsis involves the local destruction of bacteria, a concept that Lister developed after learning about their presence and control from the great Continental investigators, Louis Pasteur and Robert Koch. The principle of asepsis extended the technique further by sterilizing instruments and surgical gowns plus ensuring total cleanliness of the operating room. The understanding that infections could be caused by tiny living organisms did not emerge until the middle of the nineteenth century, however, despite introduction of the idea by the Roman encyclopedist Varro in about 100 BC and its reconsideration during the Renaissance. In 1679 in the Netherlands, a draper, Anthony van Leeuwenhoek, ground a magnifying glass powerful enough to visualize tiny "animalcules" floating in fluid, including bacteria from his mouth and his own sperm. Regardless of technical improvements, however, naturalists were unable to identify the minute forms of life until Joseph Jackson Lister, father of the surgeon, invented the compound microscope with achromatic lenses in 1832.

Discoveries then came in rapid succession, with the appreciation that microorganisms were ubiquitous and played a critical function both in the balance of nature and in disease. Pasteur in France and Koch in Germany opened the new area of knowledge. Pasteur was a chemist who had described the role of bacteria in the putrefaction of animal and vegetable matter in 1857, then showed that grapes could neither ferment nor decay in their absence, nor could milk and butter spoil. Of composed temperament and influenced by his experience with French agriculture and the wine industry, Pasteur and his small French school viewed the world of tiny organisms as part of the natural ecology.[37] He confirmed the germ theory of disease, became interested in immunization, and developed a vaccine against rabies and other scourges. He and his group also discovered bacteria in the blood of animals dying of anthrax, a fatal disease of sheep and cattle that cost the agricultural economy of the time millions of francs.

Shortly thereafter in Berlin, Robert Koch, the other towering figure in the new field of microbiology and winner of the Nobel Prize in 1905, devised means to grow anthrax organisms in artificial medium. Inoculated into experimental animals, they were fatal. He subsequently identified and cultured the tuberculosis bacterium, which was responsible for 5 million deaths worldwide each year, and the microbe producing cholera, another devastating cause of disease. He became an increasingly authoritarian figure, favoring surgery over other methods and prejudiced in his views through treating the wounded in the Franco-Prussian War. Supported both by his own substantial contributions in the role of specific agents in disease and those of the powerful German school of bacteriology, he stressed that bacteria were pathogens responsible for the ubiquitous wound infections that almost inevitably followed surgery. As such, they should be eradicated. Despite overwhelming evidence, however, it took years until his colleagues accepted the results of his investigations and appreciated the role of bacteria in operative sepsis.[38]

Between 1846 and 1865, anesthesia and the means to control infections were introduced. Working together, these two revolutions in surgical practice quickly opened the way for the introduction of more and more effective operative interventions and treatments.

four

Steps Forward and Steps Backward

Although the benefits of operative hygiene gradually became obvious to most practitioners, surgical practices per se were slow to change. During Harvey Cushing's internship year at the MGH in 1896, for instance, operations consisted predominantly of amputation of damaged limbs, removal of breast cancers, excision of superficial tumors, and minor skin repairs. Spectators in street clothes often entered the operating rooms, and techniques and safeguards now taken for granted were not yet in place. Cushing enjoyed his internship and held several of the faculty in high esteem, but he was less sanguine about the rapid, rough, and imprecise methods of some of the others, who continued to believe that speed, a holdover from preanesthetic days, was a measure of ability.[1] Despite adherence to Lister's principles of antisepsis, surgeons still considered an incision exceptional that healed without infection. They and their assistants now washed their hands before beginning the procedure, but few bothered to change their stained clothes between cases.[2] Masks and rubber gloves were not universally accepted, and sterilization of instruments with dry heat was a novelty.

The senior faculty treated the administration of anesthesia equally casually, often relegating inexperienced and unqualified medical students, residents, and nurses to the task. Observing an operation as a third-year student, for instance, Cushing was pulled from his seat in the amphitheater and ordered to a side room to put to sleep an elderly man with a bowel obstruction. Coached only by the orderly, he dripped ether onto a cloth, which he held over the patient's nose and mouth. Repeated calls from the surgeon urged haste. Wheeled into the theater for his surgery, the unconscious patient suddenly vomited, aspirated the stomach contents into his lungs, and died. Shocked and disheartened, Cushing considered quitting medicine but was informed by the professor that this event was an expected complication and was advised to forget about it. The young student never forgot. One of my teachers at the Brigham recalled a similar instance during his own internship four decades later. With the staff anesthesiologist rarely present and nurses in charge of the bulk of scheduled cases, untutored and unsupervised house officers were expected to give anesthesia for emergencies. The trainees finally refused to comply unless a senior person was present, feeling correctly that the risk to the patients was too great.

Despite anesthesiology's obvious benefits and its establishment as a highly regarded medical specialty in Great Britain, the field became accepted in the United States only just before World War II, one hundred years after its introduction. Stimulated by Ralph Waters, a visionary pioneer on its faculty, the University of Wisconsin created a chair of anesthesia in 1915 that uniquely offered scientific postgraduate education in the subject. Few other institutions followed this example. Harvard, for instance, established its first chair two years later, but the position seemed unimportant and remained vacant until 1936.[3] The presence of an anesthesia specialist at an institution was a rarity; Walter Boothby filled the role at the Brigham. Only a small coterie of physicians had become interested in the subject.

As operative techniques improved over the course of the twentieth century, interventions slowly became more routine. Surgeons entered the abdominal cavity more and more often to correct a variety of visceral conditions not requiring an emergency procedure. The Mayo brothers, for example, performed only fifty-four elective abdominal operations between 1889 and 1892 in their new clinic, but they carried out 612 in 1900 and reported 2,157 five years later.[4] The results, however, were often tarnished by dangerous anesthetic practices and frequent infections. Cushing's somewhat pessimistic outlook toward his craft lightened during his residency at Johns Hopkins when he witnessed the difference between Boston surgeons' haste and the slow, gentle, and meticulous dissections and painstaking control of bleeding advocated and practiced by William Stewart Halsted, chief of surgery at Johns Hopkins. This contrast in philosophy and approach as it related to the removal of a breast, for instance, was a revelation. A case the young trainee saw in

Boston was completed in twenty-eight minutes. A similar operation in Baltimore took four-and-a-half hours. Instructed by Halsted not to touch the incision for ten days, he skeptically recalled his earlier experiences with wet, malodorous, and infected wounds in Boston, but became a believer when he finally removed the dressings and found the site to be perfectly healed. Convincing skeptics around the country took longer. In considering what he felt was Halsted's excruciatingly slow technique, William Mayo (of the Mayo Clinic) later suggested, tongue in cheek, that the patients had usually healed their incisions by the time the procedure was completed.[5]

Such improvements in asepsis and in anesthesia concepts, training, and technique broadened the scope of surgical activities. Improvement in the treatment of acute appendicitis is an important example. For years this common disease had been unrecognized or disguised in such nondescript categories as "gastric attack, gastric seizure, cramp of the bowels," and the like. Most considered the involvement of the organ to be the result, not the cause, of some other ill-defined event that began in adjacent areas. In 1839 a London physician, Thomas Addison, first correlated the clinical picture with postmortem findings. Four decades later Reginald Fitz, a pathologist at Harvard Medical School, established the concept that appendicitis (he coined the term) was an inflammatory process beginning in the organ itself. Regardless of cause, however, the majority of surgeons adhered to long-term practices and delayed operation until perforation or rupture had occurred, believing that formation of a localized abscess would prevent the free spread of infection throughout the abdominal cavity. They could then drain the walled-off area. When an abscess failed to form, in contrast, fatal peritonitis often ensued. It took surgeons years to accept that they should promptly remove the inflamed but intact appendix.

The postponement of a royal coronation brought the ongoing debate about the optimal operative approach to public attention. The new king of England, Edward VII, was to be crowned on June 26, 1901. All was arranged. Heads of state, the royalty of Europe, assorted dignitaries, and a glittering multitude of other guests had assembled. Unfortunately, two days before the event, Edward developed abdominal pain, vomiting, and fever. His surgeon, Sir Frederick Treves, an anatomist and author of a well-known surgical text, diagnosed appendicitis. Still under the assumption that the site became secondarily infected from involvement of nearby structures, he advised deferring any operation for five days until an abscess had developed. Supported by Lister, he waited, drained the abscess, and removed the appendix.[6] Edward survived. The coronation was rescheduled. But in his later classic review of the subject in which he analyzed the anatomy, signs, symptoms, and operative treatment of the disease, Treves reversed his position and concluded that early surgery was the better option.[7] Faced with the improving results, surgeons everywhere increasingly agreed.

With symptoms and signs sometimes less than obvious, differentiating the condition from others that might mimic it, like a ruptured or twisted ovarian cyst, a kidney stone, or acute gastrointestinal disorder, entailed careful ongoing evaluation of the patient. In that not uncommon situation and because of the potentially grave consequences of waiting too long, the operator often explored the abdomen without a specific diagnosis. Indeed, the threshold of suspicion had to be so low and the threat of missing a potentially dangerous process so important that it was considered correct during my residency for about 20 percent of removed appendices to be normal on microscopic examination. Making a small incision in the lower abdomen directly over the area of tenderness, we were often rewarded with an enlarged, hot, and discolored organ. The operation took half an hour, an unforgettable learning experience for the intern allowed to take the case. The results were gratifying. The patient, who had been in severe distress the night before, was smiling and hungry the following morning.

In contrast to the smiling and hungry patient whose inflamed appendix had been safely eliminated, those with a rupture presented a different picture. Localized but worsening abdominal discomfort would often disappear when the swollen area burst, to be replaced within a few hours by generalized pain exacerbated by movement. Rising fever and chills ensued. In time, bacteria might grow in the blood and shock might develop. At operation, instead of an easily removable finger of inflamed tissue, we would be greeted with foul-smelling cloudy fluid dispersed throughout the abdomen and matted white exudate gluing together loops of bowel.

The leaking appendix would be small, often black with gangrene. We often had to enlarge the incision to wash out the entire cavity. The patient might then spend several days in hospital, receiving fluids and antibiotics intravenously. Many would not fully recover for weeks.

Despite the overall excellence of the results, the current availability of sophisticated imaging technology such as CAT scans or MRI visualization has changed the diagnostic procedure substantially. The residents now barely examine the patient before sending him or her for one of these definitive but costly tests. With the accurate images confirming the clinical impression, many surgeons remove the organ through a laparoscope, a less traumatic approach that may take somewhat longer than the traditional procedure. But regardless of method, the patients do well if the disease is caught in time. About 10 percent of appendectomies are still expected to be negative.

The success of immediate intervention for appendicitis became a double-edged sword throughout the United States in the early decades of the twentieth century. Indeed, the procedure became so popular that a multitude of partially trained practitioners often carried it out for less-than-obvious clinical indications. The excessive numbers of normal appendices they removed led to the formation of hospital tissue committees to control such unwarranted surgical enthusiasm, an early form of peer review and an example of operative "fads" that have recurred throughout the centuries.[8] Effective treatment of this feared and sometimes fatal condition, however, has become one of the triumphs of surgery, so much so that in modern times we may scoff at its importance. However, in the 1930s acute appendicitis was still the fifteenth most common cause of death. Even in 1973 more than 1,000 patients reputedly died of the disease. Although the current mortality rate is a fraction of 1 percent, it remains a danger unless correctly diagnosed.[9]

Unfortunately, some regression in treatment patterns may be currently occurring. This trend may be a result, in part, of overconfidence in the ability to recognize a condition apparently as mundane as appendicitis. Or it may be influenced by a sometimes-misguided faith in the power of antibiotics or by efforts of the insurance companies to reduce costs. A healthy young man of my acquaintance recently experienced some of these vagaries to his detriment. Overnight he developed loss of appetite and abdominal discomfort. By the next morning, the pain was worse. Lacking a family doctor, he called his insurance company and was instructed to go to the local emergency room. There he sat uncomfortably for several hours before a nurse interviewed him, prescribed antacids, and told him to go home. Another six hours went by. With worsening pain, he returned to the emergency room and received the same advice. No one examined him or performed laboratory tests. Finally, in desperation and in increasing distress, he came back a third time and demanded to see the surgeon. Shocked at what he saw, the doctor operated quickly, removing and draining a ruptured appendix. My acquaintance remained in the hospital for a week, receiving intravenous antibiotics during his slow recovery. He did not feel well for an additional six weeks. If his condition had been diagnosed and treated promptly, he would have felt better in a few days. In this instance, the shift from proven practices to short cuts in care arose through the efforts of the third-party payer to control expenses. The results saddled the patient with inconvenience and hazard and the insurance company with an unnecessary financial burden.

With surgical expertise increasing during the early decades of the twentieth century, those staffing the teaching hospitals in Boston, New York, Philadelphia, Baltimore, and in major cities to the west were able to define more precisely indications for operation, refine their methods, and improve patient outcomes. Important centers unaffiliated with medical schools were also forming. One eminent institutional contributor to the development of surgery arose in the cornfields of Rochester, Minnesota, far from any university. The operative results achieved by William and Charles Mayo, who were sons of a successful rural practitioner and had trained with surgical notables in Chicago and New York, achieved a renown that drew colleagues and younger trainees not only from the Midwest but from throughout the United States and Europe to observe and to learn.[10] With their success as a model, similar medical enterprises opened, including the Crile Clinic in Cleveland (1921), the Lahey Clinic in Boston (1923), and the Ochsner Clinic in New Orleans (1942). With experts dedicated to a variety of specialties, these private centers not only became important as postgraduate training programs but harbingers of future prepaid group practices. Even in smaller communities, well-trained surgeons were making their presence felt. Despite providing better access to services, however, surgical practice still faced certain obstacles. We must not forget that the lack of muscle relaxants with anesthesia made exploration difficult, blood transfusions were virtually nonexistent, intravenous fluids not used, and the pharmaceutical agents we currently accept as routine were undreamed of. Mortality associated with operative invasion of the peritoneal cavity, often from infection or hemorrhage, remained significant.

Wilhelm Roentgen's introduction of his cathode ray in Paris late in 1895 spearheaded the more accurate diagnosis of disease. Although physicists and engineers had used these vacuum tubes in their researches for several years, the passage of an electrical current across them with exposure of a photographic film to the resultant rays allowed practitioners the means to differentiate dense bodily structures from those of lesser opacity. They could now determine the shape of the heart, see the shadow of tuberculosis in a lung, and visualize a fracture of a bone. Using the new fluoroscopy machine on subjects who had swallowed radio-opaque dye, they could appreciate the activity of stomach and intestine and identify ulcers and cancers.[11] Radiology departments formed and interest grew as radiologists, surgeons, and physiologists spent hours peering at normal and abnormal anatomy. The further discovery that prolonged exposure to Dr. Roentgen's rays could shrink tumors in animals and then in humans evoked much excitement. Enthusiasts treated a variety of conditions indiscriminately and without appreciation of any untoward effects. In consequence, doctors and patients alike sometimes developed fatal cancers induced by the radiation. Despite their limitations and risks, however, radiology and radiotherapy transformed the face of medicine.

Less obvious advances were also important. The availability of hollow needles of various sizes provided effective means of removing blood from patients, administering fluids intravenously, and carrying out other invasive measures. Although the ancients had used quills to enter veins and bleed patients, and had occasionally inserted metal tubes between the ribs to drain fluid from the chest, the sterile needle did not enter general use until well into the twentieth century. Disposable needles were not available until the 1970s. Indeed, when I took a clinical clerkship as a medical student at a large city hospital in New York in 1961, one of my responsibilities was to collect all the needles at the end of each day, wash them out, sharpen their points, wrap them separately in towels, and sterilize the lot for use the next morning. It was then our job to draw blood from the patients, pushing a cart up and down the thirty-bed open wards for this purpose. On the cart lay a large open basin of "sterile" saline, a supply of needles, one large glass syringe, and an array of tubes labeled with the individual's name and the laboratory tests needed. We stopped at each bedside, placed a fresh needle on the syringe, drew blood from an arm vein, and transferred it to the appropriate container. We then removed the needle, put it aside, and flushed out the syringe in the basin so as to be ready for the next patient. In those days, relatively little was known about the types and spread of hepatitis and the risks of illicit drug use. Acquired immune deficiency syndrome (AIDS) was completely unknown. No one considered that we might be transferring disease.

William Stewart Halsted was primarily responsible for many of the changes evolving in modern surgery and in the education of young aspirants. A complex individual, he was one of the foremost figures of the time. Educated at Yale and at Columbia's College of Physicians and Surgeons, he traveled to Europe in 1878 to study with renowned professors of anatomy and surgery. There he was caught up in the new revelations of antisepsis and the value of applied biology in the diagnosis and treatment of disease. Returning to New York in 1880, he began a notably successful professional career. Gaining reputation for his operative refinements and effective techniques, educational leadership, and laboratory contributions, he was invited to join the original staff of the new Johns Hopkins Hospital. Eventually named head of surgery in 1889, he attracted a coterie of brilliant residents.

Two personal crises firmed his reputation for original thought and creativity. In 1881 his sister lay near death from hemorrhage after a delivery. Although those caring for her had given up hope, the young surgeon took over the case, controlled the bleeding, and transfused her quickly with a volume of his own blood. Two decades before the discovery of blood groups and without the existence of drugs to prevent clotting, this direct transfusion was not only successful but was the first undertaken in America.[12] How fortunate it was that by happenstance he and his sister were of similar blood type! Months later his mother became seriously ill with jaundice, high fever, and severe abdominal pain. Her consultants advised that operation was too dangerous. As a last-ditch effort, Halsted dissected free her distended and inflamed gallbladder. Pus under pressure boiled out from the organ as he removed seven gallstones. She recovered nicely. It was his first operation for gallbladder disease, successful because of his knowledge of anatomy and adherence to surgical principles. His supplemental step of leaving an external drain in place for several days to remove residual contamination became standard procedure during the next century.

A few years after Halsted's return from Europe, an article appeared, written by Carl Koller, a Viennese ophthalmologist and colleague of Sigmund Freud. He described the action of a few drops of the drug cocaine, which could completely anesthetize the eye when applied locally. Excited by the possibilities of a safer alternative to the persistent hazards of general anesthesia, Halsted soon administered the cocaine solution for dental procedures and was among the first to instill it between the vertebrae to provide spinal anesthesia. Within a decade his assistant at Johns Hopkins, Harvey Cushing, still wary of the dangers of ether because of his devastating experience as a medical student, began to repair hernias and amputate legs by injecting cocaine into the nerves supplying the affected areas. As the news spread, surgeons everywhere grasped the concept of local anesthesia as potentially valuable for some operations, just as general anesthesia was for others. Unfortunately, Halsted and three young colleagues had initially experimented with the novel agent by blocking their own peripheral nerves before trying it on patients. The price of this activity was that the professor became seriously addicted, a problem that affected him for the rest of his life.[13] Despite the substitution of morphine to treat the cocaine addiction, a widely used strategy at the time, the problem worsened. His personality changed from cheerful and flamboyant to stern, introverted, and mean-spirited.

Despite this burden, Halsted was responsible for a spectrum of important surgical innovations during his thirty-year tenure at Hopkins. He added applied gross and microscopic anatomy, pathology, and details of operations to the medical school curriculum. After demonstrations of specific procedures, the students repeated them on cadavers or on animals under the critical eye of their preceptors. Perhaps most important, they learned by spending considerable time on the wards observing and treating patients. Resident training began to take years of focused commitment. Halsted was one of the first in the United States to adopt Lister's antiseptic techniques and initiate the preventive principles of asepsis. He introduced rubber gloves into operating room routine, initially to protect the hands of his scrub nurse (later his wife) from the strong antiseptic solutions of the time, and eventually insisted on their use for all operations. He perfected new and effective procedures in laboratory animals based on careful physiological and anatomical observations. Many of these had direct clinical application. The impact of his contributions peaked between 1910 and 1940, when his highly talented disciples and their own disciples in turn assumed leadership positions in American surgery. They spread his beliefs, standards, and tenets throughout the profession, forcing the maturation of the field.

One of Halsted's most important technical approaches was careful dissection with minimal blood loss. The control of bleeding had concerned practitioners since antiquity. Healers in ancient India in 1500 BC tied off the umbilical cord after birth. The Greeks ligated open vessels with linen thread. Galen described a spectrum of techniques to staunch hemorrhage in injured Roman gladiators.[14] For first aid, Galen placed his fingers into the wound and compressed the site. For more definitive control, he twisted the torn edges of the vessel with a hook. If it continued, he tied off the affected area with silk. He stopped less-consequential bleeding with "styptics," commonly made of frankincense, aloes, egg whites, and a pinch of clippings from the fur of a hare, although the application of a snug pressure dressing on an oozing site of injury was more likely effective. Pouring boiling oil mixed with treacle on a fresh wound to coagulate open vessels became a later and less efficacious alternative. Vitriol (sulfuric acid), an even more corrosive substance, came into favor in seventeenth-century

Paris for the same purpose.[15] These materials, of course, only increased the extent of the injury.

The long-standing concept that "diseases not curable by iron are curable by fire" made the cautery a primary feature of the surgical control of bleeding until well into the 1800s.[16] Twelve centuries earlier, Arab sages had extolled "the nobility" of fire in stopping hemorrhage, preferring glowing iron implements over softer metals, such as bronze. Some seventeenth-century operators used a red-hot knife for amputations, and the horror of both patient and surgeon can only be imagined. Indeed, a basket of fiery coals containing appropriate instruments routinely sat on the floor beside the operating table.

Although use of the ligature ultimately replaced these brutal methods, new investigations ultimately channeled the indiscriminate searing of wounds into a controlled and effective tool. The discovery of the uses of electricity stimulated a few late nineteenth-century surgeons to try electrocautery to reduce bleeding, but its possibilities were not realized completely until 1926, when Cushing first used an electrosurgical unit successfully on one of his neurological patients. Developed by William Bovie, a physicist working at a nearby hospital in Boston, the device could both open tissue with an oscillating cutting current and coagulate small vessels with continuous amplitude.[17] By chance, Cushing first saw a demonstration of its ability to cut a block of beef at a conference in Atlantic City. Contacting Bovie upon his return to Boston, he arranged to use the apparatus on a patient. Its utility became quickly apparent. Three days before he had tried to remove a highly vascularized tumor from the skull of a 64-year-old man but had to discontinue the operation because of uncontrollable hemorrhage. He decided to try again using Bovie's new instrument. Conditions were less than ideal.[18] The room was crowded with French visitors sneezing with colds. The student serving as a blood donor fainted and fell off his stool. At one point an electric shock from the machine traveled through Cushing's metal headlamp out his arm, an unpleasant experience to say the least. That the spark did not cause the volatile ether anesthesia to explode remains a source of wonder. But with the new technique of diathermy, as it was called, he was able to remove the tumor with minimal bleeding. This innovation ultimately provided surgery with a critical and indispensable component of operating room equipment, now used throughout the world.

With safety for patients undergoing operations increasing, surgeons became more adept in manipulating, removing, and rerouting tissues and organs, often treating conditions they had not faced before. They used techniques that Halsted had introduced to perform radical mastectomies for cancer of the breast and to repair groin hernias. They cleared stones from the gallbladder and common bile duct. They removed portions of the stomach to treat peptic ulcer disease. They took out the uterus, resected tumors of the intestine, and rejoined the ends of the bowel together precisely. Indeed, these and similar operations have become part of the lexicon of all well-trained general surgeons who perform many of them routinely to this day.

The need to provide optimal and consistent standards of care became obvious as the Hopkins methods were recognized and adopted during the early years of the twentieth century. With the prevailing culture still allowing anyone to operate regardless of training and experience, a few concerned surgical leaders organized the American College of Surgeons in 1913 to improve existing levels of education and competency of practice. They based the tenets of the new body upon those of the three Royal Colleges in Britain. Begun under royal edict in the sixteenth century, these had long ruled that only persons properly apprenticed in surgery could practice the craft. Comparable reforms of the American College, however, took several decades to become accepted. While some inadequately educated individuals continued to practice, particularly in rural areas, the new American Board of Surgery, founded in 1937, tightened credentialing by mandating appropriate years of training, setting the numbers and range of supervised operations that should be carried out, and assessing clinicians with formal examinations. Specialty boards with comparable requirements appeared after World War II.

Part of this ongoing effort was to encourage formal professional preparation during a period when, it should be recalled, one could still buy a medical degree by mail. Publication of the *Directory of Medical Specialists* in 1940 did much to promote general recognition of those confirmed by the board.[19] Surgical leaders formed regional and national specialty societies and associations and introduced the concept of continuing education. By the latter half of the twentieth century, the great majority of surgeons had become board certified, a prerequisite both for licensure and for membership in the College of Surgeons. At the present time, all practicing surgeons must recertify themselves by fulfilling stipulated hours of education each year and by passing a board-orchestrated examination every ten years. Halsted's vision of standardized levels of education for surgeons, the third revolution in the history of surgery, had finally reached maturity.

The American Board of Surgery is an independent and nonprofit body that credentials surgeons who have completed a minimum of five years of organized postgraduate education with documented operative experience. The board examinations comprise two parts: the first includes two three-hour multiple-choice sessions that residents undertake after their third year of training; the second is a series of oral examinations administered toward the end of the fifth year. To pass is critical to a future career and job prospects. If unsuccessful, the trainee may retake them, although the failure rate is higher.

I remember the experience well. I took the first part in rather unusual circumstances. I was on a research fellowship in England in the late 1960s and had to travel to an American military base several hours away. Having already spent some time abroad, I was struck by the sudden appearance of a less-than-attractive piece of my own country in the midst of the beautiful British countryside. As I approached the entrance, the side of the road suddenly seemed to fill with used-car lots, billboards advertising a variety of goods, and fast-food shops. Chevrolets and Fords sat next to each other, each with a price on its windshield. As I entered the gates, I seemed surrounded by large automobiles, which were driven predominantly, it appeared, by women in hair curlers. The guards and soldiers looked as if they had just stepped out of any military facility in the United States. I felt somewhat alien. Several American surgical residents working in hospitals or in research laboratories in Britain and Europe, some of whom I knew, had gathered for the examination. We were directed to our desks by a staff sergeant barking orders. All of us had spent much time and trouble studying surgical textbooks in preparation because we knew that the failure rate was about 15 percent. Despite our care, however, many of the questions covered topics unfamiliar to us. By the end of the day, after six hours of answering multitudes of short questions, we were exhausted.

Three years later and again living in Britain, I flew to Boston for the oral examinations. We residents were instructed to report to a hotel early in the morning. The examiners were lofty figures in academic surgery whose books and chapters we had read many times. Meeting at six monthly intervals at the headquarters of the American Board of Surgery in Philadelphia, they create a broad range of questions and provide appropriate answers for the examinations held throughout the country each year. Groups of three examiners interviewed us individually in three different sessions throughout the day. Their approach was businesslike and objective; there was little small talk. Using the board questions to cover an array of relevant topics, they could quickly detect the extent of one's knowledge. Applicants giving imprecise, diffuse, or poorly considered answers encountered skeptical looks and raised eyebrows. Although stressful, the experience is remembered by most of us as a positive one, particularly so if we passed.

The ability to carry out a range of operations safely and effectively was a critical step in improving standards of patient care. Elliott Cutler, who succeeded Cushing as departmental chair at the Brigham in 1932, was a major proponent of structured residency education, exhorting his faculty to build a sound foundation of surgery for the residents based on Halsted's principles. A master technician, convinced that a qualified surgeon should be well versed in all existing techniques, he felt equally at home operating in the brain as operating in the chest or abdomen. His own enthusiasm, productivity, and broad conversance with his discipline inspired many of his trainees to enter academic careers. Using Halsted's philosophy as a model, a preponderance of these individuals became heads of departments in major teaching hospitals throughout the United States in the decades after World War II, spreading the educational precepts they had acquired to their own residents. These latter individuals, in turn, instilled the precepts in the next generation of trainees.

One of Cutler's major contributions was the 1939 *Atlas of Surgical Operations*, coauthored with a younger colleague, Robert Zollinger.[20] Its aim was to bring greater safety to the surgical patient by promoting well-considered and standard operative approaches for all in the field to follow. Available surgical textbooks described disease states and physical abnormalities, but they gave cursory attention to details of the operations themselves. Cutler and Zollinger's unique compendium showed every step of a given procedure through clear and accurate pen-and-ink drawings by an experienced medical artist who stood on a stool at the operating table and sketched each case. Included was a concise description of every step, with a brief discussion of indications and preoperative preparation. The prototype for the many specialty atlases that have since emerged, the book went through six editions and taught the fundamental techniques of the craft to generations of young surgeons.

An important section of the *Atlas* featured operations for peptic ulcers. I will discuss this subject in some detail because it was of major surgical concern throughout much of the twentieth century. Overall, its study and treatment symbolize many of the lessons, benefits, and failures of modern surgery. This sometimes annoying, often debilitating, and occasionally fatal disease has troubled a significant proportion of the population at one time or another. Long associated with emotion, stress, and with rigid and aggressive personality types, ulcers have been a stereotypic illness of executives, financiers, and other hard-driving figures in positions of power, responsibility, and unfulfilled ambition. Shakespeare, for instance, memorably describes the tense, scheming, and untrustworthy Cassius as having "a lean and hungry look" in his dealings with Julius Caesar. Portraits of Napoleon Bonaparte show him with his right hand inside his waistcoat, pressing on his upper abdomen. A stomach ulcer that eventually became cancerous caused his death. James Joyce, distressed and unhappy that his book *Finnegans Wake* received less than enthusiastic public acclaim, died of a perforated ulcer.

The properties of gastric juice were long recognized.[21] John Hunter originally noted that the material could destroy the stomach wall after death. Others commented on its ability to digest tissues outside the body. William Beaumont, a United States Army surgeon, was the first to study gastric physiology in 1825 by initiating a decade-long series of observations on his patient, Alexis St. Martin. This Canadian voyageur, an uncooperative and irresponsible figure, had been shot in the abdomen with a shotgun years before. The huge injury left him with a permanent fistula running from his stomach through the overlying abdominal wall and skin. With St. Martin's only occasional cooperation, Beaumont was able to examine the fluid escaping to the outside through the defect. It contained considerable amounts of hydrochloric acid, and both emotions and ingested food influenced its secretion.[22] By inserting his finger through the opening, he could also feel that the pylorus, the muscular ring at the outlet of the stomach, could contract or relax to control the rate of emptying of gastric contents into the small intestine.

Caused by secretion of excess acid, a peptic ulcer is a localized concavity that may extend deeply into the stomach or intestinal wall. Though gastric ulcers were apparently more common in the nineteenth century, their presence in the duodenum, the initial portion of small bowel leaving the stomach, assumed endemic proportions as the twentieth century progressed, a shift in disease pattern that is still unexplained. Despite traditional treatments of rest, bland diets, and milk supplements, large numbers of patients, usually males, experienced discomfort and intractable pain for years. Some developed serious complications that included perforation, bleeding, or obstruction. In the 1960s and 1970s we admitted three or four such individuals to the Brigham surgical service each week. We operated immediately upon those with a perforation to prevent the corrosive gastric juice from spreading throughout the abdominal cavity. If the patient was vomiting blood, my fellow residents and I would spend hours pulling out clots via a large plastic or rubber tube we inserted through the nose into the stomach and instilling iced saline in hopes of controlling the hemorrhage. These attempts, strenuous for patient and doctor alike, were often futile. Many, still bleeding, went to surgery. When the outlet of the stomach was obstructed, we placed the tube on constant suction to drain the acid and allow the acute swelling to subside. Intravenous nutrition had not yet been introduced, so many of these patients lost dangerous amounts of body mass if the ulcer did not resolve or if we delayed operation too long. Occasionally, some died.

Whereas obstruction at the pyloric junction may improve with conservative treatment, perforations and acute hemorrhage are surgical emergencies. In such cases, once we had made the incision and retracted the abdominal wall, the stomach came into view, a large pinkish-tan, thick-walled, muscular sac. By moving the overlying colon, we could see the pyloric ring separating the bottom of the organ from the duodenum. The source of trouble was often easy to locate. A perforation, where the ulcer has eroded through the front of the stomach or duodenal wall, looks as if it were made with a paper punch. With the escaping acid burning adjacent viscera, the patients cannot move without severe pain. Lacking prompt intervention, they could go into shock. We used robust stitches to close the hole, then copiously washed out the peritoneal cavity. Such afflicted individuals returned quickly to normal, just like those whose inflamed appendices had been removed. Fearing potential infection, we allowed them to recover from the acute event for several weeks before moving on to more definitive treatment. In those days, this usually involved removing part of the stomach.

The stomach and bowel of individuals hemorrhaging from an ulcer are dark in color as the blood within has turned black from its interaction with acid. On occasion we knew from prior X-rays where the bleeding ulcer was. In other instances we had to guess. The most likely source was the duodenum. After opening its front surface and suctioning out the blood and clots, we were usually rewarded by seeing a jet of red blood squirting from the back wall where the ulcer had eroded into the large artery lying directly beneath. With the finger of the assistant controlling the bleeding, we closed the vessel with sutures. Again, it was the policy to allow the patient to recover before we carried out anything more permanent.

Surgery for peptic ulcer disease has had a long and problematic history. Theodor Billroth, one of the most famous surgeons of all time, and also mountaineer, musician, and friend of the composer Johannes Brahms, performed the first successful gastric operation to excise an obstructing tumor in Germany in 1881. Embracing Lister's new doctrine of antisepsis and using chloroform as an anesthetic, he removed the bottom half of the organ and sewed a portion of small bowel to the remnant. This was his third attempt; his previous two patients had died. Indeed, an outraged citizenry had allegedly nearly stoned him to death following the initial fatality. This surgical precedent, however, both stimulated an onslaught of studies of alimentary physiology in the laboratory and sustained the interest of surgeons in treating ulcers in patients for the next nine decades. Yet many of the investigative conclusions were incorrect and led to the wrong operations performed for the wrong reasons. Indeed, it took research workers much time to realize that there is no relevant animal model for the condition; humankind is apparently the only species that develops ulcers spontaneously. Treating a disease such as peptic ulcer without understanding the normal function of the organ involved was not one of the proudest examples of surgical progress.

Pyloric obstruction is a nonmalignant but serious and occasionally fatal complication of peptic ulcer disease. Some of Billroth's European colleagues simplified his more extensive resection and retained the entire stomach in a procedure to bypass the blockage by suturing a loop of small intestine to the most dependent portion of the sac. Gastric contents could then empty directly into the small bowel. This arrangement, gastroenterostomy, not only appeared to correct the problem but was considered a conceptual advance. Alkaline bile from the intestine could now enter the stomach and neutralize its acid. Although the theory was reasonable, it could not account for unrecognized reality. The procedure was carried out in large numbers between 1890 and 1930. It was, in retrospect, like the too-frequent performance of appendectomy that we have discussed, "an operation ideally adapted to mass application with a minimum of individual discrimination."[23]

While relatively effective in older patients whose acid production was diminished, the gastric contents that drained directly through the newly created junction between stomach and intestine of younger individuals not infrequently produced an unanticipated problem, the "marginal ulcer." With acid digesting the thin bowel wall and its underlying vessels, the resultant ulcer often produced serious bleeding. An even more sinister complication of gastroenterostomy arose when the marginal ulcer and its accompanying inflammation burrowed deeply into and through the adjacent colon, forming an abnormal fistulous connection. Through this fistula, undigested food from the stomach would then bypass the entire small bowel, enter the colon directly, and be evacuated. Unless surgically rectified, the patients starved.

Dismayed by these complications and still unclear as to the dynamics of acid production, surgeons, who were increasingly expert in sewing hollow structures together, embarked upon more radical means of rearranging gastric anatomy.[24] Between 1935 and 1945, they designed a variety of strategies to remove the acid-bearing area of the stomach, thought to lie in its lower third.[25] What they failed to understand and what exhaustive laboratory experiments could not tell them, however, was that cells in that area do not themselves elaborate acid but secrete a hormone that stimulates other cell populations in the upper part of the organ to produce the material. Thus, if the stomach already contains high concentrations of acid, little hormone is formed. Conversely, the more alkaline the gastric contents, as encouraged by milk-based bland diets or by the entrance of contents of the small bowel via a gastroenterostomy, the more hormone is secreted and the more acid is formed. The acid-producing cells continued to function even when the hormone-secreting part was removed surgically, as most of the new operations were designed to do.

An understanding of gastric physiology finally improved treatment in the latter half of the twentieth century. The behavior and location of the various cell populations lining the stomach were defined, and the function of the vagus nerves, two large trunks that originate in the brain and run along the vertebral bodies through the chest and into the abdomen, were better appreciated. The vagus nerves form part of the autonomic nervous system, which influences intrinsic bodily activities such as swallowing, heart rate, and gastric and intestinal movement and function. By the middle of the 1940s surgical physiologists had shown that dividing the two nerves as they enter the abdomen decreased acid secretion substantially.[26] They also noted that the pyloric sphincter constricted shut when the nerves were cut. Interrupting the vagi to inhibit acid production, then dividing the pyloric muscle to ensure gastric emptying became the operation of choice for intractable peptic ulcer well into the 1970s. Large numbers of patients benefited from this relatively simple procedure.

In contrast to the discrete ulcers and their complications that I have just described, gastritis is a less common but more serious, poorly controllable, and potentially fatal type of peptic disease. Inflammation of the entire lining of the stomach may result in diffuse and massive bleeding. Although the cause is sometimes unknown, it most commonly develops secondary to excess alcohol intake, the overuse of aspirin, or the swallowing of poison or caustic compounds. Those with bleeding and clotting abnormalities are also at risk. A patient hemorrhaging from gastritis presents one of the most difficult problems in surgery. I still remember a night I, then a young attending surgeon, and the residents spent in the operating room trying to control Elliott Berman's massive hemorrhage. He was a 54-year-old publisher who had been on dialysis for three months because of failed kidneys. Patients sustained by the mechanical kidney are particularly prone to gastritis because acid-producing metabolic wastes can be neither excreted normally nor fully removed artificially. Not only are their clotting mechanisms also impaired but the stress of total dependence on a machine for their very existence may contribute. In addition, during the thrice-weekly six-hour treatments, anticoagulant drugs must be administered to prevent coagulation in the plastic tubing that connects the vessels to the apparatus. The potential risks are substantial. Mr. Berman had passed occasional blood in his stools and once had vomited bloody material. The X-rays showed no ulcer, but the dialysis staff were so suspicious about early gastritis that they arranged for a specialist to view the inside of the stomach through an endoscope. Her report was unequivocal. Although no bleeding was apparent, the lining of the organ was red and swollen. The patient remained stable for several days on antacids and a milk-based diet before suddenly vomiting large quantities of bright red blood. Following accepted practice, the residents sedated him and began to irrigate his stomach with iced salt solution. The bleeding seemed to slow for several hours, then the rate again increased sharply. Transfusions were started.

We discussed the situation with Mr. Berman and his frightened family, emphasizing that immediate operation was the only realistic choice, even though it might entail removal of all or most of the stomach. This radical step would alter his dietary habits irreversibly for the rest of his life. But at least he might survive. We entered his abdomen quickly. The stomach was hugely distended with clotted and liquid blood despite the hours of washout. After opening the sac and removing its contents, we could see bright blood oozing briskly from the entire lining. The situation was terrifying for the team, though there was little debate about what to do. We had no choice but to remove the entire organ. We dissected stomach and lower esophagus free from their surroundings, then divided the duodenum near the pylorus and closed its end. We initially left a teacup-sized segment of upper stomach behind that we hoped would provide an adequate reservoir for food and give us more substantial muscular tissue to sew to the small bowel than the rather fragile esophageal wall. On opening the remnant, however, we were again greeted with brisk bleeding. The difference between the hemorrhaging lining of the remaining stomach and the dry, normal esophagus leading directly into it was striking. When we finally detached this last piece, all bleeding ceased instantly. The patient had received multiple transfusions but had never gone into shock and seemed remarkably stable. The sense of relief from all involved was palpable. Yet the entire organ, like the liver one of the largest in the body, was gone. We restored continuity to the alimentary tract by sewing a loop of small bowel to the esophagus. Mr. Berman recovered without incident. No bleeding occurred during dialysis. His incision healed. After a week of intravenous fluids, we gradually allowed him to eat. Although he could sustain only small amounts at a time and lost some weight, he recovered well. Several months later we transplanted a kidney. The last I saw him, after several years, he was back at work and doing well. But it was a close call and reminded all of us why we spent years in training!

Regardless of all the time and effort put into surgical treatment of peptic disease and its complications, continuing debate about new operative concepts in the laboratory, and decades of designing and carrying out often ill-conceived and poorly followed-up procedures in patients, the incidence of peptic ulcer disease inexplicably began to decline in the population at large during the 1970s. At the same time, the introduction of potent pharmacologic inhibitors of hydrochloric acid production reduced many of its symptoms and complications. Even more significantly, investigators a decade later demonstrated that a bacterium, *Helicobacter pylori*, the only recognized organism that can survive in the highly acidic environment of the human stomach, was responsible for many cases. Although the majority of individuals who carry the bacterium rarely experience problems, some develop ulcers or gastritis. Robin Warren and Barry Marshall, two pathologists in Perth, Australia, isolated and cultured *Helicobacter* from biopsies of human stomachs.[27] In their first publication on the subject they suggested that the organism might be an important cause of peptic ulcers. The medical profession around the world greeted this unique contribution with a deafening silence that lasted for several years. Subsequent reports, however, included the news that Marshall had swallowed some of the cultured material, developed gastritis, and had recovered the organism from his stomach. Finally acknowledged universally, the two investigators received the Nobel Prize in 2005 for solving the puzzle of an important problem and providing opportunities for its successful control.[28] Treatment strategies that kept so many busy for so long now often involves a course of antibiotics.

It is interesting that surgeons today use some of the same gastric rearrangements implemented unsuccessfully nearly a century ago for peptic ulcer to treat morbid obesity, an entirely different condition that also affects a relatively large proportion of the population. Mrs. Laverne and patients like her with one condition have benefited by serendipity from the older work to correct another.

– *five* –

War and Peace

Improvements in the treatment of disease and increasing knowledge of associated basic and applied sciences poured forth in a torrent between the end of World War II and the mid-1980s. The benefits were broad. Public health measures improved. Vaccination against the infectious diseases of childhood became ubiquitous. Precise laboratory assays emerged to enhance diagnosis and provide information about normal and abnormal states. Novel radiological methods allowed the viewing of hitherto inaccessible sites in the body. Differential function of the heart was defined. Some cancers could now be cured. Dialysis began to prolong the lives of patients with nonfunctioning kidneys.

The promise of surgery also increased as surgeons, returning from the military and seasoned by their responsibilities for the wounded, broadened the scope of their craft to treat the ills of the general population. It has long been said that surgical care of the injured is the only human activity that benefits from war.[1] Because of the importance of this subject in the evolution of the modern field, I will discuss in some detail how human conflict has stimulated the expansion of surgical knowledge and has served as a focal point for a spectrum of important advances, including treatment of severe burns, blood banking and the management of intravenous fluids, and the sometimes profound alterations in the composition of organs and tissues that may develop after acute physical hurt.

The postwar period was also a time of explosive growth for the pharmaceutical industry. A better understanding of anesthesia, of antisepsis and asepsis, and the implementation of standardized care had revolutionized patient outcomes by the middle of the twentieth century. In an equally dramatic manner the growing pharmaceutical industry transformed the field during and after World War II with a cornucopia of agents for a variety of medical and surgical conditions. Energized by the prospects of better health, the citizenry and their political leaders were unstinting in their enthusiasm and support.

For centuries surgeons in combat had removed arrows, set fractures, and cared for spear and sword wounds.[2] Death was inevitable if a weapon penetrated a vital structure. In contrast, the majority of flesh wounds healed with little more than bandages and local care. The situation changed substantially, however, when Philip VI of France introduced small firearms and cannon at the Battle of Crécy in 1346 (although the English yeomen still carried the day with their longbows). Even superficial flesh wounds inflicted with firearms became potentially fatal as bacteria entered and thrived in the dead and dying tissues. The incidence of tetanus and other fast-moving infections soared. Believing that some poison in the gunpowder produced these catastrophes, surgeons resorted to pouring boiling oil on the affected site or removing the involved area outright with the red-hot cautery.

Decrying the ubiquitous use of both hot oil and the iron as inhumane and ineffectual, Ambroïse Paré, the renowned military surgeon of the Renaissance, reintroduced the technique of tying off bleeding vessels with thread, a concept popularized by Celsus 1,500 years earlier in Rome. With the ability to occlude major arteries and veins with ligatures, amputations through the thigh, where heat alone was insufficient to sear the large vessels shut, became possible. Paré also dressed gunshot wounds with a bland turpentine mixture that encouraged primary healing, a gentle, tissue-sparing approach. At the same time, he continued to use the hot iron selectively to sterilize infected wounds and remove local areas of dead or gangrenous tissue, a relatively effective practice that continues to this day.

The development of ever more deadly armaments, such as the breech-loaded rifles that replaced the commonly used but unwieldy muzzle-loaders in the nineteenth century, worsened damage to flesh and bone. Machine guns, introduced during the Franco-Prussian War in 1870, evolved into the more portable Browning automatic rifles in World War I, the Thompson submachine ("tommy") guns of World War II, and the rapid-firing M14 rifles of Korea and Vietnam. Each new generation of armaments not only became more deadly but produced more horrific wounds.

With armies enlarging as wars intensified, infectious disease began to account for more fatalities than the injuries received in battle. The conditions during the Crimean War in the early 1850s, for example, were representative of many conflicts of the time when cholera, dysentery, and malaria caused five out of every six deaths.[3] The care was horrific. The infected and the wounded lay next to each other in overcrowded, filthy wards. Blankets and decent food were in short supply. Basic sanitation was nonexistent. Numbers of deaths from communicable disease were overwhelming. Surgical treatment was rudimentary, although the occasional use of anesthesia began to instill an element of mercy into long-established norms. Many of the wounded who survived their operations died of unrelenting infection after days of agony. Septic wounds with "hospital gangrene" remained all too common and were primarily responsible for a mortality rate of about 25 percent following amputations of arm and shoulder, rising as high as 90 percent after removal of the leg above the knee.[4]

Yet bright spots emerged. Against the objections of the military establishment and in spite of obstacles that the discouraged but doctrinaire physicians in charge raised, a new force swept in. Granted permission by the British government to travel to the Turkish war zone, Florence Nightingale and her team of twenty-eight nurses initiated a series of necessary and lasting reforms in the military hospitals near Istanbul, particularly basic measures of hygiene, cleanliness, and elementary care.[5] She and her fellow nurses demanded that the fetid wards be cleaned. One of her first directives was to commission 300 scrub brushes. She ordered towels and toothbrushes, much to the annoyance of the superintendent, who thought such fripperies excessive. She complained loudly enough that the Turkish Customs House released 27,000 shirts to cover the shivering patients. The nurses quickly reorganized the laundry so that sheets, bandages, and other linen could be washed in hot, not cold, water. Forks and knives came next. They insisted that the kitchens be rearranged and bones removed from the meat. Until that time, one patient might receive an edible portion while the person in the next bed would be served nothing but bone. During the same period, J. H. Dunant, a Swiss banker appalled by the carnage but cognizant that changes were possible, suggested formation of the Red Cross to improve standards of care. The Geneva Convention adopted international guidelines for its organization a decade later in 1862.

Acceptance of these obvious but important changes moved slowly. On the other side of the Atlantic, more soldiers died during the American Civil War than in any war in the nation's history. At least some doctors produced qualitative improvements in the medical and nursing services of the Union army by adhering to the reforms that Nightingale had described in her 1859 book on the architecture and administration of hospitals, *Notes on Hospitals*. These centered primarily around organization and standards in medical units, the keeping of comprehensive records, design of pavilion hospitals, and formation of a trained ambulance corps.[6] But regardless of these administrative advances, typhus, typhoid, and dysentery were responsible for about two-thirds of the nearly 600,000 deaths. The remainder succumbed from wounds and their operative treatment.[7] Hospital gangrene from dirty and infected wounds was the primary cause.

The American "surgeons" were generally untrained country doctors who learned their trade on the battlefield. Chloroform was their choice for anesthesia, primarily because of its fast action.[8] They managed to reduce somewhat the death rate of soft tissue injury from low-velocity musket bullets, bayonet thrusts, and saber slashes compared to that of the Crimean experience. Many adopted the novelty of antisepsis (at least sporadically), applied clean, fresh dressings, and kept the tissue defects open to allow healing from the bottom up. The introduction of the Minié ball in the midst of the war, however, added to the destruction. The effects of this new bullet, which expanded upon impact by a powder charge at its base, were usually irreparable. Overall, the American Civil War represented the last time in human combat that the existing state of medical care was generally inadequate to deal with the challenges the wounded posed.

Acute care of those injured in battle improved gradually in the twentieth century. Having spent months in a field hospital in France during World War I, Cushing described in detail the head and facial injuries that soldiers received while peering imprudently over the edge of the trenches. He was disheartened about the destruction of their lungs from poison gas and discouraged by the loss of their feet from unremitting exposure to cold and wet. The relatively accurate bullets, the missiles exploding at close range, and flying shrapnel increased tissue destruction. Mud and dirt from the surrounding farmland filled the wounds. Although large numbers of soldiers died waiting for help, wound treatment advanced with practical measures of asepsis, surgical removal of dead tissue, and delayed closure. An antiseptic chlorine-based solution introduced by a French surgeon, Alexis Carrel, and an English chemist, Henry Dakin, enhanced substantially the care of wounds. Abdominal operations to remove segments of destroyed bowel or to close penetrating injuries became more common. In prior conflicts, interventional surgery had been limited primarily to amputations. Care of head and eye injuries improved. The emerging technique of blood transfusion was lifesaving, but only for a few. Sir Almroth Wright, a London microbiologist who had also worked on improved local treatment of wounds, orchestrated mass immunization against typhoid, protecting many of the allied troops from this dreaded and previously ubiquitous infection. His efforts evoke Napoleon's insistence a century before that all men in his Grand Army be vaccinated against smallpox. Wright later directed the department in which the young Alexander Fleming was to discover penicillin.

One of the relatively early wartime innovations was transportation of the injured. Surgeons often performed operations on the battlefield during the Napoleonic Wars. Baron Larrey and his colleagues introduced specialized "ambulance soldiers" to carry some wounded from the front lines. Horse-drawn "flying ambulances" then removed them to more distant field hospitals for more definitive treatment.[9] While the French used these light wagons effectively during the Crimean War, the British continued to rely on less-efficient stretchers. The American Union army designed and used a series of ambulance wagons to move injured soldiers away from the fighting. Despite the presence of a well-organized ambulance corps staffed by volunteers who transferred large numbers of men to field hospitals after major battles of World War I, many were left lying on the ground for hours and sometimes days until the overworked medical staff could get to them. They not infrequently died waiting.

World War II corpsmen carried out emergent care in the field and moved the casualties to clearing stations, where surgeons stabilized them as much as possible. The wounded were then transported by jeep, truck, or ambulance to larger hospitals. However, the pattern of injury in that conflagration changed as projectiles of higher velocity produced massive injuries and flaming gasoline created severe burns. The resultant death rate from shock was high. Attacks on civilians and noncombatants, a devastating new military strategy, increased the human cost. With better control of infectious disease, however, this war was the first fought by the United States in which more soldiers died of their wounds than from infection. Surgical intervention, often by those whose training was incomplete, saved many with abdominal and chest wounds. Transfusions of blood and plasma, the introduction of sulfanilamide in 1935, and the eventual availability of penicillin were additional critical gains.

During the Korean War, mobile army surgical hospitals (MASH units) were set up near the front lines. Surgeons controlled hemorrhage and stabilized acute conditions before helicopters removed the wounded to more substantially equipped field hospitals. More aggressive operative procedures, particularly involving wounds of the heart, saved lives. Reconstruction of injured vessels with stored human arteries, a novel intervention often against official policy, preserved limbs and decreased numbers of amputations.[10] However, despite a ready supply of blood, delays and inadequacies of fluid resuscitation pushed many patients into shock and ultimately into kidney failure. By the end of the war, the new dialysis treatment sustained some of the afflicted.

In Vietnam, fully trained surgeons rapidly and effectively controlled bleeding and maintained blood pressure, repaired tissue disruptions, and managed life-threatening injuries in well-equipped units. These definitive interventions plus the availability of powerful antibiotics and other pharmaceuticals reduced the mortality rate substantially. The incidence of acute kidney failure following shock declined because of an aggressive policy to treat deficient blood volume with salt solutions. However, some of the severely wounded developed acute respiratory distress from fluid overload. It took some time before surgical scientists arrived at more moderate resuscitation strategies.

The majority of us in medical training during the late 1960s and 1970s were called into the military. Individuals in the earliest stages of residency were sent to Southeast Asia as general medical officers, and those more senior operated in MASH units or other acute-care facilities. Some in the middle years of residency entered the National Institutes of Health to carry out research on shock, hemorrhage, resuscitation, wound healing, and other combat-associated topics, but most of us in that category were assigned to military hospitals in the United States, caring for the injured who had been stabilized in the field and transferred within days to facilities near their homes for definitive repair, reconstruction, and convalescence. We covered soft tissue defects with skin grafts, closed colostomies, controlled leaks of body fluids, amputated hopelessly destroyed limbs, and aided in long-term recovery. For the first time I saw the horrific effects of land mines. I treated soldiers with one or both lower extremities blown off. One marine officer who I will always remember was transferred to our small naval hospital in Portsmouth, New Hampshire. He had lost both his legs at the hip. Despite our best efforts, we were never able to control the burrowing infection. I recall feeling how difficult it was to remain objective and dispassionate about these wounded soldiers, who were younger than we were, often had wives and children, and whose lives had been forever changed. The politicians responsible little seemed to appreciate or even comprehend the human consequences of their international adventures. These sentiments have only sharpened as I have become older.

While injuries to chest, abdomen, or the extremities, once repaired and healed, leave scars that may be hidden beneath clothes, destruction of the face and its features can ostracize the victim permanently from normal social contact. Attempting to reconstruct such defects in the beginnings of human history, surgical practitioners launched the modern field of plastic and reconstructive surgery. Correction of nasal deformities represented the earliest recorded instance of facial repair, stemming from practices in ancient India and later depicted in Egyptian papyri. As in other cultures of the time, the authorities punished wrongdoers and occasional prisoners of war by amputating their noses. Sushruta, a surgeon who practiced around 600 BC, described a technique of tissue replacement in his monumental treatise, *Sushruta Samhita*, by raising leaf-shaped skin flaps from the forehead and sewing them around the nasal defects. He formed new ears in similar fashion using flaps from the neck.[11]

These sophisticated maneuvers were lost for centuries until necessity demanded their resurrection. Repair of damaged noses became particularly important in sixteenth-century Italy. This was a time and place when swordplay was rife, prisoners were punished with facial mutilation, and the new scourge of syphilis, which Columbus's sailors had brought to Europe from the New World, was endemic. One of the complications of this disease was the destruction of nasal cartilage, so large numbers of desperate individuals with this obvious deformity sought help. A Bolognese professor of surgery, Gasparo Tagliacozzi, reintroduced Sushruta's operation in his 1597 textbook, *De Curtorum Chirurgia per Insitionem*, the first devoted to reconstructive surgery. His most lasting innovation, however, was to create a pedicle of skin from the upper arm of the patient and attach it to the defect of the face. With the immobilized arm anchored to the head with splints, the segment could regain blood supply and heal. Once it was firmly attached, Tagliacozzi divided its site of origin at the arm and tailored the healthy transferred tissue into a new nose. The effectiveness of such vascularized skin flaps to reconstruct faces continued to evoke interest. In the early nineteenth century, a London surgeon, having practiced on cadavers, achieved success in patients and popularized the method.[12] About the same time, a German surgeon coined the phrase "plastic surgery" while describing a variety of repairs to eyelids, lips, and noses.

The modern specialty of plastic and reconstructive surgery was a product of the terrible facial injuries that soldiers sustained in the trenches of World War I. Harold Gillies, a New Zealand Rhodes Scholar, is given much of the credit for founding the field. After receiving his medical education at Cambridge University, he served in the Royal Army Medical Corps and experienced firsthand the devastation among those fighting on the front. Eventually, he persuaded the authorities to open a hospital in England devoted to the problem. Queen Mary's Hospital and its convalescent unit provided care for the flood of wounded whose faces had been shattered or burned, admitting over five thousand patients between 1917 and 1921. Many other plastic surgical units throughout the world arose as a necessity in wartime.

Gillies originally worked with dentists, then learned how to create skin flaps from a French cancer surgeon. He used this technique to reconstruct a broad array of severe wounds of the face, mouth, and jaw. His often striking results were welcome alternatives to the masks that many of the severely disfigured wore in public for the rest of their lives. As an artist, he was concerned with creating the most normal face possible and was the first to produce a pictorial record of the initial injury and the results of his reconstructions.[13] Always desirous of the most optimal benefit and concerned with the final outcome, he spent much time before each operation designing on paper, or with wax or plaster models, the flaps of skin he would use to cover the defects and relating them to the existing blood supply.

He and his increasingly expert team introduced several innovations into standard practice. One was the transfer of bone grafts from the hip to replace missing jaws. Like Tagliacozzi centuries before, they transferred pedicle tube grafts raised from the chest or shoulders to correct defects of the face. Unrolled, these tubes of skin and fat were large enough to provide extensive coverage for burns or missile destruction of lips, noses, and other features. Holes for the eyes and mouth made in the newly transferred tissue allowed the patient to see and eat until the graft regained blood supply, healed in place, and could be more precisely tailored. His method of creating new eyelids for burned soldiers unable to close their eyes because of scarring was a further advance that found later use in treating individuals disfigured by leprosy. Gillies influenced generations of adherents through his writings and by teaching his meticulous procedures. He stressed that the intricate techniques needed in the reconstruction of faces after trauma or in radical cancer surgery take much time and often involve several grafting operations.[14] Plastic surgeons faced with similar patients during World War II and subsequent conflicts have refined and embellished his methods.

An intriguing and futuristic corollary to this and subsequent advances in the field has been the recent success of face transplants. The first patient was a young French woman who had had the bottom half of her face bitten off by a dog, losing much of her nose, cheeks, and lips.[15] Eating was difficult. Saliva dripped from between her exposed teeth. A potential solution to her difficulties, a face transplant, generated much debate among plastic surgeons about the efficacy of administering powerful immunosuppressive drugs to those with nonfatal conditions. Substantial criticism was fielded from ethicists, professional peers, and the media about whether the patient would resemble the donor. In 2005 the surgical team transplanted a matching portion of a face from a cadaver to the young woman's lower face. To accomplish this, they had to join tiny arteries, veins, and nerves that they had isolated from both donor and recipient. Years later, the graft remains healthy. The woman has regained movement and sensation and looks essentially normal. Based on this remarkable success, at least five more transplants have since been carried out. They have provided such patients, hitherto socially isolated and unwilling to move outside their houses, the opportunity to become normal members of society.

A severe burn is one of the most devastating injuries that an individual can experience, regardless of whether it occurs in wartime or in civilian life. In addition to destruction of body surfaces by the acute thermal insult, massive amounts of fluid and salts (electrolytes that include sodium, potassium, chloride, calcium, and others) rapidly leave the circulation to enter the injured tissues or evaporate to the outside from the denuded areas. These complex and ongoing dynamics stimulated both clinical surgeons and surgical physiologists to pursue broad and sustained investigations into effective treatment: means of coverage, intricacies of body composition, appropriate fluid replacement, and means of intravenous nutrition.

One disaster in particular called attention to a subject that had previously evoked little scientific interest. On the evening of November 28th, 1942, fire erupted in the Cocoanut Grove nightclub in Boston. Nearly a thousand patrons, soldiers on leave and civilians alike, were inside. Toxic smoke billowed from burning furnishings, curtains, and artificial palm trees. Tables blocked the emergency exits. People were crushed trying to escape through the narrow, revolving front door. Other doors opened inward, making escape difficult. The place became an inferno. Within a short time a desperate multitude packed the corridors of all nearby hospitals. Francis Moore, later to become a distinguished chair of surgery at the Brigham, was a surgical intern at the MGH when it happened. Called to the emergency room, he and his colleagues were greeted with 114 victims filling all available space. Every bed was taken. Many of the afflicted lay on mattresses on the floor. The first task facing the doctors was to triage those obviously dying from those with a chance of life, differentiating between the categories by tying different-colored labels to wrist or ankle. They then had to administer fluids, arrange for blood transfusions, and provide acute wound care. But many manifestations of the burns were unexplored territory, particularly the severe respiratory failure that a significant proportion of the patients exhibited after breathing in the fumes from the smoldering plastic and paint.[16] Only thirty-nine remained alive after the first few hours. And when the overall numbers were finally tabulated, the incredulous citizens of Boston learned that 492 people had died. Hundreds more had sustained severe burns.

No one was prepared for such a disaster. The few advances in burn management since ancient times were limited to local application of substances such as silver nitrate to prevent fluid loss, or dyes like gentian violet to reduce infection. Little information about treatment was available in the textbooks. Antibiotics were nonexistent. No one in the 1940s had considered the profound and potentially lethal results of such a trauma. Burns involving over 30 percent of body surface area were invariably fatal.[17] But the Cocoanut Grove experience stimulated studies of burn physiology and the effect of comparable catastrophes on the chemical components of the body. In Moore's case it stimulated a sustained interest in the changes in body composition after injury that opened several avenues for clinical research and application. The scientific data that he and others produced over the following decades improved patient care to such an extent that today half of those with burns covering 80 percent of the skin surface survive. The information also became crucial in treating patients with significant trauma from other causes, including extensive surgical operations.

Although care of burned patients continued to provide many challenges in the 1960s and 1970s, I and my fellow residents were helped by the results of the groundbreaking research.[18] The unfortunate individuals were in severe pain. Those with burns of their mouth, throat, and lungs often required respirators. We had difficulty finding normal veins for intravenous access. To keep them from sliding into shock from water, salts, and proteins from the circulation flooding the injured tissues and evaporating from the burned surface, we monitored urine volume and blood levels of electrolytes hourly during the first day and nearly as often in the days thereafter. We replaced electrolytes as accurately as we could by administering appropriate solutions.

At the same time, the burned skin surfaces needed attention. We removed the dead portions surgically and tried to prevent or delay infection in salvageable areas using intravenous antibiotics and topical applications of antibacterial ointment. Because of constant external seepage from the open areas, bandages needed frequent changes. Deeply burned surfaces required coverage with skin grafts from unburned areas of the body, a lengthy operative process repeated as necessary to ensure complete closure. Long-term care was equally important. As the grafts covering the underlying tissues began to heal, contractures developed and joints stiffened despite stringent efforts by the physiotherapists. We eventually needed to release many of the contractures surgically and regraft the open areas. Multiple reconstructions were often necessary. Repair and rehabilitation lasted for months.

It became increasingly clear that changes in the body economy of patients that followed burns, severe trauma, or major operations required accurate definition and well-considered supportive measures.[19] Becoming an integral part of surgical care in the years after World War II, these included prompt transfusions of blood or plasma to replace losses from the circulation, intravenous infusions of water, salts, and sugar to maintain body balance during the acute phase of injury, and adequate nutritional supplements for more chronic care. Before surgical investigators addressed and standardized these issues, patients often died within hours from loss of body fluids or slowly starved during the ensuing days. No one understood the significance of an imbalance of electrolytes during and after injury, prolonged vomiting, diarrhea, or other abnormal states. Without means to measure blood volume or to determine fluid shifts, replacement was carried out in an empiric and inaccurate fashion. If inadequate amounts were given, the patient would go into shock; with excessive quantities, the lungs would fill and he or she would essentially drown. If the correct concentrations of electrolytes were not maintained, sometimes fatal cardiac arrhythmias or other important metabolic complications might develop.

Defining the composition of the various body compartments (bone, muscle, fat, blood, and so on) was a major advance in patient care. With the introduction of the cyclotron in 1937 and the subsequent availability of a variety of radioisotopes, investigators had the ability to tag accurately the individual components. Moore and his colleagues were the first to use these novel labels during the following decades to map patterns of distribution of body water, define the concentrations of electrolytes in specific areas, understand their relationship to acid-base balance, and calculate changes and dynamics in normal and abnormal states.[20] They determined that muscle mass may decrease substantially with inactivity, serious infection, or significant injury, but that it can be regained during convalescence. Their data established the standards we rely on today for the highly sophisticated support of the severely injured or infected.

Transfusing blood routinely, safely, and without incident was also of great interest to medical researchers in the first part of the twentieth century. This vital fluid has been a subject of fascination and awe throughout human history. The ancients endowed it with mythic properties because of the obvious correlation between its loss from the body and death. The poet Ovid, for instance, tells that the enchantress Medea rejuvenated Aeson, aged father of one of the Greek heroes, by injecting intravenously a mixture of blood from a black ewe, semen, and the entrails of a wolf.[21] In Rome, individuals seeking spiritual rebirth bathed in and drank the blood of a newly sacrificed bull in a ceremony called *taurobolium*. The encyclopedist Celsus took this further, noting that drinking the hot blood from the cut throat of a gladiator would cure epilepsy. Perhaps as an extension of the enduring practice of bloodletting to restore balance to the body and to treat disease, the administration or replacement of blood into the circulation of those requiring it was an obvious next step. In 1492 physicians transfused the blood of three young boys to Pope Innocent VIII (by mouth as no alternate route was then available) in an effort to save his life. All died, donors and recipient alike. Disregarding this and similar misadventures, a few seventeenth-century Italian physicians attempted transfusions between animals and humans, and from human to human. Such undertakings were rare and probably unsuccessful, although little information exists about the results.

These modest departures stimulated more directed considerations. William Harvey's discovery of the circulation in 1628 had suggested that substances entering the bloodstream from the outside could spread throughout the body. About five decades later, the English architect, mathematician, and astronomer Christopher Wren broadened this novel concept by injecting fluids intravenously into dogs. About the same time in London, Richard Lower, a physiologist who was the first to show that air in the lungs was responsible for turning blue venous blood bright red, transferred blood directly from one dog to another. He also hypothesized that canine blood could replace that lost by patients after injury, and that it might be useful in treating "lunatics and arthritics."[22] Others had the same idea. Satirical cartoons portraying blood transfusions between animals and humans appeared. Samuel Pepys whimsically suggested the transfer of blood between humans, conjecturing ecumenically that "the blood of a Quaker could be let into an Archbishop and such like."[23] In 1667 Jean Denis, Louis XIV's physician, transfused a young boy with the blood of a sheep, then administered calf's blood to a patient who died after the third treatment. Although the widow of the victim accused the doctor of murder, it appeared more likely that she had dispatched him with arsenic. Because of adverse publicity surrounding the subject, however, officials in England and France called a halt to subsequent attempts.

The halt lasted well over a century, until in 1811 James Blundell, an English obstetrician, showed that dogs could survive transfusions from other dogs but not from sheep. He then administered blood from human donors to several young women dying of hemorrhage following delivery, using a leather funnel and pump, then gravity, to direct it into a peripheral

vein via a sharpened quill, bone, or silver tube. The subsequent development of the sterilizable hollow needle, introduced by an Irish physician
in 1844, and the glass syringe, developed by a company in Birmingham,
England, in 1946, were substantial technical improvements that allowed
removal of quantities of blood from one individual for placement into
another. It also obviated the necessity for direct exchange, an unhandy
method, used occasionally into the 1930s, of connecting surgically an
artery of a donor to a vein of the patient.

A much better understanding of the successes and failures of blood
transfusion was provided by Karl Landsteiner, who discovered in Vienna
in 1900 that the serum of given individuals would cause the red blood
cells of some but not others to clump together when combined in a test
tube. His research led to the definition of the major ABO blood groups
and comprehension of the importance of matching precisely the blood
donor with the potential recipient. The related observation that the
addition of small amounts of an anticoagulant could prevent clotting of
blood collected in containers outside the body improved the possibilities of transfusion. But even this approach took years to be implemented.
One of the early anticoagulants, hirudin, came from the saliva of leeches.
Unfortunately, the supply ceased abruptly with the beginning of World
War I. One British investigator complained: "When the Great War came
it was no longer possible for us to get leeches as [they] were imported to
us in quantities of 1500 or more from Hungary. Shortly after the outbreak
of the war I had a consignment of 1500 leeches lying in Copenhagen. The
English Foreign Office ruled that this consignment was 'of enemy origin'
and the leeches were left to die."[24]

About the same time, the introduction of sodium citrate, a compound
that also prevents bottled blood from clotting, opened the way for modern
blood banking. This was particularly important in World War II, when
transfusions saved many lives. Agents that could be given to the patient
intravenously to prevent clotting were soon introduced, an important
advance from the relatively ineffectual transfer between individuals of
blood in paraffin-coated glass tubes. Initially isolated from the liver, the
anticoagulant heparin allowed the eventual development of more ambitious surgical operations that included open-heart procedures using an

oxygenator pump and the reconstruction of diseased arteries. Warfarin, a drug that can be taken by mouth, was originally discovered when cows died of internal bleeding after eating particular types of clover. Because of its potent anticoagulant properties, it was first developed as rat poison, then eventually adapted for sustained use in patients at risk from stroke, heart attack, or venous emboli.

Like blood transfusions, accurate intravenous replacement of water and salts is critical for the immediate support of individuals who cannot eat or drink following a physical insult. While some nineteenth-century practitioners administered milk for nourishment and castor oil to cleanse the blood by vein, infusion of these and other unsterilized materials into the circulation was associated with such a high incidence of infection that many departmental chairmen forbade treatments by this route until well into the 1930s.[25] As a result, surgeons routinely instilled fluids into the fat beneath the skin or ran volumes of saline into the rectum of the patient at the end of an operation. At least some of the liquid from both sites was eventually absorbed into the bloodstream.

A variety of practical hurdles had to be transcended before intravenous treatment became routine. Because of the potential threat of sudden fevers, chills, and occasional shock from retained bacterial products in the solutions formulated in overextended hospital pharmacies, commercial preparations made under strict, controlled conditions became increasingly available. Stored in reusable glass bottles, the infusions flowed into the patient through rubber tubing attached to a nondisposable needle placed in a vein. Although the equipment was cleaned with steam, contamination remained a constant problem. Not until after World War II were sterilizers perfected, accurate thermostats devised, and aseptic techniques involving all phases of intravenous use improved and refined. The disposable plastic blood bag was developed in 1947 and eventually replaced glass containers for all liquid substances administered to patients. Flexible plastic tubing and progressive improvements in sterility and storage of fluids have been enduring contributions to patient safety both inside and outside the operating room.

Such accouterments were and are still inadequate in some areas of the world and under particular political regimes. During the Cold War in the early 1970s, I visited a hospital in Warsaw. There were many short-ages. Unable to order plastic tubing from the West because it was used in nuclear submarines and was "classified," my hosts had to use their limited supply again and again. With repeated sterilization, the material became opaque, brittle, and fragile. I saw a similar situation when I arrived in China a decade later, shortly after the end of the Cultural Revolution. Reusable rubber tubing carried blood and fluids to the patients from glass bottles because the hospital bureaucracy was unwilling to import plastics from abroad. In spite of these difficulties, however, the patients usually did well. One of my long-term colleagues, Professor Robert Sells of the University of Liverpool, reported a similar impression on a visit to China in 1995.

> The surgical block contained 20 operating rooms, each filled 8 AM to 8 PM with elective procedures, at least two consultants involved in each operation, with four often needed for extensive cases. This is a poor provincial area, 1500 miles northwest of Beijing, a different country really. But the operations I saw for prostatectomy, varicose veins, and thyroid disease were highly impressive with low infection rates, few later recurrences, and no patient staying in for more than two days. Students washed and sterilized the rubber intravenous tubing between cases. Yesterday's dried pus was still on the floor. Theater and wards were cleaned once a week on Wednesdays; at 1 PM a hooter sounded, everyone stopped their clinical work, picked up a mop or a cloth and bucket, and started cleaning. The Secretary of the local Communist party, my constant companion during my visits to the hospital, said the reason for this was ideological. When I said that back home in Britain the cleansing of hospital rooms was given sufficient priority to justify the salaried appointments of specialist cleaners, he shrugged. With low infection rates and waiting lists no more than two weeks for any common operation, who can blame him?

Those of us accustomed to disposable plastics and more obvious measures of cleanliness, however, remain relatively unconvinced.

Although effective modern blood banking technology and fluid and electrolyte management had become integral parts of acute patient care by the 1960s, the nutritional requirements of persons with prolonged surgical illnesses were more problematic. Following a significant physical disruption of any sort, all higher organisms mobilize protein from muscle and convert it to rapidly accessible carbohydrate-based energy to keep their tissues intact, their organs functioning, and their wounds healing. Sick and debilitated patients, those with extensive burns, severe or chronic infections, or lasting complications of trauma or surgery are unable to meet the extra nutritional demands. If additional calories are not forthcoming, they may die from starvation. An alternative strategy was needed to replenish body stores.[26]

In 1968 a group at the University of Pennsylvania stunned other surgical investigators by reporting that puppies sustained solely by intravenous nutrients grew and developed normally.[27] The researchers had to solve a broad array of problems to achieve their remarkable results. They spent considerable time formulating a variety of protein supplements and fat emulsions to meet normal or increased energy requirements, and calculated the exact concentrations to supply adequate calories and prevent fluid overload. They needed to ascertain why many of the mixtures produced fever or abdominal pain following administration and to discover the necessity for trace elements and vitamins. Just as important, they had to work out many practical aspects of the new concept of parenteral nutrition (food given to the subject by routes other than by mouth), particularly proving the efficacy and safety of long-term continuous intravenous infusion devices. They designed plastic tubes that could remain within a vein for prolonged periods, an approach rare at a time when needles were used almost universally for short-term use. The type of tubing posed an unforeseen difficulty. The indwelling plastic often hardened and cracked over time, as my Polish colleagues had experienced. Alternative materials such as silicone had to be identified and tested. The investigators found that they should not use a surgical incision to isolate a large vein in the neck for catheter placement but should insert the tube through a large-bore needle. This technique would prevent infection from tracking internally from its site of entrance in the skin. By trial and error they showed that the end of the catheter should lie optimally in a major vessel near the heart to dispense the thick nutrient fluid effectively through the circulation and avoid clot formation. Arranging a harness so that the puppies could remain fully active in the kennel without stressing the tubing or interfering with the infusion from the bottle containing the solution took much ingenuity. Finally, they had to invent pumps that could accurately control the volume needed each day.

Slowly the system began to work. Enthused by the accruing experimental data, desperate pediatricians in the hospital asked the team to see a newborn infant whose bowel had failed to develop. After removal of the functionless tissue, only about two inches of normal small bowel and half her colon were left, not nearly enough to absorb sufficient nutrients taken by mouth. She was starving to death. With the parents' endorsement, the investigators went ahead with the experiment, using the techniques and equipment they had devised for the puppies. They positioned the end of the intravenous catheter in a major central vessel. To decrease the risk of infection, they used a knitting needle to tunnel the external portion of the tube beneath the skin so that it exited next to the ear. Despite the efforts, unforeseen issues inevitably arose. Lack of essential elements such as magnesium produced metabolic problems. Behavioral development was limited. A fungal infection eventually proved fatal. But almost miraculously during the 22 months she survived, the baby experienced relatively normal weight gain and growth. She had never tasted food.

This unprecedented experience led to the use of total intravenous sustenance in children with similar conditions and then in adults who, for one reason or another, had become nutritional cripples. The results were gratifying. Patients put on weight and regained muscle mass. Skin incisions that had either failed to heal or had reopened during the period of starvation closed normally. Chronic fistulae that had developed between leaking bowel and the skin narrowed and shut. Systemic infections cleared. With news of the procedure spreading quickly, groups formed in teaching hospitals across the country and became expert in the techniques. Specially trained nurses dealt solely with the intravenous lines and fluid management. Not only could many patients receive their treatments at home, but lives were saved.

It should be noted, however, that in the present era of cost cutting, many involved with such nutritionally challenged individuals are increasingly concerned that specialized care is becoming abridged and attention to detail is diminishing. Reimbursements by third-party players do not keep up with expenses. Existing quality of care is not always maintained, and persons inadequately schooled in the discipline are replacing expert nutrition teams. One result is that the rate of complications is rising among sick and fragile patients. But despite the current administrative restrictions, total parenteral nutrition has provided a major advance in the care of the surgically ill.

The possibility of removing operatively a site of inflammation or a cancer, correcting a disabling deformity, or treating a severe injury or catastrophic burn stimulated clinical and scientific advances across a broad front. We have discussed three of the most significant revolutions in modern surgery: the effects of anesthesia, the importance of antisepsis and asepsis, and the implementation of uniform professional standards. The introduction of antibiotics and other effective pharmaceuticals is arguably the fourth. Few of us can remember what life was like before antibiotics. Women died after childbirth from puerperal fever. Chronic urinary infections following multiple pregnancies eventually caused kidney failure in young mothers. Children died from communicable diseases and uncontrolled sepsis. Red streaks running up the arm from an infected cut on the hand or the development of "erysipelas," or cellulitis, on the face evoked dread. The high incidence of venereal disease among the soldiers during both world wars became a subject of national concern. The poor were under constant threat from tuberculosis, diarrhea, and typhus. Untreatable pneumonia at the end of life was called "the old man's friend." It was fatal even for Sir William Osler.

While adherence to the principles of asepsis plus improvements in the operating room paid substantial dividends, surgical wounds still became infected. There was little treatment except to apply heat to the affected area, drain abscesses when they formed, and hope that the bacteria would not spread into the bloodstream. Indeed, some patients escaped the threat. Cushing's meticulous technique and careful preparation of the operative site, for instance, produced a rate of infection among his neurosurgical cases of 0.3 percent, an incidence almost unique at that time and comparable to modern standards. In 1925 his mortality rate for operations on the brain was 8.4 percent compared to that of other leading figures in the field, whose operative death rate varied between 38 percent and 50 percent.[28] The control of contamination by compulsive attention to detail was the primary reason for the differences. The excellent results that Cushing, the Mayo brothers, and other surgical innovators accrued may have stimulated the later efforts of the American College of Surgeons and other credentialing bodies to raise the overall quality of surgical care throughout the United States.

Tragically, lives continue to be lost despite the blessings of an array of antibiotics against a variety of organisms. One important reason is the emergence of resistant strains from overuse of antibiotics. During the 1970s and 1980s in particular, doctors prescribed many of the available drugs enthusiastically and indiscriminately. Patients were no less temperate, demanding the agents for colds and other nonspecific inconveniences. As many of these minor conditions were of viral origin, the medicines were ineffectual. Surgeons over-administered "prophylactic" antibiotics before operation without sufficient cause and continued them unnecessarily in the postoperative period. As a result of these and other factors, hospitalized patients developed dangerous infections from evolving bacterial strains that became resistant to standard treatment. We now hear of individuals in intensive care units dying from contaminated respirators or with rare fungi or viruses. Newspaper headlines currently shout about untreatable "flesh-eating bacteria." And more recently, a few patients who have traveled to India and other distant sites for inexpensive operations are returning to the United States and presenting with infections completely resistant to all known antibiotics. These recent developments have become of universal concern.

Modern surgeons must occasionally deal with septic conditions so relentless that they are powerless to control them. Such an experience makes one appreciate all the more the frustrations and feelings of complete helplessness that our predecessors commonly faced before the modern miracle of antibiotics changed medical care. One such instance remains etched in my mind. Mrs. Singleton was a 75-year-old woman from a Boston suburb, living in comfortable surroundings with her daughter and son-in-law. One of my roles at the time was to provide surgical care for patients on chronic dialysis. I had known Mrs. Singleton distantly and used to greet her when I passed through the unit. Loved and well cared for, she led a relatively pleasant existence despite her kidney failure. Unfortunately, a significant proportion of such patients develop an intolerable itch, probably due to the deposition of salts beneath the skin that cannot be excreted by their nonfunctioning kidneys or removed by the dialysis machine. Indeed, it is common to see the legs, arms, abdomen, or chests of these individuals covered with scratches as they try to gain relief with their fingernails. Mrs. Singleton had this problem.

Clostridium is a class of bacteria that all surgeons dread. It lives commonly in nature, particularly in the soil and in the bowel. It can enter the skin through puncture wounds, lacerations, or scrapes. It does not need oxygen to survive or multiply, and it acts by giving off powerful toxins. One of its variants causes the intense and often fatal muscle spasms of tetanus. The development of tetanus toxoid vaccine in 1924 allowed vaccination of the allied troops in World War II against this terrible disease and saved innumerable lives. With subsequent universal protection, tetanus is now rarely a problem in the West; neither those in combat nor vaccinated children and adults in civilian life are at risk. A further type of Clostridium produces a potent (botulinum) neurotoxin, one of the most lethal substances known. Minute amounts of the material are sold as Botox, a drug used to correct crossed eyes, smooth frown lines, and reduce facial wrinkles. An additional feared clostridial variant causes gas gangrene. Also rare, this condition is unforgettable in its virulence. The organism may enter and grow readily in injured fat and muscle, particularly if the blood supply to these tissues is compromised after trauma or other disruptions. The infection spreads rapidly, producing gas as it dissolves the tissues. Antibiotics are often started too late and are usually ineffectual. The only treatment is emergency surgery to eliminate completely the entire affected site. This may involve amputation of an extremity or removal of large amounts of skin and underlying tissues on the trunk or other areas. The end result may appear as if the patient was hit with a bomb.

Stable for months on chronic dialysis, Mrs. Singleton suddenly developed a fever. One of the nurses noted that a small patch of skin on her abdomen surrounding one of the scratches had become discolored, swollen, and tender. As I happened to enter the unit a short time later, she asked me to have a look. The area in question had become the size of a golf ball, thickened, reddish brown in color, and beginning to blister. To my horror, as I pressed on it, I felt a crackling sensation from gas beneath. I knew immediately what was happening. By the time I had explained the situation to the patient and her family and scheduled emergency surgery, the site had enlarged perceptibly. Her fever was increasing and she was becoming cold and pale. We rushed her to an open operating room. By the time she was placed on the table, intravenous lines started, antibiotics pouring in, and anesthesia given, about half an hour had passed. As we washed her abdominal wall and prepared to remove as much tissue as necessary, we saw that the involved area had now spread toward her chest and onto both flanks. Blisters had coalesced. We cut through what looked like normal skin beyond the edge of the process to be greeted with foul-smelling gas and liquefied fat. No matter where we explored, we were unable to find uninvolved tissue. Her blood pressure began to decline despite intravenous replacement and massive antibiotic coverage. Within an hour she died as we watched, totally unable to do more.

Antibiotics can control the majority of infections. The presence and availability of these agents have become so important in the evolution of patient care that the story of their discovery and development is worth reviewing. The concept that natural or chemical substances might limit the growth and activity of micro-organisms arose early in the twentieth century.[29] Although Robert Koch had asserted that his discovery of tuberculin (an extract of cultures of the responsible bacteria) would cure tuberculosis, his claim was unfounded. The first real possibility of effective treatment for an infectious disease came from Paul Ehrlich, a German microbiologist. Applying findings from the emerging field of experimental pharmacology to his extensive knowledge of bacteria, Ehrlich discovered in 1909 that an arsenical compound, Salvarsan, could selectively destroy the organism causing syphilis. Although ineffectual against other conditions, his "magic bullet" became established as a relatively successful treatment for that common disease and served as the first example of the curative powers of a chemical agent.

About the same time a young Scot from a small village south of Glasgow traveled to London to join his older brother, a medical practitioner. After graduating from medical school, Alexander Fleming trained in surgery and passed the examinations of the Royal College of Surgeons but eventually became a bacteriologist at St. Mary's Hospital, one of the city's premier teaching institutions. He remained there throughout his career. Inquisitive and innovative, he not only carried out routine bacterial cultures for the clinicians but was a passionate investigator, experimentalist, and close observer of natural events. In 1922, while fighting off a head cold, he made an interesting and serendipitous discovery. Out of sheer curiosity, he plated some of his nasal secretions onto a culture plate. Among the various bacterial colonies that grew on the medium, he saw that one had completely dissolved. He transferred the colonies to a fresh plate, repeated the experiment, and arrived at the same answer. Christening the presumed antibacterial substance from the mucous *lysozyme*, he broadened his investigations, identifying the material in tears, saliva, and egg white. Noting that it could destroy a variety of different organisms in the test tube, Fleming considered that it might have a practical use in controlling infection in patients.[30] Despite several attempts, however, he was unable to realize this hope and dropped the subject.

By 1928 he was concentrating his studies on staphylococci, bacteria responsible for several human infections. It was his habit to leave culture plates from many experiments lying around his cluttered desk in apparent disorder. Some were uncovered. Upon his return from a short vacation, he noticed that spores from a fungal mold had contaminated one of the plates on which the staphylococci were growing, and that the colonies adjacent to the mold had disappeared. Conjecturing that the contaminant produced an antibacterial substance, he cultured it and found that it destroyed several varieties of bacteria, even in highly dilute form. At the suggestion of a colleague, he called it *penicillin*.

The lore surrounding this discovery has it that the contaminant blew onto the uncovered culture plate through an open window. More likely, it drifted over from an adjacent bench where another investigator was culturing fungi. The same end result opened a critical new chapter in the treatment of disease. Publishing his observations, Fleming then applied the culture broth of the mold to local infections in a few patients. A few improved. Others did not. With the clinical results inconsequential, the biochemistry of the material difficult to define, isolation difficult, and departmental interests concentrating on other projects, he apparently lost enthusiasm. Others in the laboratory did nothing to encourage him. Regardless of the success of Salvarsan, their prevailing opinion about the potential of chemotherapy (Ehrlich's term) against bacteria was pessimistic.

Despite the inertia at St. Mary's, interest in the potential importance of "antibiosis" was taking root elsewhere. In 1932 Gerhard Domagk, a research worker at the I. G. Farben Company in Germany, noted that a red dye, synthesized previously by company chemists, could control some infections in mice. Probably because of patent issues, Domagk did not report his findings for three years. Belatedly recognizing the potential significance of the discovery in treating human infections, several clinical groups then tested the material against a spectrum of bacteria. The results were striking. At the same time, a French scientist confirmed that sulfanilamide, the parent compound of the red dye, was equally effective. Word about the effects of this and related agents spread throughout Europe and the United States, even as war loomed. Quickly manufactured in bulk, the sulfa drugs saved the lives of many wounded soldiers. Although Domagk was awarded the Nobel Prize for his work in 1939, Hitler refused to allow him to go to Sweden to receive it and even had him arrested by the Gestapo. He finally collected the prize after the war, but the associated monetary reward had by then been redistributed.[31]

Others were slowly becoming interested in bacteria-fighting substances. Howard Florey, a Rhodes Scholar from Australia, was named professor of pathology at the University of Oxford in 1935. Florey had already developed an interest in the antibacterial possibilities of lysozyme. Once established in his laboratory at the Sir William Dunn School of Pathology, he and his collaborators began to search for additional natural substances that could destroy specific bacteria, something akin to Ehrlich's "magic bullet" and Fleming's lysozyme. Ernst Chain, a chemist who had fled Nazi Germany, soon joined Florey in his Oxford laboratories. Both scientists had become so intrigued by the possibilities of controlling bacteria with chemical compounds and so curious about the presumably related antagonistic or inhibitory effects of one microorganism on another that they decided to prepare a review of the subject. Although a few laboratory workers on both sides of the Atlantic had pursued these themes for some years, published information was sparse. Florey and Chain collected enough suggestive data for their review, however, that they initiated formal researches into the subject. Fleming's decade-old paper describing penicillin was among their references.

Britain was on the brink of war and research funding was scarce when they began their investigations. Neither scientist seemed particularly concerned about possible clinical application. Rather grudgingly, therefore, the British Medical Research Council granted them £25 for the project. Florey then persuaded the Rockefeller Foundation to donate £500 over five years. Gathering together a small staff and beginning work, Florey and Chain identified penicillin as the most interesting of the materials then recognized. The crude mold juice was not difficult to produce, but as Fleming had found before them, isolation of its active portion and prevention of contamination presented enduring problems. By 1940 the team had managed to extract small amounts of relatively pure material for study. They determined that, at least in the test tube, penicillin was effective against the common and serious invaders of war wounds, particularly staphylococcus and streptococcus. It also destroyed the organisms responsible for gonorrhea, pneumonia, and meningitis. In addition, they found that it was not toxic when injected into mice and had no effect on their white blood cell count. It was excreted by the kidneys and could be reclaimed virtually unchanged from the urine. American investigators later demonstrated the important activity of the material against syphilis.

Florey and his group continued their investigations despite the dark realities of war. The Nazis had overrun Europe. The London Blitz and the Battle of Britain were underway. German planes continuously flew over Oxford on their way to bomb the industrial cities to the north. Under difficult conditions, the team performed the definitive experiment with the precious substance on May 25, 1940. They injected eight mice with a lethal dose of streptococci, then gave small amounts of penicillin to four. Sleep was impossible as the tension built. By the next morning, every control animal was dead of overwhelming infection. All the treated animals remained alive, although one died two days later. With additional extract, they treated more mice. The results were unequivocal. From the lab's published reports, the scientific community began to hear about the activity in the Dunn School. Fleming traveled up from London. The data were changing medical history.

Although the investigators could produce only small amounts of the substance, using bedpans as culture vessels, they collected enough to try it in several patients. One, a 43-year-old policeman, was near death with a combined staphylococcal and streptococcal infection. He improved markedly during the four days he received penicillin, but declined and died after the supply ran out despite efforts to recover the substance from his urine. Several children with severe infections were treated and survived. Local application cured four patients with infected eyes. The results were clear, but the question of how to produce sufficient quantities remained the primary consideration.

The Oxford laboratory became a factory. Even with gradually improving methods, however, it was obvious that only large pharmaceutical firms could synthesize enough penicillin for the war effort. Florey tried to interest British companies in the project. With incessant German bombing threatening their facilities, they could not take up the challenge. As a result, representatives from the Dunn School traveled across the ocean to present their data to American companies. By 1944, Pfizer, Merck, and Squibb were producing penicillin in bulk using refined culture techniques. There is still controversy about the interpretations of patent law by the parties involved. Whereas the Oxford team felt that restricting particulars about their discovery for commercial gain in time of war was unethical, the Americans felt otherwise and quickly patented their culture process. As a result, British firms making penicillin after the war had to

pay royalties. Regardless of the bruised sentiments and differing philosophies, the discovery, production, and clinical introduction of penicillin
was one of the most notable achievements of the twentieth century, for
which Fleming, Florey, and Chain deservedly received the Nobel Prize
in 1945.

Several of the younger members of the team remained at the Dunn
School throughout their careers. During the years I spent there in the
1960s and 1970s, I got to know several of them and learned the details
of their work. I remain incredulous that they managed to carry out what
they did during the dark days of war and with minimal support, technology, and equipment. On my intermittent trips to Oxford, I still visit
a plaque in one of the gardens that is dedicated to the effort. The accomplishments of these individuals under near-impossible circumstances
remain a triumph of the human spirit.

The success of penicillin stimulated the development of other antibiotics. In 1944 Selman Waksman, a microbiologist working at Rutgers
University in New Jersey, discovered streptomycin.[32] This product of
a soil bacterium was significant, for unlike penicillin, it was effective
against the organism responsible for tuberculosis, a significant public
health hazard. The investigator saw his drug gain substantial popularity through consultation and cooperation with scientists of the Merck
Company, although accelerating disagreements about patents, royalties,
and the priorities of discovery between Merck, Waksman, and Rutgers
University resulted in a damaging series of lawsuits. Despite it all, he
received the Nobel Prize in 1952 for his contributions. Other compounds
emerged. A few years later, one of Florey's colleagues at the Dunn School,
E. P. Abraham, identified a particularly important family of antimicrobial
agents, the cephalosporins. Most significant, these agents killed several
bacterial species that had become resistant to penicillin. Additional varieties of antibiotics were introduced during that period, targeting a wider
range of bacteria. By the time we were residents in the 1970s, we had
several effective agents to use.

Medications that could actually influence disease processes rather than
merely assuage symptoms multiplied as the decades of the century

progressed. German enterprises, with extensive experience with coal tar products and aniline dyes, had exported drugs to the United States for many years. A few local scientific entrepreneurs in academic laboratories began to form pharmaceutical companies to produce their own synthetics and biologicals, often through licenses on German patents; the American Cyanamid Company and Abbott Laboratories are examples. An increasing array of effective remedies available to a population long besieged by quacks hawking their nostrums created much excitement among researchers and the public alike and stimulated further activity.

An account of the evolution of modern surgery would not be complete without considering the benefits of several pharmacological adjuncts to patient well-being and safety. Companies on both sides of the Atlantic introduced increasingly influential and powerful medicaments in the years leading up to and following World War II. Several derivatives of sulfanilamide improved the treatment of infection, not only among the injured but by tempering the spread of dysentery and other communicable diseases. Others quickly followed, including agents that inhibited inflammation, improved the activity of the heart, and increased urine flow. The value of vitamins, factors needed in small amounts for normal body growth and function, became recognized. The influence of vitamin K on blood coagulation and of vitamin C on wound healing advanced operative success. The advent of anticoagulants, antihypertensives, and anticancer agents aided care of the surgical patient.

In some cases, the availability of novel and effective agents plus associated public health measures obviated the necessity for long-established surgical treatments. The elimination of tuberculosis by careful testing of cows, the widespread use of pasteurized milk, the introduction of streptomycin, and selective removal of portions of involved lung largely eliminated the need for deforming operations of the chest wall or corrective procedures on infected joints and bone. Such nonsurgical advances are similar to those in the story of peptic ulcer disease. The discovery that iodine taken by mouth prevented the development of thyroid goiters virtually precluded the need for their removal. Reconstructive procedures on deformed or paralyzed limbs became obsolete with the availability of a vaccine for polio.

Another class of drugs, corticosteroids, were a product of war-related research. An erroneous rumor had circulated that the Germans had developed an adrenal hormone that could enhance the performance of soldiers above existing levels of stress and fatigue. At the same time, physiologists were defining ever more precisely the normal function of the secretions of the endocrine system and the pituitary gland ("the master gland"). Surgical investigators identified the role of this organ system in injury. A scientist at the Mayo Clinic and research workers at Merck and Upjohn eventually produced a series of endocrine products, the steroids. They found, particularly, that they could isolate one steroid compound in large quantities from a Mexican yam and could synthesize another from it. Used in the treatment of many disease states, this class of drugs became important in a variety of surgery-associated activities, from chemotherapy of cancer patients to immunosuppression of transplant recipients.

The pharmaceutical industry, "Big Pharma," exploded in size and power, transforming itself from small drug houses producing and selling patent medicines to a dominant and lucrative global enterprise that provides treatments for a broad array of conditions. Not infrequently initiated through collaborations with investigators in academic laboratories and with clinicians orchestrating patient trials, drug research, discovery, and design evolved via highly sophisticated technologies able to define the selective effects of chemical structures on the machinery of the cell itself. All fields of medicine have benefited.

A growing economy and the accelerating growth of clinical and scientific information in the decades following the war enhanced the lives of large segments of the population. Success in treatment of a range of diseases improved further with the advent of federal funding to pay the bills of the underserved. In combination with other technologies and disciplines, advances in medicine and surgery increasingly offered relief from existing ills, betterment of lifestyle, and confidence in the future. The patients were appreciative; doctors were happy with their careers; hospitals were solvent. One of the most substantial promises of this optimistic time was that even better results would arise through basic and applied research.

Attracted by the advances, young people of the postwar generation viewed medicine as an intellectually stimulating and socially rewarding profession that could provide both autonomy and a generous salary. With applications to medical schools increasing, new university-affiliated teaching institutions formed to keep up with the burgeoning demand for training opportunities. Well-qualified aspirants, many from abroad, entered academic clinical programs or joined research laboratories. A widening array of innovations from the academic hospitals and medical school laboratories stimulated clinical studies and investigative endeavors. As a result of these dynamics, residency programs enlarged in number and quality. Despite the challenges of prolonged and demanding periods of training, more and more fledgling doctors desired to become part of evolving specialties and research endeavors that concentrated on individual organ systems and their abnormalities, or on clusters of related disorders.

six

The Promise of Surgical Research

I had always planned a career as a clinical surgeon, and so my early involvement with the emerging area of kidney transplantation was serendipitous. It was unknown territory. While some organ recipients did relatively well, larger numbers developed problems with which we were completely unfamiliar or which hadn't even been described. Question after question arose that ranged from the meaning of obscure, obvious, or frightening physical abnormalities to the possible application of emerging data from research laboratories. We had few answers, and many of the patients died. Because scientists in Great Britain were providing much of the basic information on the subject at that time, I moved with my family to the University of Oxford to learn from the biologists and participate in their experiments. Such collaborations were common at the time. Many of the investigators lacking a clinical background welcomed interested surgical trainees for their energy, technical capacities, and ability to design and exploit appropriate animal models of human conditions and disease. The experience provided a resident, already possessing extensive patient background, the chance to think, read, and concentrate on specific areas of interest.[1] For a century or more, enthusiasts from Europe and North America transferred themselves and their families across continents, oceans, and hemispheres, where they not only gained new knowledge and expertise but met new personalities, saw new sights, and sampled new cultures.

Similar to my peers from Britain and the Continent who came to the United States and Canada as research fellows, my experience in the Oxford laboratory was far different from my life as a surgical resident. Things moved slowly. I assimilated the scientific literature. My colleagues and I carefully planned each of our experiments. We checked and rechecked the results. If they were interesting, we repeated them.

Gradually, I mastered a variety of techniques using small laboratory animals, transplanting skin and organs, and isolating, identifying, and transferring cell populations. I obtained, interpreted, and presented results in what I hoped was a meaningful way, and heard the comments, criticisms, and suggestions of my peers. We discussed the significance of the data and their place in the order of things. We met visiting scientists from around the world and listened to their lectures. We hobnobbed with Nobel Prize winners.

After three years I returned to surgery at the Brigham and began my own investigations. But even with this background, it took much time before I could ask appropriate questions in the laboratory and devise experiments convincing enough to answer them. It soon became glaringly apparent how much thought and effort goes into establishing a single, tiny fact. It was a demanding apprenticeship, for wresting information from nature takes time, patience, and perseverance. "Eureka moments" are vanishingly rare. However, those of us who became both surgeons and investigators were rewarded with stimulating professional careers in university hospitals. On the one hand, we could care for patients, operate, and teach the house staff and medical students. On the other, we could formulate a hypothesis to answer a basic question and then design an experimental plan to prove it. If the results were interesting, we could publish them. Individuals from an array of countries whose papers we studied and who we met at national and international conferences became lifelong friends. We accepted research fellows from each other's programs, trained them to write and present data, and molded them into clinician scientists.

To spend a year or two in a research laboratory during one's surgical training was common in academic programs during the latter half of the twentieth century. Some took the opportunity to broaden an interest in a particular subject, others to gain a place in a crowded senior residency, and still others to pursue a faculty position in a teaching hospital with hopes of eventually heading a specialty division or department. But as few practicing surgeons had the additional energy to further an area of interest by assessing and amassing convincing clinical data or to pursue an elusive fact in the laboratory, a significant proportion of those initially desiring to follow such a path found that they were not equipped, personally or logistically, for quiet contemplation of a problem or lengthy consideration of theories or concepts. Their active, decision-making personalities often demanded more rapid results than research projects could usually provide.

There were significant drawbacks to becoming a career surgical scientist. Time was inevitably limited. Academic surgeons who spent many hours each week in the operating room had difficulties getting to the laboratory, orchestrating discussions with students and fellows, or scheduling and attending meetings with collaborators. Those who persisted in their studies as junior faculty members had to ensure that their department chairs encouraged and supported their efforts. Earning adequate income to support one's family was an additional problem. Although salaries during the years of residency had improved substantially from times past, few could afford to spend additional time as research fellows at a considerably reduced pay scale. In addition, university stipends would never match income from private practice.

Another hurdle that all surgical researchers continue to face is skepticism from full-time scientists. These doubters often feel that clinicians can neither be conversant with the emerging biologies nor dedicate sufficient time to pursue their applied studies. In a well-known quote, Francis Moore summarized the challenges inevitably present for the academic surgeon, even in the halcyon years of the 1960s and 1970s. "The surgical investigator must be a bridge tender, channeling knowledge from biological science to the patient's bedside and back again. He traces his origin from both ends of the bridge. Those at one end of the bridge say he is not a very good scientist, and those at the other say he does not spend enough time in the operating room."[2] Despite these challenges, those individuals able to balance the two disciplines have contributed much.

Hip replacement surgery is an example of "bridge tending" that has improved the lives of a large number of patients. It has been estimated that arthritis of the hip inconveniences or incapacitates 20 million people in the United States.[3] Orthopedic surgeons currently perform about 300,000 total hip replacements each year, with significant benefit to the previously crippled patients.[4] However, it took decades of failure before this treatment improved enough to be accepted as routine. In the 1920s occasional surgical researchers attempted to reconstitute the roughened surface of the diseased ball-joint portion of the hip in dogs and humans using materials that ranged from pig bladders to sheets of gold or zinc. Some fitted a hollow hemisphere of glass over the bony ball to provide a smooth surface; not surprisingly, this fractured with weight bearing and walking. A covering of chromium and cobalt alloy, introduced in the 1930s, showed early promise but eventually failed. By the 1950s, investigators had devised a prosthetic ball on a metal stem that could be thrust into the bone of the thigh. However, this device inevitably loosened because there was no satisfactory means to anchor it.

A decade later, a surgeon in Manchester, England, began to consider the problem. John Charnley trained as a general surgeon, carried out research in a physiology laboratory, then spent time learning to use a lathe to make small medical apparatuses. Becoming increasingly interested in orthopedics, a minor and rather unappreciated specialty at the time, he began to study joint function. Some of his senior colleagues felt his evolving ideas about replacement of the diseased bone to be so radical that they forced him to carry out much of his initial work in an old tuberculosis sanatorium that had been converted into a hospital. Testing some of the new plastics, he introduced an additional novelty by creating a socket to accept the metal ball device, and then glued both parts of the new joint to appropriate sites of pelvis and femur with a recently introduced bone cement he had acquired from dentists.[5] Introduced in 1962, his operation is performed throughout much of the world with ever-improving results and with constant advances in materials and techniques. Always inventive, Charnley went on to reduce the possibility of infection in the new joints by carrying out his procedures in sterilized and sealed facilities, specialized techniques of asepsis used to this day. The remarkable effectiveness of the operation, one of the most commonly performed in the world, has proved its worth; it is now considered on a par with coronary bypass surgery in enhancing quality of life.[6]

Just as Charnley's innovation was based on his study of joint function, many scientists have sought to understand natural phenomena by direct observation. Some individuals of a more curious bent went further and carried out experiments on living subjects to define the anatomy of the body and to understand the function of various organs and tissues. This was followed by application of operative procedures to reproduce, control, or correct physical abnormalities or disease in laboratory models. To explain these activities more fully, I turn now to the controversial subject of the use of animals in understanding physiology and in the evolution of surgical research. In my view they remain an integral and indispensable resource for scientific advancement.

Scholars of the ancient world were the first to describe experiments on animals. Galen, as noted, based all his anatomical descriptions on studies of species other than humans, despite his voluminous writings that exclusively concerned mankind. Indeed, many of his original observations were erroneous or became erroneous as they were translated and retranslated over the next millennium and a half. In contrast to the decline and virtual cessation of scientific investigations during the Middle Ages, interest in practical matters revived during and after the Renaissance. Science gained status during the Enlightenment, and by the turn of the nineteenth century, the new field of experimental biology arising in France and Germany began to yield significant discoveries about the functioning of the body. The accruing knowledge also provided opportunities for students hoping for scientific careers to work in universities with interested and enthusiastic professors.

A few natural philosophers led the way in applying the scientific method and inductive experimentation to the study of disease. The most important member of this group was John Hunter, the foremost surgical experimentalist of perhaps any age. Using findings based firmly on physiologic and pathologic data from both the laboratory and the autopsy room, he transformed surgery from a hitherto primitive field to one based on hypothesis, clinical findings, and the use of applied animal research. He has been called, along with Ambroïse Paré and Joseph Lister, one of the three greatest surgeons of all time.[7] As a young man Hunter traveled from his village in Scotland to London in 1748 to join his brother, already a highly regarded anatomist. The younger Hunter's talents at dissection and preparation of human material in the school of anatomy soon became apparent. He studied the craft of surgery under the foremost figures of the time, treated casualties of the Seven Years War in France and Portugal in 1762, and cared for the famous as his reputation spread. An inveterate collector of natural specimens and fascinated by all living things, he compared and documented anatomical differences in over five hundred different animal species, gathering together a myriad of details and subtleties of normal and abnormal structure and function. His dissections of human cadavers allowed him to describe a spectrum of disease states. The investigations ranged from shock to the transplantation of teeth, from studies of inflammation to details of digestion, and from venereal disease to the action of the lymphatic system. His realization that a deer's antler could survive via its collateral circulation after he had tied off the primary vascular trunk led to his successful occlusion of the major artery in the thighs of patients to control enlarging aneurysms behind the knees.

François Magendie was a high-profile scientist of the early nineteenth century. He was interested in all aspects of biology, creating a variety of pathological states in animals and using the recognized principles of chemistry and physics to explain the activities of organs and tissues. The first of a new generation of experimental physiologists in France, he identified selective behavior of specific areas of the brain and spinal cord, ascertained that the pumping power of the heart caused blood to flow in the veins, and investigated the mechanism of vomiting. His public demonstrations of operations in awake animal subjects, however, evoked well-deserved criticism among peers and public alike. In contrast, following the availability of anesthesia, detailed studies in experimental creatures became more common. Pain could be controlled and related variables diminished. Toward the end of the century researches on the gastrointestinal tract by one of Magendie's best-known pupils and successors, Claude Bernard, encouraged surgeons to address a variety of human conditions, particularly involving the stomach. Vivisection was becoming an important means of biologic definition and discovery, revealing information pertinent to human ills.

Unlike their Continental peers, most British doctors, traditionally strong in human anatomy and physical diagnosis, eschewed laboratory investigations until the 1870s, when several physiologists formed major research schools and prepared scientific texts for public consumption that included important observations on experimental subjects. About the same time, a group of physicians from some of the London teaching hospitals accentuated Hunter's original premises by performing immediate postmortem examinations on their deceased patients to correlate symptoms and signs with any abnormal findings. This contribution to diagnostic medicine, particularly of diseases involving the lung, heart, thyroid, and bowel, was important. Although few treatments were forthcoming, an additional result of the emerging knowledge was that the Royal College of Surgeons began to insist that those taking their qualifying clinical examinations be more conversant with bodily functions. Studies on anesthetized animals, along with increasingly stringent controls and restrictions on their use, increased sharply as students entered laboratories to confirm and expand their clinical observations.

Investigations to understand human ills through the application of experimental models also germinated in the United States. Surgeons were the obvious group to carry these forward. One of Halsted's lasting contributions to surgical education was his introduction of a surgical research laboratory at Johns Hopkins in 1895 to study clinical problems in living animals, a departure from the established medical curricula that taught human anatomy almost exclusively through dissection of cadavers. Using the subjects as models for patients, he instructed his trainees about operative techniques and the scientific method, and emphasized the importance of accurate and detailed record keeping. The new professor developed original and effective techniques in dogs to suture together segments of bowel, to stabilize fractures by screwing a metal plate across a broken bone, to create experimental hydrocephalus (abnormal amounts of fluid collecting in the spaces of the brain causing the organ to atrophy and the heads to enlarge), and to examine the effects of removing various endocrine glands. The important information and operative innovations that he and his team produced proved that academic surgical departments could rise to the same levels of scholarship and prestige as those in more basic fields such as pathology or physiology.

Cushing also became an important force in the new area of surgical research, having acquired a thirst for investigation from his sojourn in

Europe. Upon the return of the young surgeon to Baltimore in 1901, Halsted gave him the responsibility for a series of lectures to the third-year medical students and the opportunity to direct a practical session in surgery using both cadavers and anesthetized dogs. The course quickly dominated the curriculum, not only because he taught operative methods but also because it encouraged direct contact between student and teacher. At the end of each session Cushing targeted the most promising individuals to participate in ongoing research projects and to apply for a surgical residency. With growing patient responsibilities limiting his own time, he appointed the best trainee to run the laboratory as his assistant. The person chosen had to possess good academic qualifications, enthusiasm for investigation, and the ability to work alone. If successful he would spend the following year in a highly sought-after position on Cushing's clinical service, a huge boost to a career. Also in 1901, J. Collins Warren opened a laboratory of surgical research at Harvard Medical School to stimulate interest among the students and house staff in carrying out clinically applicable scientific projects. Arriving in Boston a decade later, Cushing expanded this initiative. The success of his innovations motivated other medical schools to form similar laboratories for applied investigations and teaching. Indeed, during much of the twentieth century many in senior academic positions had taken full advantage of the experience such enterprises offered.

Although advances in biology potentially useful to humans were impossible without the study of living subjects, objections arose. The abuse of animals had long been a sensitive topic, particularly in the United Kingdom.[8] Public sentiment began to resist the cruel and well-established customs of dog and cock fighting and bull baiting. Questions were raised about breeders and care of farm animals. Reforming zeal and moral crusades involving causes from the political to the social and religious filled the second half of Queen Victoria's reign and reflected the public's burgeoning interests in humanism, evangelicalism, romantic poetry, and fiction. Arguments about Darwin's theories raged. In addition to ecclesiastical and moral disagreements concerning evolution and its associated sciences, the coincident use of experimental subjects to advance biological knowledge evoked passion and sometimes exposed obvious antipathies.

Distinguished writers and artists decried the practices with tracts, pamphlets, short stories, and magazine articles, sometimes on humanitarian grounds, sometimes from an anti-intellectual stance. In the eighteenth century the diatribes of Joseph Addison, Alexander Pope, and Samuel Johnson against such "barbarous treatment," and the abusive scenes that William Hogarth depicted in his paintings, *The Four Stages of Cruelty*, are examples. Eminent figures of the latter nineteenth century continued the pressure. In art, Sir Edwin Landseer pleased a sentimental public with his portraits of endearing animals with human qualities. Literature was filled with innuendoes against scientific experimentation. Sir Arthur Conan Doyle, on a break from Sherlock Holmes, described an unfeeling and over-directed physiologist who dispassionately considered the workings of the lachrymal glands as his wife wept on his shoulder. In his poem *In the Children's Hospital*, Alfred, Lord Tennyson described, perhaps rather harshly, the surgeon who "was happier using the knife than in trying to save the limb." Wilkie Collins, a prolific novelist and friend of Charles Dickens, portrayed the suicide of a research worker after antivivisectionists had thwarted his experiments. Robert Louis Stevenson whetted public suspicion of science and scientists by characterizing the nefarious Dr. Jekyll as a vivisector. Although a vocal proponent of education and the author of a popular text on science, H. G. Wells pictured his antihero, Dr. Moreau, as a dark and driven torturer who anthropomorphized his animal victims by reconstructing and transplanting their bodily features without anesthesia. His book, *The Island of Dr. Moreau* (1896), is both a parody of Darwinian selection and an uncomfortably accurate description of the older techniques of physiologists.

Alongside these protests by writers and artists, the antivivisectionist movement evolved into a national and international force that gradually spread from Britain to the Continent, and then across the Atlantic. Suspicion toward teaching hospitals that were opening animal laboratories and the human experimentation allegedly ongoing within their doors inflamed public antipathy. Even the microbiologists and vaccinators did not escape notice. Koch's inoculation of farm animals against infectious diseases evoked adverse comment. Complainers loudly derided Pasteur's work on rabies vaccine, although many presumably were dog lovers. Even

Charles Darwin was ambivalent. "Physiological experiments on animals is justifiable for real investigation, but not for mere damnable and detestable curiosity. It is a subject which makes me sick with horror so I will not say another word about it else I shall not sleep tonight."[9]

The United States became equally caught up in the cause. In 1866 individuals in New York, distressed at the maltreatment of horses, established the American Society for the Prevention of Cruelty to Animals. The movement spread, encouraged by its success abroad, by adverse publicity about animals used in research, and by religious and secular prejudice toward the emerging sciences. In Massachusetts, public hearings on the subject captured so much attention that several distinguished scientists, physicians, and leaders, including President Eliot of Harvard, attended to support the aims of the experimentalists and to speak forcefully about academic freedom and education. "He [his antivivisectionist opponent] said he was here to represent dumb animals. I represent here some millions of dumb human beings. It is for them that the scientific biologists are at work."[10]

Such arguments continued unabated in the new century. Scientists, concerned physicians, and a preponderance of the public itself took the side of "academic freedom and education." A minority of reformers and private practitioners remained opposed. Concerned about loss of income from competition with university faculties, the latter were a highly vocal group whose stance against experimentation in nonhuman subjects began to interfere directly with advances in medical treatment. Objections arose about perfecting in animals the innovative technique of lumbar puncture to diagnose meningitis in children, trials with antisera in rabbits to develop diagnostic tests for syphilis, and the tuberculin test to assess prior exposure to tuberculosis. Even Alexis Carrel, who had won the 1912 Nobel Prize for his work in vascular surgery and transplantation, became a target of the antivivisectionists. The media pushed emotions further. The *Washington Post*, for instance, published a headline in 1913 entitled "Doctors of Death," an exposé of clinical practices based on animal work.[11] The subheadings included: "Humans Murdered by Vivisection; Victims of Poison; Girls and Little Children Inoculated with Germs of Loathsome Disease in the Name of Science; Practices Like

Spanish Inquisition." With this type of hyperbole, rational dialogue was problematic.

While irregularities undoubtedly arose, the great majority of biological scientists were seriously concerned with animal welfare and conscientiously ensured that those in their laboratories acted responsibly toward their charges. Interested in advancing medical science in the United States during the early years of the new century, organized medicine prepared guidelines for animal use, although not until 1966 were minimal standards formulated. These standards evolved into the current regulations from the National Institutes of Health (NIH) and other federal bodies, which are now as stringent as those involving patient trials. The restrictions became even more severe in Britain, Germany, and other European countries, where research projects are screened carefully, and laboratory licenses are difficult to obtain. Such uncompromising precepts are still not enough for relatively small groups of activists who liberate animals from laboratories, destroy results of investigations, break equipment, and burn buildings. These individuals have occasionally threatened the lives of research workers, vandalized their homes, and planted letter bombs in post boxes and explosive devices in cars to cause injury.

Despite such harassment, those working in the laboratory sciences have improved the lot not only of ill patients but of animals as well, with significant advances in veterinary medicine. Positive changes have been made that affect the comfort and quality of life of laboratory animals. The cosmetics industry, for instance, no longer uses rabbits to test its products. Because of professional and public pressures, the pig and the sheep have for the most part replaced the dog in large-animal experiments. Nonhuman primates are used more discriminately as subjects of investigation than in previous decades as ethical questions surrounding studies of AIDS, risks of viruses transmitted with organs transplanted across species, and other issues are debated by both researchers and concerned citizens. Still, few facets of medical biology could have progressed without animal experimentation. The advances in physiology and surgery are prime examples. While thoughtful individuals continue to hope that biological knowledge can be gained without the use of laboratory subjects, the prospect seems unlikely in the foreseeable future.

Stimulated by Halsted's successes at Hopkins, research by surgeons broadened appreciably as the twentieth century progressed. Some of their investigations remain important to our present understanding and practices. Others disappeared from consciousness or led to human benefit by more circuitous and delayed routes. Many failed completely. Although the Peter Bent Brigham Hospital was still unfinished when Cushing arrived in 1912, he and the two research fellows he brought with him from Baltimore immediately began work in his new Surgical Research Laboratory across the street at Harvard Medical School. Their most important and lasting contribution during that period involved the discovery that the cerebrospinal fluid bathing the brain and spinal cord continuously recirculates, a conclusion contrary to accepted dogma that had long portrayed it as a static and unchanging substance. Lewis Weed, a young investigator who later became a professor of anatomy at Johns Hopkins, carried out a still-unique series of experiments on dogs to prove the point. In his detailed publications, he reviewed the multiple existing theories about the origin and fate of the fluid, then showed that specialized cells lining the spaces of the brain produce it while other cell populations absorb it.[12] Weed's elegant, complete, and irrefutable studies in the early years of the twentieth century stimulated later treatment of hydrocephalus in children and raised the image of research by surgeons substantially among the medical school faculty. Then, as now, the underlying value of these investigative efforts in animals was their potential clinical application.

A broadening spectrum of relevant and applicable information from both clinical and laboratory investigators was gradually garnering public and professional attention. Accumulating interest in and knowledge about the "ductless glands" in particular was to become so significant that I shall discuss the subject in detail. The glands comprising the endocrine system secrete a variety of specific hormones into the bloodstream to modulate activities and behavior of distant organs and tissues. Physicians were beginning to appreciate the manifestations of hormone deficiencies at the same time that surgeons began to clarify individual functions by selective removal of glands from experimental subjects and from patients. The thyroid evoked particular scrutiny because its diseases were so common.

By the end of the nineteenth century, medical practitioners understood that inadequate thyroid hormone, often from lack of iodine in the diet, was responsible for cretinism among children and myxedema in adults. The children showed stunted mental and physical development, characteristically coarsened facial features, and bony distortion. Often with coincident goiters, adults with myxedema experienced swelling of the face and hands, thinning of the hair, progressive lack of energy, lethargy, and intellectual deterioration. Over time, the puzzle of these symptoms was resolved. Physicians began to ensure that all affected patients received adequate amounts of iodine or, in extreme cases, of thyroid extract for the rest of their lives. They also realized that operative removal of the entire gland for goiter caused progressive slowing of activity, decreasing energy, profound physical changes, and eventual coma. Surgeons learned to leave small remnants of functioning gland in place as well.

In 1893 Sir William Osler wrote a definitive report describing the critical necessity of administering thyroid hormone to sixty afflicted children, and showing photographs of many of them before and after treatment. One case was representative. "M. has been under my observation from January 1892, at which time she was two years old, and presented with a typical picture of [cretinism]. The thyroid extract was started in March 1893, and she grew four inches in the first fourteen months. She learned to walk and talk, and lost altogether the cretinoid appearance. She has continued to grow and develop, and now nothing peculiar is to be noted about her."[13] Adults too were transformed from somnolent invalids to vital members of society. The differences were miraculous. Osler embellished the theme in a follow-up paper:

> Whom has suffering humanity to thank for this priceless boon? As with many great discoveries, no one man, indeed, no set of men. The points in the development of our knowledge of the function of the thyroid gland have been worked out in almost equal shares by physicians, surgeons, and physiologists. To [them] we owe directly the experimental evidence which made possible the successful treatment of myxedema and sporadic cretinism. That I am able to

show you such marvelous transformations, such undreamt-
of transfigurations, is a direct triumph of vivisection, and
no friend of animals who looks at the "counterfeit present-
ments" I here demonstrate will consider the knowledge
dearly bought, though at the sacrifice of hundreds of dogs
and rabbits.[14]

The endocrine function of the pancreas became a second area of investigation. The control of diabetes with the pancreatic hormone insulin is
a triumph of perseverance in surgical research, arguably on a par with
the discovery of penicillin for its contribution to patient health and well-
being. The pancreas is a soft organ that straddles the aorta and vena cava
deep in the upper abdomen. Several large blood vessels enter and leave it.
When stimulated by the presence of ingested food, it secretes fat-digesting
enzymes into the small intestine via the pancreatic duct. Physiologists and
surgeons had long studied this external "exocrine" activity by tying off the
duct and assessing the subsequent nutritional status of the experimental
subject, whose dietary fats were expelled unchanged in the stool. What
they did not realize until the end of the nineteenth century, however, was
that the gland had an additional activity critical to life itself, the internal
"endocrine" manufacture of insulin.

The ancients had recognized that some of the ill exhibited extreme
hunger and thirst coupled with a massive urine output. Arataeus, a
second-century Greek physician second only to Hippocrates in reputation, described the condition as "a melting down of the flesh and limbs
into urine." For centuries thereafter clinicians diagnosed diabetes mellitus
(the word *diabetes*, from the Greek meaning "pipelike" or "siphon," implies
an overproduction of urine; *mellitus* is the Latin word for "honey") by
recognizing its symptoms and signs and by tasting the urine and finding
it sweet.[15] However, understanding of a direct association between the
disease and the pancreas lagged far behind. In 1869 a medical student
in Berlin, Ernst Langerhans, noted clusters of peculiar-looking cells scat-
tered randomly throughout the gland substance, apparently unrelated to
its exocrine role. The function of these "islets of Langerhans," as they were
later christened, was not known. Twenty years later two investigators at

the University of Strasbourg excised the pancreas from a healthy dog to test whether its juice was necessary to digest fat. Allegedly curious that a puddle of the dog's urine attracted large numbers of flies, they confirmed it to be filled with sugar. This observation led them to show in a long series of animals that removal of the organ not only created deficiencies in digestion but was inevitably fatal. Finding additionally that the condition did not develop if they only blocked the flow of pancreatic juice by tying off the duct, they and other investigators postulated that some unknown factor in the gland seemed selectively responsible for normal sugar metabolism. In 1901 a pathologist at Johns Hopkins, Eugene Opie, associated the sugar derangements with abnormalities of the islets, noting that these cells were responsible for the production and release of the "unknown factor," later recognized as insulin, into the bloodstream.[16]

"Sugar disease" or the "pissing evile," as seventeenth-century physicians called it, occurs when the body is unable to metabolize food into energy. During its progression through the gut, meals are normally broken down into complex carbohydrates, proteins, and fats. With further digestion, these nutrients are absorbed through the bowel wall into the portal venous system that drains, in turn, into the liver. This large organ transforms them into simple sugars, fueling its own functions with some, storing others for later need, and releasing the remainder into the circulation to nourish cells throughout the body. If insulin is reduced or lacking, transfer of sugar from the bloodstream into the cells that need it for energy cannot occur. The excess builds up to high levels in the blood and is excreted in the urine. The elevated concentrations of sugar in diabetic urine also cause a large increase in daily volume.

Only in modern times have clinicians recognized two distinct forms of diabetes mellitus. In the childhood or juvenile onset Type I disease, the islets are destroyed by an autoimmune process or viral infection. The patients endure fatigue and weakness with progressive loss of weight as the body futilely depletes its own fat and muscle to produce energy for adequate cellular activity. Essentially starving to death, they lapse into a coma and die. Without control of these events by frequent injections of insulin to allow sugar to leave the blood, enter the tissues, and restore normal metabolism, the expected survival of these unfortunate individuals may be as short as a year after diagnosis. Type II maturity onset diabetes, in contrast, occurs in older people whose islets produce insufficient amounts of insulin either because of aging of the cells or by excess body mass that outpaces the existing supply; we recall how Mrs. Laverne became diabetic as she gained weight. These persons require either insulin or oral medications that stimulate their islets to produce more insulin. Even with adequate control of blood sugar, however, both forms may over time lead to blindness, infections, accelerated arteriosclerosis, gangrene of the lower extremities, kidney failure, and other complications. Indeed, diabetes is becoming a public health hazard. The incidence of the disease in 2000 was 2.8 percent of the world population (171 million people).[17] In 2008 in the United States 24 million persons had been diagnosed, a number increasing further during our current epidemic of obesity. Indeed, recent figures suggest that over one-third of the population will be diabetic within a few years.[18]

Treatment was useless before the introduction of insulin. Until the middle of the nineteenth century, patients were bled and blistered. Opium was widely administered, perhaps primarily to dull the feeling of hopelessness; Osler still advised its use in the 1915 edition of his textbook. The ingestion of large amounts of sugar became popular for several decades— an ill-conceived notion that worsened the symptoms and accelerated the complications. Starvation became a slightly more successful alternative, based on the observations of French practitioners that the amount of urinary sugar declined in some of their diabetic patients when food was scarce during the siege of Paris in the Franco-Prussian War in 1870.

Frederick Allen at the Rockefeller Institute in New York was the best known of several physicians in the United States specializing in the care of diabetics in the years before World War I. Re-examining the French data, he concluded from confirmatory studies in a variety of animal species that stringent restriction of food was the most effective treatment for severe diabetics. If they did not eat, they excreted less sugar in their urine. In a book published in 1919, *Total Dietary Regulation in the Treatment of Diabetes*, he discussed seventy-six patients who had undergone his "starvation treatment." The demands that this stern and rigid scientist laid down were terrible for the hungry and thirsty diabetics who entered the hospital to starve.[19] He and his assistants sometimes took the practice to extremes by locking the patients in their rooms for weeks or months at a time. Many desperate emaciates escaped to their homes, gorged, and eventually died. The few who adhered closely to the regimen gained an extra year or two of miserable life. Allen's staff was continually on the alert for "forbidden food." One patient illustrates the extreme measures taken. The urine of Case Number 4, a twelve-year-old blind diabetic boy, always had some sugar in it, presumably from food he had eaten. The nurses could never discover the source. "It had seemed that a blind boy isolated in a hospital room and so weak that he could scarcely leave his bed would not be able to obtain food surreptitiously when only trustworthy persons were admitted. It turned out that his supposed helplessness was the very thing that gave him opportunities that other persons lacked. Among unusual things eaten were toothpaste and bird seed, the latter being obtained from the cage of a canary that he had asked for. These facts were obtained by confession after long and plausible denials."[20] He weighed less than forty pounds when he died.

The results of laboratory investigations were equally frustrating, although assays gradually emerged that could measure levels of sugar in the blood. These rudimentary determinations encouraged occasional researchers to try to treat the condition with pancreatic extract. While the results of the majority of studies were relatively inconsequential or were interrupted by the war, two investigators made some progress. One in particular was Nicolas Paulesco, a Romanian who demonstrated that elevated blood sugar levels in dogs made diabetic by removal of their pancreas would fall to normal and that sugar in their urine would disappear after he gave them an intravenous injection of gland extract in saline. By 1921 he had published several reports in French journals.[21]

About the same time, a young surgeon and University of Toronto graduate, Frederick Banting, became involved. Returning wounded from the conflict in France and trying to start a clinical practice, he took a part-time position as a junior faculty member in the Department of Surgery at the University of Western Ontario, in London. As one of his new duties, the professor asked him to give a lecture to the medical students on carbohydrate metabolism and diabetes, subjects about which he knew little and cared less. In reading about the subject in preparation for his talk, however, he found descriptions of a technique to tie off the pancreatic duct. It occurred to him that if he blocked the exocrine secretions of the gland in such a manner, its substance would gradually shrink and scar. If he waited long enough, these changes might allow him to "obtain the internal secretion free from the external secretion."[22] He could then prepare an extract and give it to a diabetic animal. Banting had translated Paulesco's writings from French during his review but misinterpreted the conclusions, not giving them the credit they deserved.[23] His concept was otherwise a novel one. Prior investigators who had described the ductal ligation technique had concerned themselves primarily with its effects on exocrine function.

Having the summer free, he traveled to the University of Toronto and persuaded the senior professor of physiology, J. J. R. Macleod, to give him laboratory space and ten dogs with which to pursue his idea. The plan was to make one group of dogs diabetic by removing their pancreas, and then treat them with an extract from the duct-ligated glands of the remainder. After much procrastination, an unenthusiastic Macleod agreed. By a toss of a coin, they chose Charles Best, a medical student, to assist in the project. The assigned space was rudimentary; no one had used the small, dirty room for ten years. The summer was hot. The operating room, immediately adjacent to the odoriferous animal quarters, was sweltering. Means of testing blood and urine for sugar were primitive. At first, little was accomplished. All those who have begun new research projects are very familiar with this stage. Some subjects died of hemorrhage, others of anesthesia overdose, still others from infection. Tempers grew short. Finally, after two months of effort, a few pancreatectomized dogs remained alive. Banting and Best removed the scarred glands from three donor animals whose duct they had occluded weeks before, macerated the tissue in salt solution, and filtered out the residue. They administered small portions of the material intravenously to three of the diabetic dogs, measuring sugar in blood and urine at intervals before and after the injections. Despite abysmal record keeping, it became clear that for several hours following the injection, levels of sugar in the blood fell toward normal and disappeared from the urine. During the same period the somnolent dogs became lively. Encouraged, the investigators broadened the scope of the experiments, finding that extract of normal pancreases was more effective than that from the duct-ligated glands. Even Macleod was becoming less skeptical. Despite no formal employment or salary, Banting moved to Toronto to pursue the experiments full time.

The picture gradually improved. The young surgeon was given a position in the Department of Pharmacology. Macleod provided better laboratory space. Best elected to defer his studies and continue work on the project. A biochemist, J. B. Collip, joined the team to devise a way to isolate pure material from their filtrate. The investigators soon discovered that extract of beef pancreas, obtained in bulk from the slaughterhouse, was effective in rabbits and other animals, and the filtrate from pig pancreas was equally beneficial across species, findings of later profound impact for patients. At a meeting of the American Physiological Society in New Haven at the end of December 1921, Banting, a notoriously poor speaker, presented the findings to the notable figures in diabetes research. Although his presentation fell flat, the smooth and practiced Macleod came to the rescue and convinced many of the audience of the potential importance of the work. A phone call to the professor after the conference then opened a new chapter in the insulin story. A researcher at Eli Lilly and Company, George Clowes, inquired whether his group in Indiana could work with the Toronto investigators to produce "insulin," as they now called the substance, on a commercial basis. Macleod did not think the project had advanced far enough for this departure, yet the future collaboration became crucial to the eventual clinical introduction of the hormone.

In spite of the intriguing results, a schism deepened between the irascible and rough-edged Banting and the urbane Macleod. Banting also felt that Collip was taking undue credit for the work. While Best seemed to ride out the storm, the rest of the group were at odds regarding contributions and priorities. Arguments also arose about when to try the substance in a patient, particularly because some animal subjects had developed serious side effects following its administration. Macleod and several of his senior colleagues considered a clinical attempt at treatment to be ill advised, precipitous, and premature, but they reluctantly acquiesced. On

January 11, 1922, the team watched a house officer give an injection of Banting's crude extract to Leonard Thompson, a 14-year-old diabetic on the public ward of the Toronto General Hospital. Having been on Dr. Allen's starvation diet of 450 calories per day for some time, he weighed forty-five pounds, was pale, listless, and obviously nearing the end.[24] The injection had little apparent effect except to produce a sterile abscess at the needle site in his buttock.

Meanwhile, Collip was purifying the filtrate with increasing success, although refusing to divulge details of his technique. The new material was so effective in diabetic rabbits and other experimental animals that a truce was declared and all participants consented to test it once again on Thompson. They gave the first dose of the new material to him on January 23. His blood sugar fell, his urine cleared, and he felt better for the first time in months.[25] Other diabetics on the ward were treated with similar benefit. In their subsequent publication, the team concluded: "These results taken together have been such as to leave no doubt that in these extracts we have a therapeutic measure of unquestionable value in the treatment of certain phases of the disease in man."[26] Thompson lived relatively normally until 1935 as an assistant in a chemical factory. When Banting enquired whether he had had any fun in his life, the answer came back that he had become drunk every weekend. The surgeon nodded approvingly.[27]

The limited supply of insulin that Collip was producing was insufficient to meet the increasing demand. Many patients died waiting for help. With a mindset similar to the later sentiments of Florey and his colleagues about penicillin, Banting and most of the others on the team agreed that patenting the new agent was not professionally ethical and that it should be free for all. The University of Toronto, perhaps more realistically, eventually obtained a patent. By May 1932, after much dialogue, the institution and its researchers came to a satisfactory agreement with George Clowes and Eli Lilly, a company well equipped to produce pharmacological agents in bulk. Gradually and not without difficulties, insulin began to save countless lives in New York, Boston, other cities in the United States and Canada, and soon in centers in Britain. Within a few years crystalline insulin was introduced. Four decades later chemists synthesized the molecule, opening the way for the current availability of genetically engineered human material. The routine use of this hormone among diabetics has been a seminal advance in medicine in this century, based on relatively primitive beginnings with a few dogs.

Although a few earlier investigators had noted an effect of pancreatic extract on blood sugar levels, the Toronto group received the credit for discovering insulin and pushing its use into clinical reality. But even the awarding of the Nobel Prize to Banting and Macleod in 1923 was not without controversy. Banting, furious at the exclusion of Best from the prize, divided his prize money with his young associate. Macleod followed suit with Collip. In his book on the development of insulin, the historian Michael Bliss summed up the troubled relationship of the investigators as follows: "It would have been like going through a whole Canadian hockey season without allowing a single fist fight."[28]

Subsequent laboratory investigations into the endocrine system concentrated on the influence of hormones on cancer. In 1941 Charles Huggins, a Canadian-born urologist working at the University of Chicago, noted that some biological substances could modify the growth and spread of cancer cells in rats. In further studies he showed that depressing the secretion of male hormones by castration could cause regression of primary prostate tumors and slow their rate of spread. His choice of the dog as the subject in these experiments was fortunate, as only that animal species develops prostate cancer. Some of Huggins subsequent clinical results were striking. Patients relegated to bed with painful bony metastases were able, often for prolonged periods, to resume essentially normal lives.

The unique observation that changing the hormonal environment of the body could control some tumors exemplifies how the flow of scientific information typically builds on existing knowledge. John Hunter had initially noted that castration of dogs caused their prostate to atrophy.[29] A half-century later, a surgeon at the University of Pennsylvania confirmed this finding in dogs and in patients.[30] At the same time, an investigator at a cancer hospital in Glasgow observed that removal of the ovaries caused metastases to disappear in some women with advanced breast cancer. With more sophisticated techniques and ongoing animal experimentation, Huggins put these earlier observations on a scientific basis and elevated them into universal clinical acceptance. The surgical removal of gonadal tissues to slow the progression of human prostate and breast cancers lasted into the 1970s. Since the advent of synthetic hormones and their selective inhibitors, however, pharmacologic strategies plus coincident chemotherapeutic agents and radiation have generally replaced extensive operative intervention. For conceptualizing an entirely new strategy in the treatment of cancer, Huggins and a colleague received the Nobel Prize in 1966, joining Banting in a group of ten surgeons so honored.

The knowledge arising from the expansion of basic and applied research in the decades after World War II improved understanding of the biology of human disease and enhanced the development of new strategies in treatment and cure. With the introduction of ever more effective pharmaceuticals and advances in nuclear technologies opening new avenues for investigation, the emphasis on the health of the country began to shift from the control of infections through public health measures to more specific treatments of cancer, heart disease, and chronic illness. Clinical residents desirous of pursuing academic careers joined the increasing number of established investigators addressing these subjects in university and medical school laboratories. Increasingly funded by a variety of grants and contracts that supported the new disciplines and innovations, research became a firmly established mission for academic institutions.

The idea of targeting funds for scientific inquiry first arose in the late nineteenth century in the United States when universities and federal agencies began to work together to improve agricultural yield and efficiency. Philanthropists such as John D. Rockefeller, Andrew Carnegie, J. P. Morgan, and others began to offer support for libraries, research institutes, and laboratories. This trend increased somewhat between the world wars, although many clinical investigators still paid out of pocket to finance their experimental studies. Support of science slowly intensified commensurate with America's growing role as a major economic and military force. In 1939 President Franklin D. Roosevelt named Vannevar Bush, a professor from the Massachusetts Institute of Technology, as Chief Science Advisor to oversee scientific endeavors throughout the

United States. In his 1945 book *Science—the Endless Frontier*, Bush laid out a comprehensive scheme for the advancement of science by promoting relations between industry, government, and academe. The encouragement of university-based research via a stable source of federal monies was to become the national strategy, with academic investigators pushing into the unknown and industry translating their discoveries into practical use. The plan was to make the United States pre-eminent in science, attracting experts from both Eastern and Western Europe and taking advantage of the "brain drain" from Britain and other nations during the 1950s. In addition, Bush wanted to enhance and refine innovations initiated in other countries less able to promote them. Obvious examples from war-torn Britain include the inventions of radar and jet engines and, as we have seen, the discovery of penicillin.

The growing American interest in the possibilities of science sharpened acutely when a beeping object suddenly appeared in the night sky on October 4, 1957. The Russians had dumbfounded the United States with the launching of Sputnik. This perceived humiliation was exacerbated by the subsequent explosion of America's first rocket on its launching pad and caused many to question the commitment of the country to serious scientific development. But commit it did. The fruits of research into human disease with the possibilities of longer and healthier lives were especially welcome. There was, for instance, universal jubilation when investigators introduced the polio vaccine in 1955. The NIH grew enormously as the government responded with generous funding. Total federal expenditure for medical and biologic research and its institutions soared from $18 million to $181 million per year during the 1950s. By 1960 the annual NIH budget reached $400 million. Money from private sponsors flowed apace. Mary Lasker organized the American Cancer Society, then went on to lobby Congress to increase support, believing that "the doctors and research scientists were too accustomed to thinking small."[31] The Lasker Foundation became an important source of awards for those increasing the understanding of prevention and treatment of human disease.

Doctors and research scientists were quick to embrace the increasing array of opportunities offered. Forming and maintaining a laboratory, however, is an enduring challenge for all investigators. Adequate funding involves the submission of grant applications to private agencies, pharmaceutical companies, and particularly to the NIH. To design and prepare a grant takes an inordinate amount of time, energy, effort, and attention to detail. For many years a completed paper document for the NIH ran to fifty pages of single-spaced type, tables, graphs, illustrations, and a plethora of relevant references. More recently, the format has been shortened and applications are made online. Regardless of format, it still constitutes an art form, a highly stylized presentation of the proposed studies that includes a concise review of the subject, detailed plans for individual experiments, and supportive pictures and diagrams. Persuasive preliminary data and relevant publications by the investigator are crucial to its completeness, and a detailed budget and biographical sketches of the principal investigator and collaborators are integral components.

The applications must be precisely presented and sometimes resubmitted before eventual acceptance. In my own experience of applying for and receiving NIH funding for nearly three decades, I purposely put aside a period of nine months in the final year of each three- or five-year funding cycle to prepare for the next proposal. During that period of gestation, I wrote draft after draft of text, constantly revising, rearranging, and refining. The final product had to be scientifically sound, original in its concepts, and clear and convincing to those who reviewed it. Meeting the deadline for submission was an added burden; I knew several colleagues who completed their forms the night before, then flew to Washington, D.C., and hand-delivered the heavy package (the original and multiple copies) to the appropriate institute to ensure its inclusion. The preparation of these documents was an enduring challenge, crucial for continuation of one's laboratory effort, of the salaries of one's research fellows, and for one's academic career. Despite all the effort, however, I sometimes could not help feeling, as the submission date approached, that I was caught in a not-very-productive ritual or some elaborate but wholly necessary game.

In 2006, not unusually, the NIH received over 45,000 grant proposals for consideration. Their processing, distribution, and ranking is a huge project for the research administrators who every year invite about 18,000 experienced scientists throughout the country to review and grade the applications in 2,500 study sections. Meeting every four months, each study section is responsible for assessing a range of assigned topics. About a month before each gathering, the twenty or twenty-five reviewers receive a stack of about fifty grants relevant to their own area of expertise. Three reviewers examine each application in detail, assessing and scoring it for scientific worth, uniqueness, and potential value to the field. During the two-day meeting they present their summaries to the entire group for general discussion and final decisions. Most of us on the review committees leave these sessions exhausted and humbled when we realize that only about 10 to 15 percent of the applications are accepted. While those chosen are superb, concern always exists that we may have missed projects of great potential value outside currently favored areas. Overall, however, the system seems as fair and equitable as one can make it.

Regardless of these challenges in applying for funding, interested clinicians and scientists took Lasker at her word and began to "think big" after World War II. Despite ongoing political and social disruptions in the United States in the 1960s and 1970s, laboratories and hospitals received encouragement and funding to advance science and improve patient health and well-being in unprecedented ways. There were many examples. The definition of the double helix and the unraveling of the genetic code gave birth to the entire field of molecular biology, the practical benefits of which are only now becoming evident. Researchers began to grow livers, heart muscle, skin, and other tissues outside the body for eventual engraftment within, define substances limiting the blood supply to developing tumors, and consider the repopulation of deficient or diseased sites with stem cells. Exploration of the function of the normal and diseased heart led to an array of operative manipulations, using open or minimally invasive approaches to correct abnormalities of that organ. Investigations into the phenomenon of rejection of genetically foreign tissues introduced the novel field of organ transplantation. I shall specifically review these two latter subjects in the following chapters as important examples of the clinical application of surgical research efforts in academic institutions.

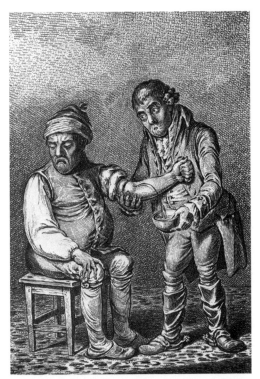

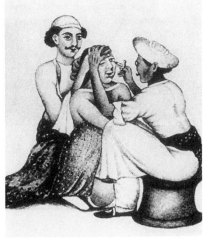

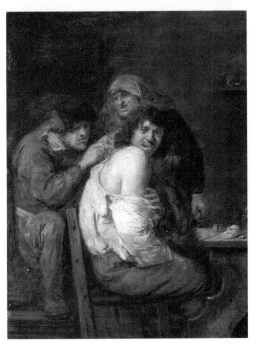

◄ Surgical interventions have been part of the human experience throughout history. The ancient Greeks introduced the drawing or letting of blood to restore bodily humors. Used to treat a broad spectrum of ills, this common practice lasted into the twentieth century. (James Gillray, 1804, *Blood Letting*, in G. Williams, *The Age of Agony*)

▲ The couching of cataracts began in India in the sixth century BC. With an attendant supporting the patient's head, the surgeon used a needle or fine blade to dislocate the clouded lens and push it backward, out of the field of vision. (H. Ellis, *A History of Surgery*, reprinted with permission of Cambridge University Press)

◄ Early surgeons drained abscesses, removed superficial tumors, set fractures, and corrected dislocated joints as the need arose. (Adriaen Brower, seventeenth century, "Operation on the Back," Städelsches Kunstinstitut, Frankfurt am Main)

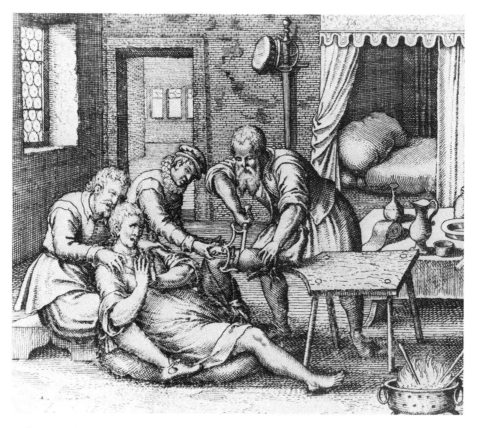

▲ The types of operative procedures broadened with growing experience. Amputation of the leg became increasingly common as battles intensified, the bullet replaced the arrow, and compound fractures led to potentially fatal infections. (Fabricius Hildanus, 1617, *De Gangraena*, National Library of Medicine)

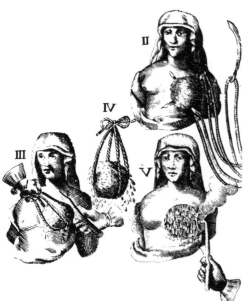

◄ Removal of the cancerous breast was carried out on women desperate enough to permit such an operative extreme. (Johannes Scultetus, 1656, *Armamentarium Chirurgicum*)

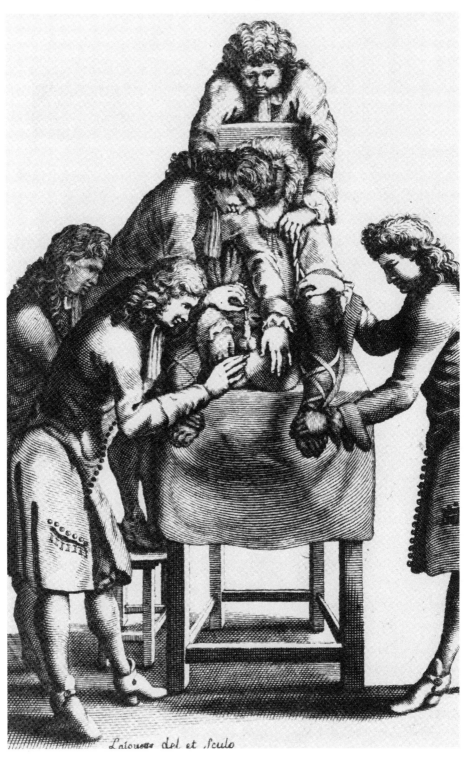

Lalouette del et sculo

▲ "Cutting for bladder stones" became an important part of the surgical armamentarium during the eighteenth and early nineteenth centuries. (François Tolet, 1682, *Traité de l'extraction de la pierre*)

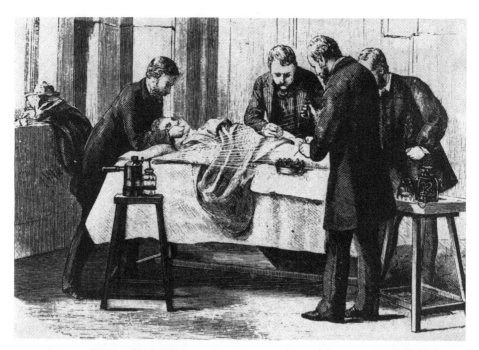

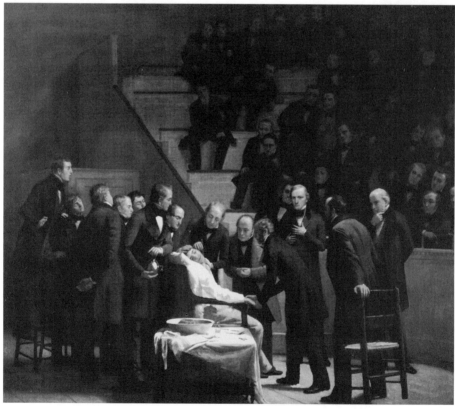

◄ Infection of any wound, open fracture, or surgical incision was ubiquitous and often fatal. Introduction of the principle of asepsis substantially reduced this threat. In 1846, Joseph Lister introduced an aseptic technique whereby the surgical incision, instruments, and hands of the surgeons were enveloped in a constant spray of carbolic acid. (*The Antiseptic Spray in Use*, in G. Williams, *The Age of Miracles*)

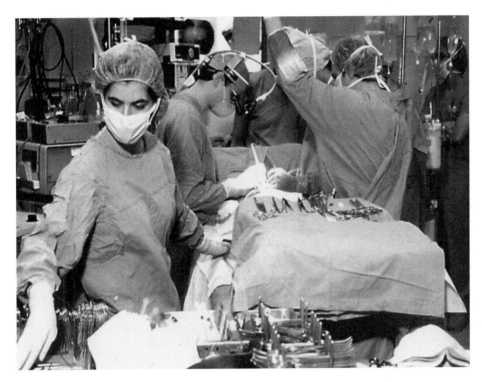

▲ After World War II, equipment, monitoring devices, and anesthesia became increasingly sophisticated and personnel more highly trained.

◄ As surgery became more complex, so did the operating room. In the eighteenth and nineteenth centuries, surgeons wore street clothes, spectators stood around the table, and students and other onlookers looked down from the tiers of an amphitheater. (R. A. Hinckley, *The First Operation under Ether*, Francis A. Countway Library of Medicine, Boston)

► Surgical operations and their safety improved during the early twentieth century. Varicose veins were a common affliction. Their removal by internal stripping allowed patients to resume normal and comfortable lives. (J. Homans, *Textbook of Surgery*)

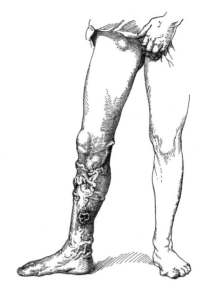

▼ Huge, disfiguring thyroid goiters occurred particularly among individuals living inland in iodine-poor regions. Their removal became increasingly routine. (T. Kocher, *Deutsche Zeitschrift für Chirurgie* 4 [1874]: 2417)

▼ ▼ Many individuals suffered with peptic ulcers of the stomach wall (A) and duodenum (B), as shown here. In response, surgeons designed a spectrum of operations that were relatively ineffectual and sometimes harmful. (J. Homans, *Textbook of Surgery*)

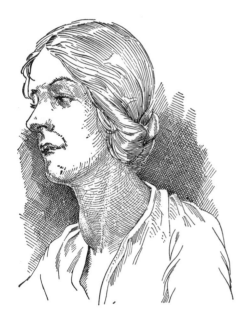

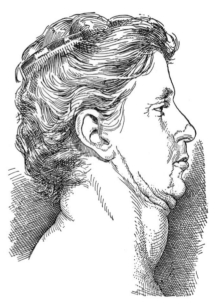

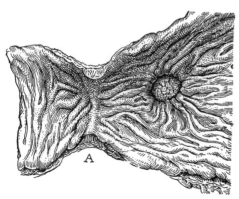

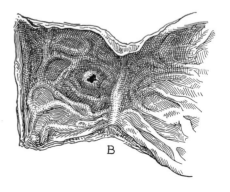

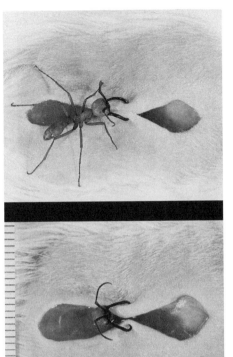

◄ The closure of surgical wounds altered markedly throughout history. Practitioners in ancient India often used biting ants to close incisions or superficial wounds, positioning the head of the insect over the skin defect, stimulating it to bite the area closed, then dislocating the head from the body. (G. Majno, *The Healing Hand*, Harvard University Press)

▼ As operations became more extensive in the decades after World War II, stapling devices gained popularity. The operator could close large skin incisions faster than by placing and tying individual sutures.

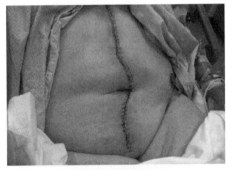

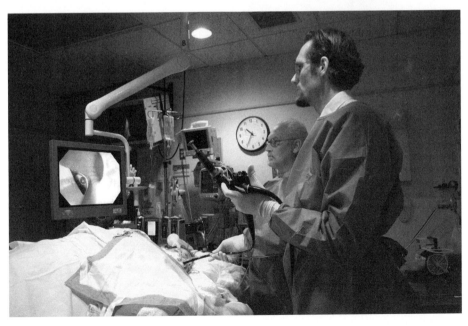

▲ The use of a body orifice such as the mouth or anus to enter the body cavity and manipulate or remove organs and tissues is under trial. There is no external incision and no postoperative pain. (*BWH Bulletin*, 2008)

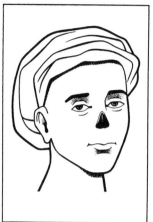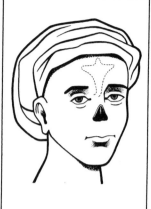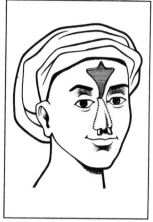

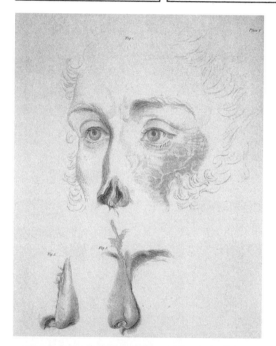

▲ Surgeons devised increasingly effective methods to repair obvious tissue deformities and loss. Using a technique noted initially in Egyptian papyri, surgeons in ancient India raised a flap of skin from the forehead to cover the defect left after amputation of the nose. (From the *Sushruta Samhita*, in G. Majno, *The Healing Hand*, Harvard University Press)

◄ Joseph Carpue in Victorian England repaired severe nasal deformities using skin flaps. The technique was first described in sixteenth-century Italy. (In H. A. Ellis, *History of Surgery*, reprinted with permission of Cambridge University Press)

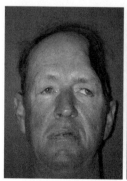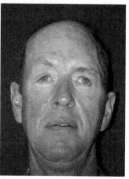

◄ Today, nonreactive materials like silicone and other synthetics are used for breast implants and as substitutes for large bony defects. (Courtesy of Michael Yaremchuk and with permission of the patient)

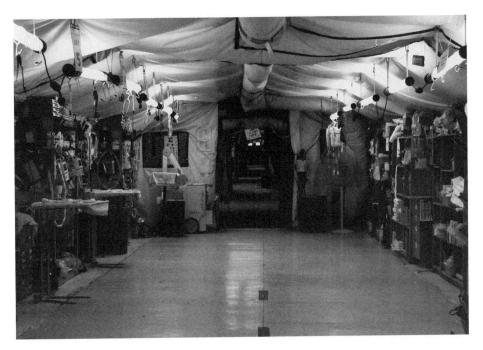

▲ Surgical advances developed during wartime, when surgeons treated the injuries sustained in battle. Surgical conditions in field hospitals improved during twentieth-century conflicts. This is a temporary Air Force Theater Hospital at Balad Air Base, a combat support facility in use during the Iraq War. Such mobile, highly sophisticated, and well-equipped units have been described as "MASH on steroids." (Courtesy of Michael Paul Mason)

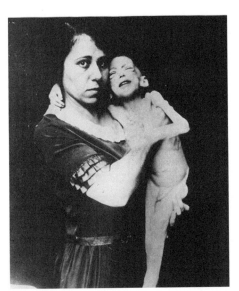 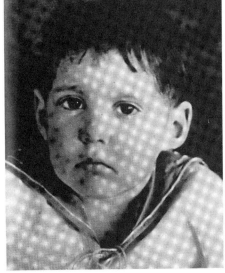

▲ Surgical investigators isolated insulin from the normal pancreas and demonstrated its use in severe diabetics. Its effects were nothing short of miraculous. Patient J. L., three years old, weighed fifteen pounds in December 1922. Following insulin treatment, he weighed twenty-nine pounds, a normal weight, in February 1923.

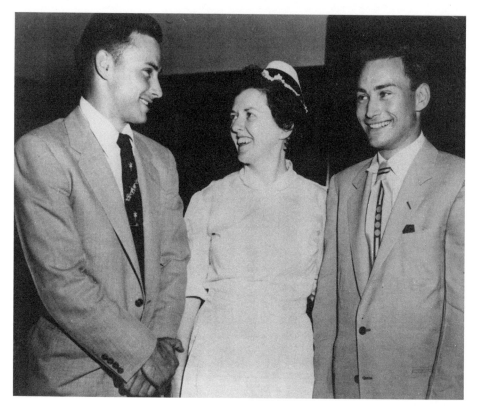

▲ Organ replacement slowly became reality during the second half of the twentieth century. The first successful organ transplant was performed in 1954 when the kidney of a healthy donor was transplanted to his terminally ill identical twin brother.

▼ ► With ever more effective suppression of the immune responses, grafts between genetic strangers became increasingly possible. This baby was dying of liver failure from a congenital absence of her bile ducts. Several years after a successful liver transplant, she was living a normal life. (Courtesy of D. Hanto)

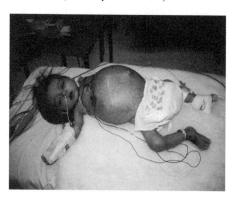

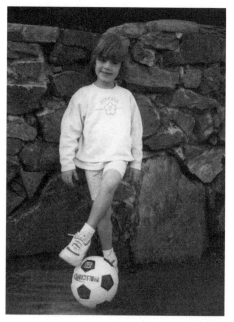

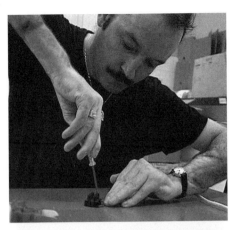

◄ Microsurgery allows the joining of minute blood vessels, nerves, and muscles under the microscope for the transfer of grafts from one body site to another. With advances in the transplantation of foreign tissue, composite grafts can be removed from a donor and placed in or on a recipient. Having lost both his hands and forearms in an accident some years before, this patient received replacements from a deceased donor. Two years later, normal motion and sensation returned with nerve regeneration. (Courtesy of J. M. Dubernard and with permission of the patient)

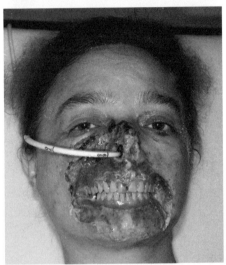

◄ A refined use of microsurgery has been in use in face transplants. A dog chewed off the bottom part of this patient's face, including her nose, cheeks, chin, and lips. (Courtesy of J. M. Dubernard and with permission of the patient)

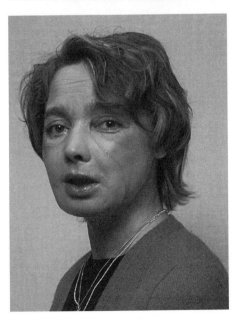

▲ An appropriate portion was removed from the face of a deceased donor with precise sparing of all structures. (J. M. Dubernard, B. Lengelé, E. Morelon, et al. *New England Journal of Medicine* 357 [2007]: 2451)

◄ One year after transplantation, the patient had regained some motion of her mouth, satisfactory speech, and improving sensation. (Courtesy of J. M. Dubernard and with permission of the patient)

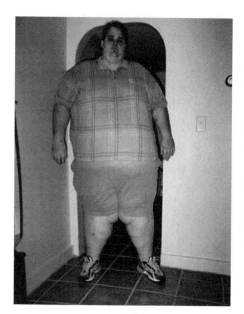
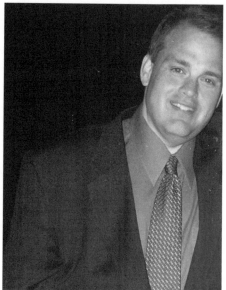

▲ Bariatric surgery has arisen as a specialty to aid those with morbid obesity, an increasing public health problem. Gastric bypass, the primary operative treatment, has become the most common operation now performed in the United States. Beneficial results are often striking. In addition, co-morbid conditions arising from the obese state, like diabetes and hypertension, may disappear with significant weight loss. (Courtesy of David Lautz and with permission of the patient)

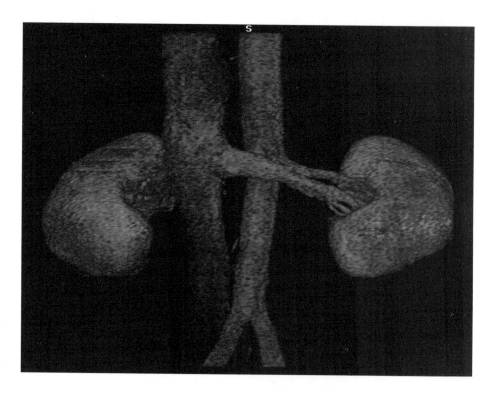

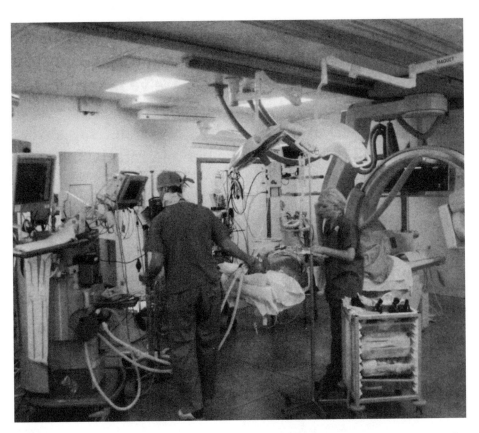

▲ Imaging in the hybrid operating room allows the specialist to manipulate catheters, balloons, and other devices within the patient's vasculature in a fully equipped surgical suite where a definitive procedure can then be carried out if necessary. (M. L. Field, J. Sammut, M. Kuduvalli, A. Oo, and A. Rashid, *Journal of the Royal Society of Medicine* 102 [2009]: 92)

◄ Increasingly sophisticated technology is allowing surgical interventions undreamed of in earlier years. Precise imaging has removed much of the guesswork from clinical diagnosis. The emergence of the CAT angiogram, for instance, produced with only small amounts of intravenous dye, provides striking detail of the vessels entering and leaving an organ, in this case the kidneys.

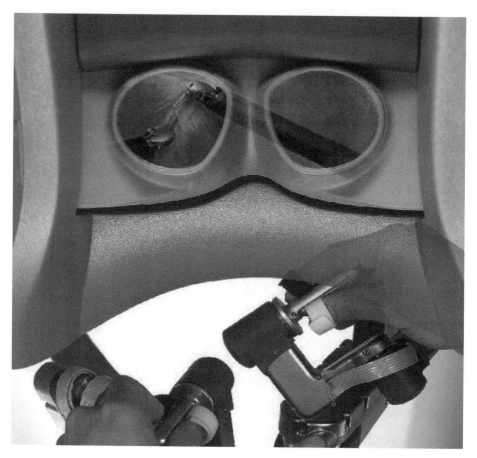

▲ Robotic surgery is gaining attention. Using sensitive and responsive instruments, the surgeon may operate at a distance from the patient. Even the finest finger movements may be translated into precise three-dimensional tissue manipulations.

seven

Operations on the Heart

L ate one winter night in 1971 the nurse in the emergency room of the Peter Bent Brigham Hospital received a call that a man had been shot in the chest. The ambulance had picked him up and was on its way. She immediately paged me from the ward where the intern and I were examining a patient. I was the senior surgical resident in the hospital at the time, in my fifth year of training. We rushed down to the emergency room while she called the cardiac surgeon at home. He said he would be there in half an hour.

The emergency room of the aging hospital was circular in shape with a central desk and ten narrow beds lining its periphery. Curtains could be drawn for privacy. The usual array of night visitors had collected, exhibiting a spectrum of complaints and conditions. Several sat on benches awaiting attention. A few lay on the narrow beds. One of these was an alcoholic we all knew well from his many prior visits. The police, finding him in a stupor, had brought him in to warm up and recover. A young woman had had a miscarriage and was awaiting the obstetrics resident. A middle-aged man had experienced a seizure on his way home on a passing streetcar. Kind passengers had delivered him to the door. An elderly lady had fallen on the ice and broken her arm; I hadn't yet had a chance to get downstairs to set the bone. It was otherwise a quiet night.

Surgical procedures that the residents carried out in the emergency room were generally limited to the suture of lacerations and comparable minor operations. Patients with pressing or more complex conditions were admitted and taken to the operating room as necessary. Bottles of plasma and several packs of instruments were stored on a shelf–just in case. One of the packs was for opening a chest. The nurse and I had enough time to undo it. The instruments were wrapped in two blue cotton sheets, an outside one and a sterile inside one. We moved adjacent beds to the side to give us more room, opened the wrappings, arranged the contents on a nearby table, and covered them with sterile towels. The intern gathered a supply of intravenous tubing, needles, and a urinary catheter. He then brought over a small tank of oxygen connected to a face mask by a plastic tube. By compressing an attached inflatable rubber bag, he could force oxygen into the lungs under pressure. I had already spent rotations on the chest surgical service and was moderately familiar with what to do. But in retrospect, the prospect of being the surgeon fully responsible for the patient was daunting. Fortunately, my training clicked in and I moved from step to step as if programmed.

Sirens heralded arrival of the ambulance. Within seconds the doors burst open and the crew rushed in, pushing the victim on a litter. The ambulance personnel of the early 1970s were restricted in what they could carry out. They checked blood pressure, controlled obvious sites of bleeding, and administered oxygen, but they could not start intravenous lines, administer drugs, or insert breathing tubes. They were not the highly trained and licensed emergency medical technicians we currently depend upon to carry out lifesaving maneuvers in their large stand-up vehicles. But the men moved fast. We moved fast too. Unlike the majority of patients, for whom there is time to perform a history and physical, make a diagnosis, and formulate a plan, those with trauma to the heart give us little chance for reflection. We had to intervene quickly and stabilize what we could until support arrived. Few situations in surgery, I was quickly learning, gave one so little leeway. There could be no delay and no mistakes.

On the cart lay a young man of high-school age wearing a uniform with the logo of a nearby fast-food establishment. He was ashen and barely breathing. His shirt was soaked with blood. We lifted him immediately onto the bed and quickly cut off his clothes, a faster maneuver than trying to remove them intact. Blood was welling from a single bullet hole in the front of his chest. Listening with my stethoscope, I could discern only distant and faint heart sounds. The nurse reported his blood pressure to be barely measurable. We could hardly feel a pulse. Preparations moved forward promptly. Unexpectedly, a medical student had arrived, and so we set him to work keeping the boy breathing by holding the mask over his nose and mouth and squeezing the rubber bag every few seconds to push the oxygen-air mixture into the lungs. Unable to insert a needle into an arm vein because the patient's shock had caused his vessels to collapse, the intern isolated a major vessel in his groin and placed an intravenous line within it. He then sent a sample of blood to the blood bank to set up transfusions. With the line secured in place, he ran in saline and plasma as fast as they would go. He then pushed a catheter through the penis into the bladder to monitor urine volume.

I knew we had to stop the bleeding immediately if we had any chance to save the boy's life. But what incision was I to make? Splitting the breast bone down the middle and forcing the two halves of the rib cage apart would give us an excellent view of the heart but would take longer. As the bullet hole was to the left of the midline and bright red blood was trickling out, opening the left chest seemed the most reasonable approach. The nurse and I turned the patient onto his right side, taped his hip to the table to stabilize the position, and secured his left arm on a frame over his head. While placing sterile drapes around the incision, I realized I hadn't painted his skin with antiseptic solution. I made a long incision between the ribs from his back around to his breast bone. Cutting down quickly through the intervening muscles, I opened the chest cavity. As air rushed in, the lung immediately collapsed.

Membranes anchoring the heart and great vessels in the midline separate the lungs from each other. These large organs, inflating and deflating as the subject breathes, normally hug the walls of their respective cavities because of the negative pressure within. Upon inhalation, the lungs expand passively as the rib muscles contract to enlarge the chest volume. Upon exhalation, the muscles relax, decreasing the size of the cavity and forcing the air out through the windpipe. If the chest wall is breached, however, atmospheric air under positive pressure fills the space around the lung, causing it to deflate like a balloon. Total collapse was beneficial in visualizing the heart in this instance. I did not have to waste precious seconds dividing adhesions that are sometimes present between lung and chest wall. The right lung functioned adequately to provide oxygen for the tissues. The next step was to insert a retractor into the incision between the ribs. Shaped like the letter C, this is one of the most critical instruments in a chest pack. Once the intern and I had it in position, I turned a crank on its handle to force the blades apart and gain an opening of about eight inches. I cut through one of the ribs using the double-action cutter also in the kit to expand the opening farther. The unconscious boy never moved.

Even in an emergency, one cannot help noticing the texture, colors, and movement of the organs. The lungs are a delicate pink in young people or in those who live in unpolluted environments. One can see a pattern of tiny air sacs beneath the smooth surface, like a fine sponge. In contrast, the lungs of city dwellers are often mottled with dark patches from impurities in the air. In smokers, they are uniformly muddy gray or black. In contrast to the expanding and deflating lungs, the heart is in constant motion, contracting and dilating strongly and rhythmically. The thin-walled, reddish upper two chambers of the heart, the atria, lie directly on top of the two muscular lower chambers, the ventricles. These are dark in color, rather like a piece of raw steak. In some people the outside of the ventricles may be covered with a layer of yellow fat. Coronary arteries, sometimes hidden in the fat, course over the surface, their small branches feeding the muscle beneath.

With the chest of the patient now gaping widely I could see the pericardium, the glistening, opaque, tough envelope that encloses the heart. Even though a stream of red blood gushed through the obvious bullet hole, the sac was grotesquely distended with dark blood and clot, completely hiding the weakly beating organ beneath. I quickly opened the membrane with scissors, taking care not to damage the large nerves running along its length or to injure underlying structures. Although the heart was abnormally soft and seemed relatively empty, blood still flowed with each contraction from obvious holes in the front and the back of one of the chambers. Reacting almost reflexively, I cupped one hand around the organ and pushed my thumb into one hole and my forefinger into the other. The bleeding stopped. We removed the blood and clots with a suction device someone had thoughtfully plugged in, and stopped to catch our respective breaths. The copious amounts of intravenous fluid and plasma now running into the patient began to raise his blood pressure. The muscular activity under my hand strengthened. Almost as an afterthought, I found the bullet lying free in the pericardium behind the heart. Although what we had done had taken only a few minutes, it seemed like a lifetime. I looked down. Although I had on sterile gloves, I had no mask and was wearing a shirt and tie, as scrub clothes were only used in the operating room in those days. I didn't even know the patient's name.

The cardiac surgeon and an anesthetist arrived shortly thereafter. The portable equipment the latter brought with him was especially welcome as the boy was beginning to struggle. Despite his movement, a tube was inserted into the windpipe and appropriate anesthetic administered. Once the patient was safely asleep, the staff surgeon helped me place large sutures on curved needles through the contracting cardiac muscle around my thumb and then my finger. The bullet, fortunately of low caliber, had traveled cleanly in and out of the left ventricle without other disruption. With the other surgeon tightening and tying the stitches, I slowly withdrew my hand. The field remained dry. We irrigated the site with saline and sewed the pericardium closed. Once we had removed the retractor and brought the ribs together, the anesthetist reinflated the collapsed lung by squeezing the bag and forcing out all residual air between lung and chest wall. With the newly arrived blood transfusions running in, we wheeled the boy to an operating room, where we completed the closure. When all was stable, we located his parents.

Tommy O'Rourke, the shooting victim, was a junior at a local high school who worked occasional evenings at a sandwich shop near the hospital. He lived with his parents and brothers a few blocks away, not far from Mrs. Turner's old house. The next morning the entire family, a priest, and two policemen gathered with us for an emotional meeting at the bedside. We filled the room. Tommy told us he had been alone in the shop when two men entered and demanded the contents of the cash register. He resisted, so they shot him, took the money, and fled. They were never caught. Considering the gravity of his condition the night before, he was alert and seemed remarkably fit. He continued to do well, developed no infection despite the less-than-routine preparation, and was discharged a few days later. For years I received a Christmas card from him.

The heart has held a dominant position throughout human history as one of life's ongoing metaphors. Perhaps uniquely among the principal components of the body, it engenders a variety of basic emotions. Poetry, literature, and the arts extol its perceived responsibility as a vital force, the site of spirituality, and a mystical place where noble sentiments are retained. Entire lexicons have been built around it, tinged with the most intense feelings: *heartache, heartbroken, heartfelt, bleeding heart, tenderhearted, heartless, heartsick, heart of a lion.* Its emotional reputation endures. As I write this, Valentine's Day looms. This is a pleasant, sentimental, and cardiocentric occasion, but difficult to separate from the associated naked commercialism.

The organ also symbolizes the traits and character of personhood. Long considered the seat of the soul, the heart was also considered by Hippocrates and Aristotle to be the center of intelligence. If violated, life was over. But evidence contradictory to this accepted dogma kept emerging. Galen noted in practical terms that gladiators often maintained their mental faculties during the hours they endured an ultimately fatal heart wound.[1] Members of learned societies of the late sixteenth century were shaken when Ambroïse Paré described a man whose heart had been penetrated in a duel but still managed to chase his adversary 230 yards before collapsing.[2] After identifying myocardial scars in subjects who had been hanged, the seventeenth-century anatomist Barthelemy Cabral conjectured that an injured heart could heal itself.[3] It was also reputed to act differently than other organs after death, a bit of lore passing even into modern times. Sushruta in ancient India was the first of many to suggest that hearts from individuals dying from poison did not burn in a funeral pyre. Legend also has it that when the body of the drowned poet Percy Bysshe Shelley was cremated on a beach in Italy in 1822, his friend, E. J. Trelawney, plucked the undamaged structure from the ashes and presented it to his wife.[4] The mythic status of the organ occasionally caused it to be buried separately from or entombed more visibly than the remainder of the body of a hero, king, or important personage. This tradition continues. For example, the heart of the revered priest Brother André, who died after World War II, currently lies in its own box near his coffin in a large basilica in Montreal.

The moment the heart stopped was traditionally considered synonymous with the end of life, a mystery permeating the collective psyches of individuals, cultures, and religions. Primitive societies considered death a kind of deep sleep, an inexplicable transformation from one state to another. Religions evoked the possibilities of an afterlife, assuaging and tempering associated fears and superstitions with ritual and ceremony. Forms and customs of burial, different in each age and society, ensured respect for the deceased before he or she was returned to the earth to lie forever beyond the ken of family, admirers, and colleagues. We still gather at funerals to mourn and remember a deceased friend or relative.

Understanding the physical transformation from life to death was problematic in earlier times, and, in some ways, it remains so today. An underlying and generally irrational terror of being buried alive arose in the Middle Ages and peaked in eighteenth-century Europe, as exemplified in an array of stories and poems. Corpses were reported to have awakened during their funerals or even after burial. Rumors of scratch marks found inside the lids of coffins after the body was exhumed fueled speculation. Morgue attendants sometimes attached a bell to a post near the grave, tying a connecting string to the finger of the deceased in case he should awaken. The "death watch" became important, a ceremony at which a group of people gathered around the bed watching as life ebbed and agreeing finally that the person had breathed his last and that all cardiac activity had ceased. More doctrinaire medical pundits considered putrefaction to be the ultimate determinant. Definition of the event became considerably more objective, however, when René-Théophile-Hyacinthe Laennec invented the stethoscope in 1819 in Paris. The early prototypes were hollow tubes of wood or metal that the listener could interpose between his ear and the skin of the patient. This important diagnostic tool magnified sounds of heart and lung and relieved the examining physician from the occasionally embarrassing maneuver of placing his ear directly on the patient's chest. An obvious corollary to such an advance was the ability to determine when all internal activity had ceased. Death could then be declared.

Certainty about the end of life became less obvious, however, as technology emerged that could support, delay, or even reverse impending death. While various breathing devices had been tried in prior centuries, and mouth-to-mouth resuscitation occasionally attempted, the mechanical support of respiration by a machine did not become reality until the

1930s when physiologists in the United States and Denmark designed the "iron lung" to breathe for paralyzed polio victims. Applying the principle of intermittent external negative pressure to cause the chest wall to rise and the lungs to fill, this unwieldy apparatus saved many lives. With ongoing ventilation mediating oxygenation of the blood and tissues, the heart continued to beat. As effective as they were, however, the ponderous iron lungs became obsolete two decades later during another polio epidemic when respirators were introduced that transmitted positive pressure directly to the lungs via a tube placed in the windpipe. An adjunctive device appeared in 1962 that could stimulate an arrested heart to beat or correct a fatal rhythm abnormality with appropriately timed electric shocks. Thus, it became increasingly clear that life was not over if the heart and lungs could be supported artificially. Only with the introduction of the concept of brain death toward the end of the 1960s was the boundary of the end of life established. The heart was not necessarily the factor limiting existence; irreversible cessation of brain activity was the final common denominator. We shall see how the advent of organ transplantation stimulated this philosophical change in attitude.

The enduring emotional and spiritual overlay associated with the heart, its rather startling motion, and its storied relationship with death did much to discourage scientists and practitioners from studying its behavior directly. Indeed, it was anathema for surgeons to touch it, as the disturbing prospect of interfering with the only organ in the body that so exuberantly moves was thought to have inevitably fatal consequences. Not only did they accept that its manipulation or repair was beyond their ability, but they believed that such a departure was ethically unacceptable. As late as the end of the nineteenth century, no less a formidable surgeon than Theodor Billroth stated dogmatically that no one might "deserve the respect of his colleagues if he would even attempt to suture a heart wound." His opinion was probably based both on the heart's symbolic reputation and on practical fear of doing harm.[5] Stephen Paget, a renowned British surgeon and author of a major 1896 textbook on surgery of the chest, noted more pragmatically that operations on the heart have "probably reached the limits set by Nature; no new method, no new discovery, can overcome the natural difficulties that attend a wound of the heart."[6] These sentiments were to change little for half a century.

Even during the early years of my residency in the 1960s, an operation on the adult heart remained a relative novelty despite efforts by a handful of surgeons in academic departments to develop the subject, first in dogs and then in occasional patients. The specialty of cardiology was in its infancy, and anatomical and functional details of the diseased heart sparse. Digitalis was the only effective drug available. Cardiac catheterization was just appearing. Pump oxygenators were rudimentary. Surgical attempts to correct advanced heart disease were generally unsuccessful and often led to death. Although we residents occasionally sympathized with Billroth and Paget when assisting on seemingly endless and futile cases, the thrill of exposing a beating human heart and the challenge of trying to repair its defects were an exciting part of our training process. I still find the sight captivating.

My experience with Tommy O'Rourke emphasized to me that the heart is a mechanical pump and that surgeons can repair or improve many of its abnormalities in a mechanical way. With this in mind, it might be well to describe its anatomy and central role in the circulation of the blood. The fist-sized organ lies in the middle of the chest, the center of the four great vessels that enter and leave it. It consists of two parallel pumps joined together by a common wall, each with two chambers, an atrium sitting above a ventricle. The movement of the chambers is exquisitely choreographed to drive the circulation forward. One-way valves prevent backflow. Both atria contract together to deliver their load of blood into their respective ventricles that dilate at the same instant to receive it. These, in turn, expel the contents into the exit vessels just as the dilating atria receive blood for the next cycle. The synchronous contraction of the atria followed immediately by the ventricular contractions produces the "lub-dub" sound of each heartbeat that one hears while listening through a stethoscope.

The two pumps regulate two separate but connected circulations, the systemic and the pulmonary. The left ventricle, the largest and most muscular chamber, governs the systemic circulation, contracting powerfully to force its contents of oxygenated red blood into the aorta under high pressure. Like the limbs and twigs of a tree, branches of this large, thick-walled, elastic vessel divide and subdivide into arterial channels of ever-diminishing size that supply all bodily organs and tissues. The tiniest tributaries form capillaries, minute and delicate tubes that lie between individual cells or clumps of cells. Oxygen carried and then released by the red blood cells traverses the capillary wall to supply energy to the surrounding tissues. At the same time carbon dioxide and other waste products move from the tissues into the blood, turning it blue.

The venous system is like another tree superimposed upon the first. The small veins arising from the capillaries coalesce into larger and larger vessels that drain all bodily structures. These have thinner walls than the arteries because the blood within them flows under low pressure. As we noted in the discussion of varicose veins, valves positioned intermittently along each vein keep the column of blood moving centrally and prevent pooling. The largest venous channels, the superior and inferior vena cavae, drain the upper and lower portions of the body, respectively. They may be as large as two inches in diameter where they join together to empty their contents into the right side of the heart.

This latter pump controls the low-pressure pulmonary circulation. The right atrium pushes the effluent from the vena cavae into the dilating right ventricle, which contracts in turn to force the blood through the pulmonary artery and its branches into the lungs. The end vessels form capillaries that lie directly next to thousands of minute air sacs. The thin walls between these structures allow efficient transfer of oxygen from inhaled air in the sacs to the red cells and carbon dioxide from the blood to the sacs to be breathed out, patterns opposite to what happens in the systemic circulation. The oxygenated red blood is directed into the arterial system via pulmonary veins of ever-increasing size that empty into the left atrium. The names are confusing: the pulmonary artery is the only artery in the body that carries venous blood, and the pulmonary vein is the only vein carrying arterial blood.

Surgical investigators were increasingly attracted to the possibilities of treating mechanical abnormalities of the cardiac chambers, valves, and great vessels. Three separate problems associated with these structures demanded operative solutions: the repair of direct injury to the organ, correction of congenital anomalies, and treatment of diseases of the adult heart. I will review each development in turn.

As discussed, war inevitably gives impetus to surgical innovations. Relief of conditions affecting the pericardium, which encloses the beating heart, came first. In March 1810, during the Napoleonic Wars, Baron Larrey encountered a situation which made him aware that blood under pressure from a heart wound could fill this unyielding covering and compress normal dilation of the chambers within.[7] A 30-year-old soldier in the Imperial Guard had stabbed himself. He was rushed to the hospital in shock, blood flowing from the site. Doctors applied tight dressings to stop the bleeding. After six weeks, however, it was apparent that pressure from fluid accumulating in the pericardial space from the dissolving clot constricted both muscular activity of the heart and the great vessels carrying blood in and out of it. Without anesthesia, Larrey opened the pericardium and removed a liter of old clot and serum. The organ immediately regained full function. Unfortunately, the soldier died three weeks later of sepsis. The message, however, was clear.

Seventeenth-century practitioners had first realized that a related pericardial condition, chronic constrictive pericarditis, could follow trauma, tuberculosis, and other infections. Three centuries later, patients also developed the disorder following radiation of the chest, a newly introduced, popular, and sometimes unwarranted treatment applied to a variety of disease states. Like pericardial fluid under pressure, the ensuing thickening, scarring, and contracture of the membrane selectively narrowed the chambers of the right side of the heart in particular, compromising the normal low-pressure flow of venous blood entering them. As a result, the left side received inadequate amounts of blood to pump through the arteries. Because of increased venous pressure, fluid built up in the legs, liver, and abdominal cavity. After prolonged misery and without surgical relief, patients died. Although German surgeons removed the scarred and tight covering successfully in a number of afflicted individuals before World War I, the treatment never achieved general popularity until the 1930s, when operations on the chest became increasingly common. It is now performed routinely on those who require it.

Occasional early attempts to repair wounds penetrating the heart muscle were also reported. In 1896, despite Billroth's imprecations, a German surgeon anesthetized a 21-year-old patient with chloroform and successfully closed a stab wound of the ventricle, a feat that may have been based upon the experimental reports of European physiologists who had sewn shut cardiac lacerations in rabbits and a dog. That the muscle would hold stitches was a revelation. Soon afterward, and with the help of Dr. Roentgen's novel X-ray, a Frenchman located and removed a bullet adhering to the surface of the heart of a young officer.[8] The prospects of operative manipulation of organs within the chest improved during the opening decades of the twentieth century. Antisepsis, anesthesia, appreciation of Halsted's principles of careful and gentle dissection, and external means to inflate the collapsed lung all contributed to greater success. Surgeons became increasingly adept at dividing ribs and removing portions of lung tissue destroyed by tuberculosis. Some of their dissections came close to the heart itself. French and British surgeons had occasionally excised bullets near the hearts of the wounded in World War I, but there was little general interest in studying the heart.[9] Not long thereafter, however, the work of one surgeon during World War II kindled a spark about the subject that became a flame.

After a residency in Boston in the early 1940s, Dwight Harken took additional training in London with one of the foremost thoracic surgeons of the time. While learning the newest techniques of lung and esophageal surgery, he became intrigued by the still-remote possibilities of operating on the human heart. Upon his return to Boston he designed techniques to explore the mitral valves of dogs via the left atrium, experiments of potential applicability to human patients. With infections of the heart valves being relatively common and inevitably fatal in that preantibiotic era, his idea was to scrape off bacterial residue and vegetations before the process destroyed them.

Harken left his investigations unfinished when the United States entered the war. He soon joined the military and was posted to an English army hospital to care for patients who had sustained severe combat injuries. With his expertise in chest surgery, he was faced with wounded soldiers with bullets and other bits of shrapnel lying in and around their hearts and great vessels. He set to work, operating on 134 of them without a fatality.[10] Thirteen of the procedures involved entering the cardiac chambers, using methods he had perfected in animals. His first patient had been badly injured during the D-day landings. An X-ray showed a metallic foreign body lodged in the heart itself. On opening the chest and pericardium, Harken discovered that it lay within the right ventricle. He described the subsequent events in a letter to his wife.[11]

> For a moment, I stood with my clamp on the fragment that was inside the heart, and the heart was not bleeding. Then suddenly, with a pop as if a champagne cork had been drawn, the fragment jumped out of the ventricle, forced by the pressure within the chamber. Blood poured out in a torrent. I put my fingers over the awful leak. The torrent slowed, stopped. I took large needles swedged with silk and passed them through the heart muscle wall, under my finger, and out the other side. With four of these in, I slowly removed my finger as we tied one after the other. Blood pressure did drop, but the only moment of panic was when we discovered that one suture had gone through my glove. I was sutured to the wall of the heart! We cut the glove and I got loose.

The soldier recovered. But many of Harken's cases were not that simple. A spectator described another. "The missile [had been] pinpointed by fluoroscopy. At operation, the patient was induced with intravenous anesthesia, intubated [with a tube in his windpipe] and maintained with anesthetic gas. To remove the missile the heart was split wide open with tremendous blood loss. Massive, rapid blood transfusions, used relatively infrequently at that time, were needed to keep the patient alive. Penicillin, which was just beginning to make an impact, was administered." Again, the soldier narrowly survived. Because of Harken's unprecedented pioneering success with this unique clinical series, many people were saved, including, years later, Tommy O'Rourke.

The operative approach to simple lacerations of the heart muscle has changed little since the initial attempts at salvage. Yet over recent decades the availability of highly equipped and staffed emergency facilities has allowed ever more routine interventions for complex and immediately life-threatening situations. Patients are transferred quickly from the ambulance with blood and fluids already running into their veins. Needle or tube drainage of chest cavities or the filled pericardium may buy some time. Transfer to the operating room occurs promptly. If the cardiac injury is immediately life threatening, such as the rupture of a chamber or disruption of the common wall between the right and left side of the heart, rapid initiation of heart-lung bypass may be lifesaving. The use of pericardial or synthetic patch grafts to repair large defects in the ventricular muscle has proven relatively effective. If there is time, ultrasound or even cardiac catheterization can be carried out to detect unappreciated abnormalities. Such aggressive diagnostic and therapeutic options have increasingly found a place in our modern urban environment, where the bullet as an instrument of violence has replaced the knife blade. Unfortunately, the tissue devastation and destruction associated with ever more sophisticated and available weaponry such as the automatic pistol, the attack rifle, and the hollow-nosed bullet have not improved the possibilities of salvage.

The surgical treatment of congenital anomalies of the heart and its great vessels was a coincident early advance. But such operations would never have evolved until surgeons developed the ability to sew arteries and veins together in such a way as to retain both their diameter and to prevent clots from forming at the site. A political tragedy in 1894 triggered the innovation. France was in political turmoil, with bombings, riots, and confrontations occurring between police and workers angry at inadequate living conditions, poverty, and social inequality. Despite the disorder, the still-popular president, Sadi Carnot, traveled throughout the country.[12] During a visit to the city of Lyon, an enthusiastic crowd surrounded his open carriage. A young baker's assistant turned anarchist, Santo Caserio, pushed to the front of the throng and stabbed him in the abdomen. Carnot bled massively and later died despite strenuous attempts at control. The knife had divided the great vein entering his liver. Although expeditious control of the severed portal vein might have saved the president, operative expertise was lacking. Indeed, during previous attempts to reconstruct injured vessels in patients, surgeons either could not control the bleeding or clotting occurred in the inadequately repaired or narrowed segment.

The death of the president stimulated a young surgeon at a nearby hospital, Alexis Carrel, to consider the problem. In preparation, he took sewing lessons from Mme. Laroudier, an experienced seamstress in the city, using silk thread. (Lyon was then the capital of the thriving silk-worm industry.) He perfected his technique in animals, separating the edges of the vessels to ensure perfect visualization. He learned to place the fine, oiled stitches threaded on sharp, straight milliner's needles, presenting as little suture material as possible on the smooth internal lining to prevent clot formation. Vascular and cardiac surgeons use Carrel's methods to this day.

Nearly half a century later, three relative strangers living far apart from each other used the techniques to open an entirely new field. Their success in introducing a novel surgical treatment for cardiovascular defects in infants and children illustrates a theme that recurs with uncanny regularity in medicine and science: research workers unknown to each other and often separated by great distances may arrive at advances and discoveries virtually simultaneously. The first of these researchers was Robert Gross of Boston, who transformed a young invalid to complete physiological normalcy by successfully occluding her patent ductus arteriosus, a relatively common congenital cardiovascular anomaly diagnosed in the days after birth.[13] Gross had trained in both surgery and pathology at the Brigham and at the adjacent Children's Hospital, performing a series of autopsies on infants and children who had died with a variety of such disorders. He became convinced that operative correction might be possible for many of them. Abnormalities of the great vessels entering and leaving the tiny hearts intrigued him.

A persistently open, or patent, ductus arteriosus is one such aberration. Because oxygen and nutrients from the pregnant mother must supply the needs of the developing baby via the placental circulation, a vascular connection between the pulmonary artery and upper aorta develops during fetal life to allow blood to bypass the nonfunctioning lungs. This shunt, the ductus, normally scars down to a fibrous band four to ten days after birth when the child begins to breathe, the lungs inflate, and venous blood flows through them in a normal fashion. If closure fails and the connection remains open, however, complications occur. With some of the aortic blood that is supposed to supply bodily tissues diverted into the lungs under high pressure through the intact channel, the heart enlarges to compensate for the excess demands placed upon it. Circulatory failure may ensue, and physical growth may be retarded. The walls of the ductus may become infected. Aneurysms may form, with the threat of rupture, thrombosis, or embolism. Uncorrected, the condition may ultimately be fatal.

Gross studied the anatomy of the heart and great vessels and their relationship to important surrounding structures in anesthetized dogs. Having become comfortable with dissecting and isolating the individual components, he worked out a precise approach to close an open ductus. Finally feeling ready, he prepared to operate on a child with the condition in August 1938. He was the chief surgical resident at Children's Hospital. The patient was a seven-and-a-half-year-old girl with progressive loss of energy and increasing fatigue. She was sallow and obviously ill. Those examining her could feel an intense vibration coming from within her chest. Her heart was enlarged on X-ray. With the goal of reducing cardiac work and preventing subsequent bacterial infection of the abnormally functioning vascular connection, Gross elected to go ahead as the diagnosis seemed clear.[14] A nurse anesthetist gave ether by mask. The young surgeon opened her chest, carefully freed the abnormal connection from surrounding tissues, and tied it off with a stout piece of silk thread. The bounding pulmonary artery that had been receiving abnormal amounts of aortic blood under high pressure throughout the child's life quieted. She withstood the operative procedure well and went home in seven days, cured. He described the events in graphic detail in his operative note, a departure from his usually brief reports.

> Palpating finger placed on the heart disclosed an astonishing coarse and very strong thrill [vibration] which was felt over the entire cardiac musculature. When the stethoscope

was placed on the pulmonic artery there was almost a deafening continuous sound like a rushing stream. When the
ductus was obliterated all of these murmurs disappeared.
The clamp was taken off and the ductus was ligated with
a single silk [strand]. After this tie had been put in place it
seemed as if everything was still in the operating field. All
of this buzzing [was gone].[15]

Gross nearly lost his position of chief resident by performing the operation. He had suggested to his departmental chair the possibility of treating such a patient several weeks before. The professor forbade him to
consider such a thing, dogmatically noting that operating in the chests of
children was not done and that surgery around the heart or great vessels
was inevitably fatal. Undeterred, the young surgeon waited until his chief
had boarded a ship to Europe, then admitted two young patients with
the condition—two, in case one died. Upon the professor's return, despite
the obvious success of the operation, he was so furious that he fired Gross.
Others on the staff who understood the usual outcome for such children
and were impressed and elated with Gross's cure implored the departmental chair to bring his resident back. Finally, he relented and allowed
Gross to complete his training.

Emboldened by the initial result, Gross performed the operation on a
series of patients. Thirteen of them did well. The fourteenth was a girl
who thrived initially but collapsed two weeks later during a party at her
house. The ligature had cut through the fragile shunt, producing massive
and fatal hemorrhage. Indeed, Gross's concern about such a possibility
had caused him to test a variety of materials to tie off the ductus in
animals, including thick silk, cotton tape, and a technique of wrapping the
occluded portion with cellophane to increase local scarring and contracture of the vessel.[16] To prevent a further disaster, he devised an occlusive
clamp that did not crush or cut the thin wall of the dilated conduit,
divided the clamped channel, and closed the ends meticulously with silk
sutures. His operation continues to save the lives of many children around
the world, although during the past few years medications have become
available to accelerate closure of the ductus in some affected newborns.

Few others had considered the possibilities of mechanical closure before Gross's first attempt. The only prior attempt had resulted in the death of the patient. Gross's initial case dramatically changed long-held surgical opinions about manipulation of the heart and great vessels. These opinions had limited treatment to occasional repair of stab wounds, relief of constriction of the pericardial sac, and rare attempts to open partially closed mitral valves. Indeed, the success of the procedure injected reality into the long-standing debate about the possibilities of operative approaches to the organ and stimulated the formation of surgical laboratories in North America and Europe to pursue related studies. It was a watershed event.

The young surgeon and a handful of investigators with similar interests began to broaden their researches on the correction of other congenital defects during the 1940s. Treatment of another important developmental anomaly, coarctation of the aorta, was particularly challenging. Babies with this condition are born with a localized constriction of the upper segment of that great vessel at or near the origin of the ductus that prevents normal flow of arterial blood downward. Hypertension of the upper part of the body may produce hemorrhage into the brain and cardiac failure. The blood pressure in the legs, in contrast, is abnormally low. Although some patients may live normally if the narrowing is not too severe, the complications of aneurysm, rupture, and infection may be fatal even in adult life. First alone and then in collaboration with Charles Hufnagel, a resident working in the surgical laboratory, Gross perfected nonslip vascular clamps to block the thoracic aorta of anesthetized dogs without crushing its wall. With blood flow controlled above and below the affected segment, the investigators could then divide the vessel and restore continuity with fine silk on small needles, as Carrel had done decades before. Testing several types of suturing techniques in the animal subjects, they ultimately arrived at one that they could employ routinely without compromising the artery. Gross carried out his first clinical repair in the summer of 1945 but did not publish the results until several years later. Indeed, he mentioned his initial two patients only in an addendum to a paper in which he described the earlier canine experiments.[17] The first child died shortly following removal of the clamps, possibly because of a sudden release of metabolic wastes into the circulation. These had built up in the tissues that were deprived of oxygen during the period of arterial occlusion. On his second attempt the following week, he removed the clamps slowly. This child and subsequent children did well.

Although Gross was unaware of their efforts, others were also working to correct the anomaly. Clarence Crafoord was an experienced professor of thoracic surgery in Stockholm and the first to sew the ductus shut instead of ligating it. He performed his initial repair of an aortic coarctation in October 1944 and his second twelve days later, publishing the results about the same time Gross's paper appeared.[18] But despite these early successes, unanswered questions remained. A potentially frightening difficulty that researchers faced was the high incidence of paralysis of the hind legs of dogs following an aortic operation. How could surgeons transfer their experimental findings to children if this complication loomed as a possibility? The answer soon became clear. Clamping the aorta acutely interrupted the circulation to the lower part of the spinal cord of the normal animals. During the hour or so it took to repair the divided vessel, nerve cells to the legs, deprived of their normal blood supply, were injured or lost. In the affected children, in contrast, the aortic constriction had been present throughout their lives, with long-established collateral channels providing adequate circulation to keep the spinal cord and other tissues intact. Transient obstruction of the already narrowed artery during its reconstruction caused little change because the accessory channels continued to supply blood. No child developed leg weakness after surgery.

Another unanswered question was how the surgeon could bridge the aortic gap left after he had removed a long coarctation. Synthetic grafts did not exist, although older investigators, including Carrel, had interposed tubes of glass, gold, or paraffin-lined silver as vascular substitutes that would not form clots. Other researchers were examining the use of sections of vena cava from the animal itself or from members of the same or different species, using metal cuffs to connect graft to artery. While sometimes feasible in experimental models, such arrangements, although of appropriate size for children, would constrict the vessels as the child grew. Aware that Carrel had transplanted fresh pieces of aorta between dogs before World War I, Gross and Hufnagel began to investigate means to preserve vascular segments for later use. They examined

the effectiveness of quick-freezing the grafts.[19] Radiation, a technology
that was becoming increasingly common in the 1950s, seemed promising. Emboldened by their experiments, Gross implanted lengths of stored
human arteries into children with extensive coarctations. In important
experiments, Hufnagel was also designing a plastic prosthesis to replace
arterial defects in dogs.[20] Other surgeons were attempting to bridge arterial defects in adults with similar material from cadavers; some of them
saved the legs of wounded soldiers with such grafts during the Korean
War. But even with the early successes both in children and in adults, it
became apparent that later constriction or aneurysm formation reached
unacceptable levels. Within a few years bioengineers had developed
prosthetic grafts from the newly emerging synthetic materials to replace
abdominal aortic aneurysms and other diseased vessels. Such improved
products have become standard in modern vascular operations.

Another surgeon-scientist was pursuing similar investigations but using
quite different strategies. Alfred Blalock moved from Vanderbilt University
in 1941 to become chair of the Department of Surgery at Johns Hopkins.
One of the projects he and his longtime laboratory technician, Vivien
Thomas, initiated was a means to treat coarctation of the aorta. Unaware
of the events unfolding in Stockholm and in Boston, they conceptualized a
less direct approach.[21] To devise a model in dogs that resembled the clinical condition, they divided the aorta at the appropriate site in the chest
and sutured the ends shut. They then isolated the subclavian artery, a large
vessel arising at the aortic arch that supplies one of the upper extremities.
They swung this vessel down and bypassed the interruption by joining
its end to the lower segment of aorta. Existing accessory channels were
adequate to nourish the foreleg of the dog, and by extension, the arm of a
child. The success of this technique, at least in animals, stimulated Blalock's
enduring interest in repair of cardiovascular anomalies in children.

Because of the burgeoning clinical and administrative commitments
of the new surgical chief, he increasingly assigned research projects to
his assistant who, in turn, devised appropriate models in dogs for the
actual experiments. Together they investigated shock, crush injuries,
adrenal function, treatment of coarctation, and correction of other cardiac

abnormalities. Thomas invented instruments, originated new techniques, and perfected old ones. He became a master surgeon, particularly expert in joining small vessels together. It may be that without his efforts and innovations, many of Blalock's substantial contributions might never have occurred. Vivien Thomas, an African American, worked at a time when and in places where members of his race were not generally welcomed or accepted.[22] Toward the end of Thomas's career, the faculty and administrators at Johns Hopkins publicly recognized his talents and contributions by commissioning his portrait to hang next to that of Blalock in an entrance hall of the medical school. They also awarded him an honorary degree. Both honors were fitting tributes to a remarkable individual.

Blalock's interests led to an important collaboration with Helen Taussig, a fellow faculty member and an authority on congenital heart disease. Prominent among her patients were a group of "blue babies" with an untreatable and ultimately fatal condition called *tetralogy of Fallot*. She was well aware that this and other abnormalities of the infant heart occur during the period of rapid change and growth in the first six weeks of fetal life. During that interval the vascular analogue of the developing heart, initially a single hollow tube, doubles back on itself and fuses together to produce two separate but parallel beating units, each with two chambers. The organ is complete by the end of the second month of pregnancy. The anatomy of the tetralogy is complex. As the name implies, it has four features: the wall separating the two ventricles never fully forms, leaving a hole; the pulmonary artery is constricted; the normally thin-walled right ventricle thickens from pushing blood under high pressure through both the narrowed pulmonary artery leaving it and into the left ventricle via the defect in its wall; the aorta overrides both ventricles and carries a mixture of oxygenated and nonoxygenated blood to the body when the lungs expand after birth. As the tissues never receive adequate oxygen, the children look blue, not pink as they would if they received fully oxygenated blood. Hence the term "blue babies." They fatigue easily and assume a characteristic squatting position to catch their breath after minimal exertion. They often die in their teens. Indeed, in contrast to children with an open ductus or coarctation who may look relatively healthy, these children live compromised and shortened lives.

Following an initial meeting with Taussig, Blalock asked Thomas to create a canine model that would resemble the clinical manifestations of tetralogy of Fallot as closely as possible. This assignment was not easy, as he first had to conceptualize how to make a dog "blue." After studying Taussig's extensive collection of preserved congenitally defective hearts to understand the abnormalities, he addressed the major species differences in anatomy between humans and dogs. In humans, membranes in the center of the chest separate the two thoracic cavities, fixing the heart, great vessels, trachea, and esophagus in relatively firm position. If one side is opened, the lung collapses. As we noted with Tommy O'Rourke, the other lung remains inflated and continues to function. In the dog, in contrast, these supporting tissues are delicate and connect the cavities. If the chest is opened, both lungs collapse. To keep at least one canine lung functioning, Thomas had to create a breathing tube that he could pass into the canine trachea and join to the anesthesia machine. The tube had to fit tightly against its wall to prevent back leakage of air and anesthetic as the lungs were inflated. Unfortunately, few such apparatuses were available either for laboratory or clinical use. He solved the problem by placing a balloon circumferentially near the tip of the tube. When blown up, it filled the space between tube and tracheal wall, allowing air and anesthetic gas to enter and exit the lungs in a controlled fashion. He first made the tubes of polished brass, then rubber, and eventually plastic.

Blalock and Thomas tried a variety of operative techniques to create a relevant canine model of a blue baby, finally settling on removing a large portion of one lung and bypassing an additional segment by creating a fistula between a branch of the pulmonary artery and its vein. With this arrangement, a significant portion of circulating blood never received oxygen. With appropriate amounts of lung removed and made nonfunctional, dogs survived but became blue with activity. The next question was how to treat the condition they had produced. The objective was to oxygenate the blue venous blood by redirecting it into the lungs. The red blood could then travel normally from the left side of the heart into the arteries throughout the body.

Taussig provided an interesting clue to her surgical colleagues by recounting her experience with several babies who had been born with severe narrowing of their pulmonary artery. They were pink and healthy-looking immediately after birth because the open ductus arteriosus directed circulation from aorta to pulmonary artery beyond its congenital constriction, allowing the blood to traverse the lungs and gain oxygen. They became blue, however, after the channel closed normally and the blood flow across it ceased. This observation intrigued the investigators. To create an artificial ductus, they modified their approach in the coarctation model by isolating the subclavian artery and joining its end to the side of the pulmonary artery. Bringing deoxygenated blood into the lungs worked well. The dogs looked and acted normally. But it took much time, ingenuity, and effort to perfect techniques to sew the two small vessels together. The surgeons needed fine needles attached to sutures as thin as horsehair. They had to devise vascular instruments to fit into tight places. Vivien Thomas was responsible for many of the innovations.

Toward the end of November 1944, Blalock announced that he was ready to try the experimental strategy on a blue baby, although he had never actually performed the operation either on an animal or on a human. He insisted that his laboratory assistant stand directly behind him during surgery to advise and monitor his every move. As nothing comparable then existed for patients, Thomas brought his special animal instruments and sutures from the laboratory to the hospital operating rooms for sterilization and packaging. The few disparaging remarks about the presence of a black man were quickly quelled as the procedure began. Blalock, the anesthesiologist, a senior resident, the intern, and the scrub nurse comprised the team. The field was limited. The patient, Eileen, who weighed nine pounds–the size of a cat–could hardly be seen beneath the cloth drapes. An especially small tube was placed in her trachea for anesthesia and oxygen. Blalock opened the left side of the tiny chest and packed the lung into a corner. He then gingerly isolated the pulmonary artery and placed a tape around it. He next dissected the subclavian artery free along its length, clamped its origin, tied the other end, and divided it. The vessels were minute, about half the size of those in the dogs. With Thomas coaching, he made a small incision in the clamped portion of the pulmonary artery and slowly sewed the open end of the subclavian to it. Clamps were removed. There was no bleeding.

Those involved remembered the event well. The first assistant excit-
edly described "the color of the blood after we made the incision; it looked
like purple molasses, this thick, black blood [oozing] from many small
vessels. Vessels in the [tissues around the heart] looked like a bag of black
dilated worms. After completion of the vascular procedure and removal
of the clamps, the anesthesiologist shouted: 'Take a look! Take a look!' Dr.
Blalock and I leaned over the ether screen and looked at the child's face
and saw the cherry red color of her lips. We were all beside ourselves
with joy."[23] Similar successes transformed two older children to glowing
health.[24] The press picked up on Blalock and Taussig's published report of
the three patients and soon disseminated the news throughout the world.
Parents with blue babies from the United States and abroad descended
on Hopkins. The surgical team carried the load, perfecting techniques,
streamlining operating-room logistics, and improving lighting and equipment as they gained experience. Outside doctors arrived to observe and
learn, and then opened units in other cities and other countries.

It should be noted, however, that Blalock's operation was not a cure
for tetralogy but a stopgap measure. While some of the treated patients
lived normally for a long time, others had to have the tiny vascular junc-
ture enlarged as they grew. Some died after a few years. We should also
remember that on occasion the surgeons discovered during the procedure
itself that the diagnosis was incorrect; indispensable tools such as cardiac
catheterization, angiography, scans, and ultrasounds did not exist, and
chest X-rays could only provide a rough idea of the nature of the problem. In addition, intensive-care units and monitoring devices would not
become available for nearly two decades, and cardiopulmonary bypass
for more definitive repair would not become routine for a quarter-century.

The work of these and other early clinical investigators during the
1940s brightened the dreary futures of those with congenital anomalies
of the heart. Gross and Blalock, both deservedly famous in their field,
had quite different personalities. Each was technically superb, a master of
anatomy and physiology, and able to operate on tiny structures in obscure
places. Both were effective chairs of their respective departments, dedicated to the education of their residents. Each acquired a coterie of loyal
and enthusiastic disciples, who in turn contributed much to the field.

Imaginative and responsible for the surgical treatment of a broad spectrum of congenital anomalies, Gross was a complex figure whose apparent distance and aloofness in the hospital covered much personal humility and compassion. Blalock confined his scientific interests primarily to the cardiovascular system. Gregarious, socially active among the well-heeled of Baltimore, he was a revered and popular figure.

Interest on the part of surgeons toward operations on the adult heart lay relatively fallow during much of the first half of the twentieth century despite slowly accumulating clinical anecdotes concerning actual repair of injured ventricular muscle: fifty-six such cases had been reported by 1904, with 40 percent of the patients having recovered.[25] In addition, a few prescient investigators were examining the effects of disrupting structures within the canine organ itself. In 1872 a German ophthalmologist ruptured the aortic valve of dogs to study the increased pulsations of the vessels in their eyes.[26] Others copied his techniques by introducing a tiny knife blade on a long stem or a whalebone rod down the major artery or adjacent vein in the neck of the animals to assess the physical effects of disruption of valves in the left and right sides of the heart, respectively. Cushing was one of the first to operate on the hearts of dogs in his surgical laboratory at Johns Hopkins, publishing his results in 1908.[27] Besides learning to manipulate the beating heart and suture its muscular walls, he created abnormalities of the valves. Not only did many of the animals survive, but physical examination of the subjects familiarized the medical students with comparable valve defects in patients.

The time appeared right for the elective treatment of abnormalities within the adult heart. Medical knowledge of these abnormalities had increased with Cushing's novel laboratory experiments and teaching aids, and there had been occasional clinical successes. Increasing numbers of individuals with potentially correctable heart problems sought relief. Surgeons could now repair accidental cardiac wounds; electively treating abnormalities seemed the logical next step.

Rheumatic heart disease was common in the years before antibiotics, with many persons who had experienced a streptococcal infection or scarlet fever as children later developing the condition. The body makes antibodies against the bacteria during the initial phases of the infection, a natural mechanism of defense. These antibodies, however, not only kill the infectious agent but years later may react against specific body tissues, particularly the mitral and aortic valves. Correction of disease of the mitral valve, lying at the junction of the left atrium and left ventricle, was the first challenge. This valve consists of two leaflets. Normally, these flatten against the chamber wall as the contracting atrium pushes its load of blood into the dilated left ventricle, then snap shut to prevent backflow as the ventricle contracts in turn to eject its blood into the aorta. With fusion, thickening, or calcification of the affected leaflets narrowing the valve orifice from its usual one- to two-square-inch size, the volume of blood flowing through the compromised aperture is significantly diminished. Conversely, if the valve becomes incompetent because the leaflets are destroyed and cannot close, blood flows forward normally when the atrium contracts but rushes back when it dilates. In both situations–the first, mitral stenosis; the second, mitral insufficiency–circulating blood backs up into the lungs, and fluid leaks through the engorged capillaries and fills the air sacs. The patients go into congestive heart failure and cannot breathe, essentially drowning in their own secretions. Individuals with narrowed valves might be improved by surgery, although nothing could be offered to those with incompetent valves until the advent of the heart-lung machine.

We saw so many patients with mitral stenosis during my residency that we could often make the diagnosis from across the room. Most were women in their thirties or forties, invariably thin as the overworked heart used much available energy just to circulate the blood effectively. Often unable to lie flat, they had to sit up to breathe because of lung congestion. Some had suffered strokes. Their lives were miserable, with death a continuing specter. Treatment options were limited. Over the short term we were able to control excess fluid by removing blood, strengthening cardiac function with digitalis, or stimulating the kidneys with diuretics to excrete more urine. The only surgical answer to this purely mechanical problem was to open the stenotic valves. The risks were great.

The ever-present possibility of an arterial embolus posed an additional hazard. Because the left atrium had to force its contents through a narrow mitral valve under pressure, the thin-walled chamber enlarged substantially in size and volume. The heart rhythm often became irregular as the attenuated muscle lost its normal intrinsic beat and moved asynchronously and in a disorganized fashion at multiple sites. As a result, blood pooled and clots formed in the dilated space. Pieces of these occasionally broke off and migrated into the arterial tree to block flow in various parts of the body. If an embolus lodged in the brain, a patient would develop a stroke, often a tragic and irreconcilable problem. More commonly, such individuals suddenly experienced a blue, cold, and numb leg. This situation was a surgical emergency. We first had to open the artery at the groin to try and remove the obstruction. This was not easy. The only instruments available were corkscrews on long handles that we threaded down the vessel and inserted into the clot, hoping it wouldn't break as we cautiously tried to withdraw it. Alternately, we raised the leg high above the body, applied a tight elastic wrap at the ankle, and slowly moved this toward the thigh, hoping we could squeeze the obstructing material from the incision. If we were unsuccessful, which occurred frequently, amputation would inevitably follow.

Introduction of the Fogarty embolectomy catheter in the 1960s emphasized how primitive and ineffectual the earlier techniques had been. Thomas Fogarty was a technician in a Cincinnati operating room when he invented the flexible catheter with an inflatable balloon on its tip. A surgeon could push this simple but ingenious device down the vessel beyond the end of the clot, inflate the balloon, and slowly extract the entire structure. Currently a professor of surgery at Stanford University, Fogarty holds one hundred patents for a variety of surgical instruments. His catheter was an important advance in the emerging field of vascular surgery.

An embolus to the abdominal viscera posed an even greater threat. I remember one such unfortunate patient well. Her youth and thinness were typical of those with mitral stenosis. Several days previously her compromised valve had been successfully reopened. Her breathing had improved and she could lie comfortably in bed. Her heart rhythm, however, was still irregular. The nurses called me to see her one night because of sudden, severe abdominal pain. Clearly, a catastrophe had occurred. It appeared that a clot had migrated from her enlarged left atrium down her aorta and into the artery that supplied her intestine. We had little choice but to operate immediately, although we couldn't prove the diagnosis because arteriography was not yet routine. On opening her abdomen, her entire small bowel was blue. There was no pulse in the pencil-sized artery at its base. We dissected this free, opened it, and were able to extract a clot about four inches long. We repaired the vascular defect with fine stitches and released the clamps. Before our eyes the bowel slowly, progressively, and pleasingly regained its natural pink color. Within a few hours we heard bowel sounds that implied returning function. It was miraculous. Despite the risk of bleeding, we administered blood thinners in order to prevent further episodes. All seemed calm for twenty-four hours until the same thing happened, like a recurring nightmare. Again we operated. Again we opened the artery, and again we removed a clot. Again she recovered. This time, however, she remained stable. The cardiologists were then able to shock her heart into a normal rhythm that substantially reduced further risk. But it was a close call.

Cushing had discussed the possibilities of reopening diseased valves in his 1908 publication, quoting a renowned British surgeon, Sir Lauder Brunton, who had previously emphasized the need for effective operative treatment: "Mitral stenosis is not only one of the most distressing forms of cardiac disease but in its severe forms it resists all medical treatment; one is impressed with the hopelessness of ever finding a remedy that will enable the atrium to drive blood in a sufficient stream through the small mitral orifice. But no one might be justified in attempting [such] a dangerous operation as dividing a mitral stenosis on a fellow creature without having first tested its practicability and perfected its technique on animals."[28] Brunton made both functional and conceptual advances in the many experiments he carried out in dogs. Showing that the heart would continue to beat after extensive manipulation, he presciently suggested that approaching the valve through the thin-walled atrium was superior to entering the muscular ventricle. Finally, he conjectured that the best way to open a stenotic mitral valve was to dilate the opening either with a finger or with an instrument. Despite the correctness of his conclusions, however, a quarter-century would pass before a new generation of surgeons would take them seriously.

Slowly, a few began to consider the possibilities of correcting valvular disease operatively. In 1913 a French pioneer in the nascent field of chest surgery attempted unsuccessfully to relieve a constricted mitral valve. A year later, a colleague visualized the aortic valve via an incision in the aortic wall but did not attempt repair. In 1922 surgeons in St. Louis unsuccessfully operated on a tight mitral valve. In London, Sir Henry Souttar, for the first and only time in his life, felt the valve directly by placing his index finger into the heart via the atrium as Brunton had suggested long before. The patient survived. His medical colleagues, however, were so appalled by his departure from the routine that they stopped their referrals. He wrote later: "I did not repeat the operation because I could not get another case. Although my patient made an uninterrupted recovery the Physicians declared that it was all nonsense and that the operation was unjustified. It is of no use to be ahead of one's time."[29]

The first relative success occurred in 1923 at the Brigham. Elliott Cutler and his colleagues had initiated a series of laboratory experiments to develop a surgical treatment for mitral stenosis. They had produced a satisfactory model in dogs by narrowing the external circumference of the valve with screw clamps, tight ligatures, or local radiation. They then designed a valvulotome to relieve the constriction, an instrument that they could introduce through the bottom of the left ventricle and push blindly upward through the leaflets. On opening the device, they exposed a semicircular punch. When they thought that the blade of the punch was in the correct position by feel alone they closed it, removing a portion of the diseased valve.[30] After extensive testing in the laboratory, they felt ready to use it clinically.

Their patient was a 12-year-old girl who had developed progressive shortness of breath after experiencing many colds and sore throats as a young child. Any activity increased her symptoms; she spent most of her time sitting up in bed, gasping. On examination she was thin and underdeveloped. Her heart rate was rapid. Her greatly enlarged heart made an obvious bulge on one side of her chest. All agreed that an operation was her only hope. After the anesthetist put her to sleep, Cutler opened her chest widely using a T-shaped incision, first splitting the breastbone along its length, then cutting perpendicularly along the ribs of each side. With

wide retraction, he exposed the entire enlarged heart. When he pulled
the organ forward to bring the left ventricle into view, her blood pressure plummeted but returned toward normal when he placed the organ
back into position. A solution of adrenalin in warm saline dripped on
the muscle restored vigorous contractions. The surgeon and his residents
took this moment of improved function to roll the heart over slowly. With
the bottom of the ventricle in plain view, he inserted the valvulotome
and pushed it upward through the tight mitral orifice. Localizing the
abnormal area by feel alone, he punched out a portion of one thickened
and calcified valve, then turned the device around and removed part of
the opposite leaflet. He withdrew the instrument and sewed the muscle
closed. There was no bleeding and the heart beat well. The operation
took an hour and a half.[31] Despite her now incompetent valve, the patient
improved considerably before suddenly collapsing four and a half years
later from recurrent stenosis. Emboldened by the initial result, Cutler
performed similar procedures on three more individuals. All died within
hours. By 1929, other surgeons had carried out nine additional but
uniformly unsuccessful operations. While those involved felt that operative intervention was warranted in particular instances of the disease
and that additional opportunities should be exploited, no further activity
occurred until after World War II.

Meanwhile, clinical investigators were discovering more about the
heart and its function. In 1929 a young resident physician, Werner
Forssmann, from Eberswalde, Germany, introduced the novel idea of
cardiac catheterization. Conceptualizing that he might be able to guide a
tube into the heart via a peripheral vessel for eventual injection of dyes
or measurement of pressures, he approached his professor for permission
to attempt such a procedure on himself. Firmly forbidden but determined
to carry out the experiment, he went to an operating room where he
isolated a vein in his own arm. When the nurse became frightened and
threatened to report the incident, Forssmann allegedly tied her to the
operating table. He inserted a long, fine catheter into the vein and fed
several feet of it upward. He then walked upstairs to the X-ray room.
A film confirmed that the end of the catheter was in his right atrium.
Furious at such a breach of discipline, the professor arranged for him

to take an unpaid position with a famous surgeon in Berlin, Ferdinand Sauerbruch. Equally disenchanted with his new charge, Sauerbruch not only fired the young man for self-experimentation but sent him elsewhere to train as a urologist. But his feat had been noticed, and two years later André Cournand and Dickinson Richards Jr., clinical investigators from Columbia University, used the technique to study the dynamics of the right heart and lungs of children by injecting X-ray dye through the catheter and measuring differential pressures between vessels and between chambers. For their joint introduction of this critical diagnostic tool, all three received the Nobel Prize in 1956, despite Forssmann's long-term membership in the Nazi Party.

This novel approach, combined with the later introduction of left heart catheterization via an artery in the arm, allowed cardiologists and radiologists to ascertain anatomical and physiological differences between normal and abnormal adult hearts, appreciate the importance of valve gradients, identify problems with selective X-rays, and consider appropriate surgical approaches. In the years after World War II those specializing in the new field were beginning to use the techniques to define a variety of cardiac conditions. Surgeons were correcting congenital anomalies in children with increasing accuracy and conceptualizing approaches to heart disease in adults.

Unbeknownst to each other and arriving at the same idea at the same time, three surgeons began to operate on stenotic mitral valves virtually simultaneously in the late 1940s.[32] Dwight Harken joined the Brigham staff in 1948, tempered by his experience with the war wounded. He had become increasingly interested in the tragic problems posed by the all-too-common disease and attracted to the possibilities of opening the valve directly. Having already shown in laboratory animals that a partially occluded valve produced progressive loss of function of the enlarging left atrium and backed up circulation in the lungs, he felt ready to move to patients. In his first operation, he split the fused mitral valve by introducing Cutler's valvulotome through the pulmonary vein. It did not go well, and Harken described the disastrous result to Cutler on his deathbed. In Philadelphia, Charles Bailey, one of Harken's enduring rivals, used a dilator to open the valves of four patients. All died. Six days after Bailey's first unsuccessful case, Harken operated on his second patient. She did well. And within a few months, Russell Brock in London reintroduced the technique that Brunton had suggested and Souttar had carried out a quarter-century before. He inserted his finger through a portion of the left atrium and opened the valves of eight patients. Six survived.

The mortality rate of the few patients undergoing the procedure did not improve appreciably for several years, and pressure from skeptical colleagues in other institutions to wait for new developments was intense. John Gibbon, a surgeon who was then developing the heart-lung machine, "urged a moratorium on surgical intervention until his cardiopulmonary bypass could render direct vision surgery available, which he felt to be on the verge of practical realization."[33] Unfortunately, practical realization of such hopes lay several years in the future. Harken and a handful of others persisted, despite obstacles. Harken published a rather bleak report of his first five cases "only to indicate the ability of such patients to withstand the operation. The evaluation of any long-term benefits attributed to this procedure must rest on objective criteria gained from hemodynamic studies."[34] Such criteria were minimal or nonexistent at that time. Indeed, the results were so bleak at the Brigham that the surgical residents petitioned the chief of the department, Francis Moore, to halt the program. Regardless of the deaths and perhaps encouraged by Gibbon's slow advances with his bypass machine, Moore encouraged Harken to continue. He believed the operation to have important potential. It was a brave and well-considered decision. Each week all of us on the surgical staff sat at Morbidity and Mortality Rounds to hear and discuss the recent complications and deaths. In those days, the pathologist brought in the actual specimens on trays for all to examine. Week after week we would view the hearts of patients who had died after the operation. Many of them passed before us. Gradually, however, the flow of specimens turned into a trickle and then into a few drops as such techniques for fracturing the fused portions of the diseased valves were refined. It is interesting to consider that although results improved slowly but progressively, such a relatively casual approach probably would not be allowed in our present age of Human Subjects Committees, litigators, and stringent administrative regulations, all carefully controlling patient participation and professional innovation. The operation, despite its early failures, opened a successful new avenue of treatment.

The number of Brigham patients with rheumatic heart disease grew exponentially. In 1955 Harken and a cardiological colleague reported the results of five hundred consecutive mitral valve finger fractures.[35] The progressive improvement was remarkable. The early mortality for the first one hundred patients was 32 percent for the sickest and 14 percent for the most favorable. For the other four hundred patients, the death rate fell to 24 percent and 4 percent, respectively. In a subsequent publication, he noted that mortality for the next five hundred patients to undergo the procedure declined to 20 percent and 0.6 percent, respectively. A decade later Harken and his colleague published a twelve-year follow-up on over 1,500 of the surviving individuals, a unique clinical experience shared by Bailey and occasional others.[36]

With success increasing and information spreading, heart surgeons in the United States and Europe began to carry out the procedures. Patients numbered in the thousands. Indications and contraindications to operation were developed. With growing confidence, surgeons accepted individuals with calcified valves, not previously thought to be operable. Complications, including the incidence of emboli, diminished. Dilators were improved for difficult cases. Devices to restore normal heart rhythm were perfected. At the same time those involved realized that the condition would recur in many patients within a few years, as had happened in Cutler's first case. Scars and adhesions made reoperation difficult and placed the patient at considerable risk. Overall, these early, strenuous, and often unsatisfactory attempts at adult heart surgery, while critical advances at the time, were limited in scope. As we shall see, the introduction of cardiopulmonary bypass, an "artificial circulation," changed the entire field. With this new tool, surgeons could stop the heart and repair or reconstruct whatever was necessary in a bloodless setting. A new chapter in the remarkable evolution of surgery of the heart would emerge.

eight

The Mechanical Heart

John Gibbon Jr., a surgical resident at the MGH in 1931, was typical of those training in prestigious programs at that time. A fourth-generation physician from Philadelphia, he had been educated at Princeton University and Jefferson Medical College. Patrician, tall, spare, and handsome, he was quietly dedicated to his career. One evening the nurses called him urgently to the bedside of a postoperative patient who had suddenly lost consciousness. Her skin, lips, and fingernails were blue, her breathing was labored, her pulse was weakening. She was dying before his eyes from a pulmonary embolus. Despite hours of support with intravenous fluid and appropriate medication, the situation appeared increasingly hopeless. Gibbon and the chief of the department, a highly regarded pioneer in the surgery of the lungs and pericardium, took her to the operating room, where they attempted to remove the clot from her pulmonary artery. Their efforts were of no avail.

A pulmonary embolus is a dreaded complication of a clot that may form in the large veins of the legs or pelvis and migrate to the lungs. These may develop after surgery, when the potential for clotting increases; if the individual becomes dehydrated and the blood becomes more viscous; when flow decreases during prolonged periods of sitting; or if an area of vein wall becomes inflamed. The site of formation acts as a base for a snakelike extension that propagates upward in the venous stream. These extensions may be many inches long and as large in diameter as the vessel enclosing it. If the entire clot floats free or if a segment breaks off, the circulation carries it to the lungs, where it lodges in the pulmonary artery, blocking blood flow. These events often end in death.

Since the turn of the twentieth century surgeons debated whether such a massive and life-threatening obstruction could be removed surgically. In 1908 a German surgeon actually opened the pulmonary artery and extracted the clot from a young calf. He then repeated the attempt on two patients; one lived for sixteen hours, the other for thirty-seven.[1] In a major address in 1933, Elliott Cutler suggested to the skeptical surgical establishment that an emergency operation should immediately be carried out in those afflicted.[2] Within months of his address, another German surgeon removed a clot with survival of the patient, an unprecedented achievement. A decade later, despite this striking success, one of the surgical leaders of the United States summarized the prevailing opinion, condemning such attempts at an annual conference. "I hope we will have no more papers on the [possibilities of] an operation which should be of historic interest only."[3] But within eight years the Europeans added additional reports to the literature. Finally, in 1958 Mr. Costello's surgeon, Richard Warren, performed the first successful pulmonary embolectomy in the country, as noted in Chapter 1. His success encouraged subsequent attempts that were enhanced by accurate radiological diagnosis and the introduction of cardiopulmonary bypass. Currently, the lives of many individuals developing the condition can be saved.

I assisted a cardiac surgeon who removed a pulmonary embolus during my residency. The patient was recovering from a hysterectomy performed three days before. She was eating and walking. Suddenly she collapsed, began to gasp, and became blue. We could barely feel a pulse. With no time to establish a definitive diagnosis and with the only bypass machine unavailable, we rushed her to the operating room and opened her chest. The heart was beating weakly. The pulmonary artery was engorged with solid matter to about the size of two thumbs. Quickly passing tapes around the vessel and making an incision through its wall, we immediately saw the large clot within. No blood could get by. With my colleague compressing the entire lung in his hands, I slowly extracted the huge embolus. It was eighteen inches long. We controlled the bleeding from the now empty pulmonary artery and repaired the defect, administering blood thinners at the end of the operation to prevent further clot formation. She did well.

Most pulmonary emboli are currently removed with the patient on cardiopulmonary bypass. The concept that a mechanical heart could take over the circulation of the body had a long gestation. In seventeenth-century Oxford, as noted, Richard Lower, a natural philosopher and early member of the newly formed Royal Society, first carried out direct blood transfusion in animals. Toward the end of the following century, Antoine Lavoisier defined the properties of and named both oxygen and hydrogen. Active in the prerevolutionary government in France, this imaginative polymath was considered "the father of modern chemistry" and a major contributor to many of the emerging sciences. Unhappily, he was guillotined during the Revolution as an aristocrat and intellectual. Early in the nineteenth century, a French physiologist suggested: "If one could substitute for the heart a kind of injection of [oxygen bearing] arterial blood, either naturally or artificially made, one would succeed in maintaining alive indefinitely any part of the body whatsoever."[4] He had based this supposition on the observation by colleagues that organs and tissues of newly dead animals could function transiently if fresh blood was instilled into the artery from an external source. Subsequent investigators developed the concept further. One enthusiast reversed the rigor mortis that had developed in the limbs of executed criminals by perfusing them with his own blood; the nonperfused limbs remained stiff.[5] German workers then built an apparatus to circulate blood through isolated organs. Others perfected a device that turned venous blood red by bubbling oxygen through it; however, air in the system precluded any practical use.[6]

Refinements continued. Jay MacLean, a Canadian medical student working at Johns Hopkins in 1916, introduced heparin, an intravenous agent that prevents coagulation.[7] This innovation increased the possibilities of propelling blood through tubing outside the body without the danger of clot formation. Others attempted bypass procedures in animals for physiologic and pharmacologic studies using improved pumps, valves, and devices for oxygenation. Even Charles Lindbergh, the American aviator, concerned about his sister-in-law's serious heart disease, became interested in producing a pump to take over heart activity temporarily and collaborated with the French surgeon Alexis Carrel. The theme of their work in the 1930s shifted increasingly toward the perfusion of organs outside the body.[8]

The promise of an effective circulatory support device lay far in the future as Gibbon sat by the bed of his patient in frustration and despair. Decades later, he recalled the circumstances. "During that long night, helplessly watching [her] struggle for life as her blood became darker and her veins more distended, the idea occurred to me that if it were possible to remove some of the blue blood from the swollen veins, put oxygen into it and allow the carbon dioxide to escape, then to inject continuously the now-red blood back into the patient's arteries, we might have saved her. We would have bypassed the obstructing embolus and performed part of the work of the patient's heart and lungs outside the body."[9] The team could then have removed the clot calmly from the motionless vessels and heart.

Gibbon and his wife, Mary, the technician on the project, pursued their elusive dream in the surgical laboratory of the MGH despite little encouragement from senior figures either within or outside the department. Money was scarce. To get enough animals for their experiments, the couple picked up stray cats off the Boston streets at night. The cats were more practical subjects than dogs because they were small and needed relatively little blood replacement. They toiled throughout the decade, perfecting and improving. Gibbon later described the results of their efforts. "The assemblage of metal, glass, electric motors, water baths, electrical switches, electromagnets, etc, looked for all the world like some ridiculous Rube Goldberg apparatus. Although it required infinite attention to detail it served us well and we were very proud of it."[10] Within a few years the husband-wife team moved to Philadelphia, where Gibbon joined the faculty of Jefferson Medical College. World War II interrupted the work. Upon his return from four years of military duty, they resumed their efforts. A fortuitous meeting followed with Thomas Watson, the president of International Business Machines (IBM) and the father-in-law of one of Gibbon's colleagues. Intrigued by the possibilities of an external heart-lung bypass machine, Watson offered the resources and engineering expertise of his company in designing and building a model suitable for eventual human use. With corporate funding, improving prototypes produced increasingly satisfactory results in open-heart operations in dogs. As the machine continuously reoxygenated blood circulating outside the body of the animal, a beating heart was not necessary to maintain life.

But it was a difficult gestation. During its later development, a group of surgical professors visited Gibbon's laboratory in Philadelphia to see how "the great machine was coming along." Francis Moore described the scene:

> We trooped in, 10 or 15 of us, and were asked to take off
> our shoes and put on rubber boots. We were then ushered
> into the operating room. At that time the pump oxygen-
> ator was approximately the size of a grand piano. A small
> cat, asleep on one side, was the object of all this attention.
> The cat was connected to the machine by two transpar-
> ent blood-filled plastic tubes. The contrast in size between
> the small cat and the huge machine aroused considerable
> amusement among the audience. Watching this compli-
> cated procedure, concentrating mostly on the cat, whose
> heart was about to be completely isolated from its circula-
> tion, opened, and then closed, we began to sense that we
> were not walking on a dry floor. We looked down. We
> were standing in an inch of blood. "Oh, I'm sorry" said
> Gibbon, "the confounded thing has sprung a leak again,"
> but his machine opened an entirely new era in surgery.[11]

Gibbon operated in February 1952 on his first patient, a 15-month-old child with what was thought to be a large atrial septal defect–lack of the common wall between the right and left atrial chambers. Like the open ductus, this "hole in the heart" is a normal feature of fetal development, allowing the circulating blood, oxygenated via the placenta, to bypass the lungs. It usually closes shortly after birth when the baby begins to breathe. If closure fails, depending on the size of the defect, then heart failure, infection, or stroke may ensue. Surgeons had attempted to close these congenital abnormalities for some years using a variety of tech-niques that inevitably involved operating blindly in the blood-filled, beat-ing organ. They were rarely successful. In contrast, Gibbon was able to use his bypass machine to stop the heart and open the still and blood-less organ of his patient to examine the area directly. Unfortunately in this case, no intra-atrial defect was present. Later, after the child had died, they found a large patent ductus arteriosus. It was unrecognized because adequate diagnostic tools were not available. The surgeon had been unable to see the ductus through the incision he had made, although the approach was correct for the operation planned.

His second attempt a year later involved Cecelia Bavolek. Eighteen years old, she had been admitted to the hospital multiple times during the prior six months with recurrent congestive heart failure. Catheterization of the right side of her heart, a method used increasingly in the early 1950s, showed a large atrial septal defect with blood from the left side of the heart flooding into the right chambers and lungs under high pressure. This technique involved threading a plastic catheter up a peripheral vein in the arm under fluoroscopy, and positioning its tip near the heart. Radio-opaque dye was then injected, allowing precise visualization of the blood flowing through the defect. With his bypass machine pumping oxygenated blood through the patient's body and with cardiac motion stopped, Gibbon could easily see the extent of the defect and sew it closed. The repair took twenty-seven minutes. When he discontinued the artificial circulation, the organ resumed a normal beat. Repeat catheterization was normal. Cecelia was cured forever. Having proved at long last the efficacy of his machine and its remarkable utility in open-heart surgery, he never again operated on a patient, feeling that younger colleagues should carry on.[12] He was thrice nominated for the Nobel Prize for one of the most important surgical contributions of all time.

Others improved the apparatus in the years to follow, refining the types of pump, perfecting the connections between the patient and the machine, devising means to oxygenate the blood without damaging the red blood cells, and designing selective bypass for either the left or the right side of the heart. The project became an important international effort with investigators from centers in the United States, Canada, Europe, Britain, and Australia introducing a variety of prototypes during the 1970s and 1980s. Much was accomplished. Surgeons could operate precisely on the functionless organ without time constraints, visualize all defects and abnormalities, and reconstruct what was necessary while a machine supplied oxygenated blood to the rest of the body of the patient. It was a major step forward.

Preservation of the myocardium is a critical adjunct to safe and effective cardiopulmonary bypass. Reducing the core temperature of the subject seemed an obvious approach to protect the heart muscle, particularly as it became clear that the organ would stop its contractions when the body temperature was brought below a certain point and would resume normal activity with rewarming. During his training at Johns Hopkins, Wilfred Bigelow, a surgeon from the University of Toronto, had witnessed the Blalock-Taussig "blue baby" operation in 1944. He realized that "surgeons would never be able to correct or cure heart conditions unless they were able to ensure direct vision."[13] Instead of relying on a complex series of pumps and tubing, he wondered if hypothermia, a general cooling of the body, might reduce metabolic demand enough that the heart could be stopped for short periods. Although he showed by 1949 that the circulation of deeply cooled dogs could be interrupted for fifteen minutes, half the subjects died. After three years of work, however, he reported complete survival of hypothermic monkeys whose hearts he opened, manipulated, and repaired. With laboratory results improving further, surgeons at the University of Minnesota first used the method late in 1952 to close a large atrial septal defect in a five-year-old girl. She recovered quickly and was living a normal life thirty-three years later. Cooling has become an integral part of cardiopulmonary technology.

The new concept of stilling the cooled heart with mechanical bypass not only allowed correction of complex congenital cardiac anomalies in children but permitted definitive replacement of defective or diseased valves in adults. Until these techniques were combined, effective valve surgery had not been possible, despite a variety of attempts. In addition, it encouraged the clinical investigators already advancing surgery of the mitral valve to consider means to operate on the aortic valve. This structure sits at the junction of the left ventricle and the aorta and consists of three half-moon-shaped leaflets. When the contracting chamber expels oxygenated blood into the artery, the leaflets lie flat against the wall. With dilation, they come together, preventing backward regurgitation of blood. As a result of rheumatic heart disease or infection, the stiff, thickened, and calcified leaflets may significantly narrow the orifice. Blood unable to escape from the ventricle of patients with resultant aortic stenosis backs up into the lungs. Other sequelae of the condition include fainting, probably caused by deficient arterial blood supply to the brain, and angina from inadequate coronary artery flow. Some with the condition die suddenly. Conversely, if the aortic root enlarges because of aging or hypertension, or a congenital absence of one of the cusps, or calcification of the valve leaflets (or their destruction by bacteria) and prevents closure, the ejected column of blood falls back from the aorta into the dilating ventricle. These patients have aortic insufficiency, developing a character-istically bounding pulse as blood rushes ineffectively back and forth in the arteries. Congestive heart failure frequently results.

Before the availability of cardiopulmonary bypass, surgeons through-out the 1950s devised several methods to correct diseased aortic valves in the beating heart. In patients with severe aortic stenosis, they inserted dilators through the ventricular wall, although the ensuing hemorrhage was often fatal. Alternatively, they controlled bleeding by sewing a cuff of cloth or vein to the side of the aorta through which they introduced the instrument or their finger to dilate the tight valve. Often the fused valves were too calcified to open; not infrequently, the diseased cusps tore apart. Some patients survived but did not improve; others quickly died. Relief of aortic insufficiency fared no better. To narrow the enlarged orifice of the incompetent valves, investigators decreased the size of the root of the aorta by banding it with steel wire or with tight cloth slings. At times, they pinched the sides of the vessel together with sutures, or placed patches or plastic baffles. As with aortic stenosis, little worked. Among all the failures, however, one interesting novelty arose. Charles Hufnagel introduced the concept of a ball valve.

In addition to his collaborations with Gross on the development of vascular grafts, Hufnagel had become expert in the dynamics of aortic insufficiency in canine models. To correct the condition, he designed and tested a series of ball valves that he placed inside the rigid plastic pros-theses he had already created to bridge excised aortic coarctations.[14] He anchored the devices in the thoracic aorta with multifixation external rings in lieu of sutures, a technique still used in cardiac surgery. The valves were like snorkels; as the left ventricle contracted, the ball floated free in the stream of blood. When the chamber dilated, the ball fell back into its socket, preventing backflow.

He implanted his first prosthesis in a patient with aortic insufficiency in 1952, eventually placing over ninety.[15] Many of the afflicted improved substantially. Despite the efficacy of the devices, however, they were hardly ideal. I remember seeing one of the patients when I was a resident. The clicking noise of the ball shooting back and forth in the bloodstream was audible to all of us standing around the bed. Indeed, the very bed frame shook. The incessant noise and activity was very distressing and led to occasional suicides among those having received the valve. Hufnagel improved the problem in later designs, allowing some patients with hitherto fatal aortic insufficiency to live for extended periods.[16] His unique contributions to the repair of valvular heart disease led the way to an entirely new avenue of treatment. Becoming chief of surgery at Georgetown University, he continued to improve on the original concept throughout much of his career with novel leaflet and disk-type cardiac valves.

The relative success of the ball-valve device positioned in the thoracic aorta stimulated others to consider substituting an artificial valve for the diseased one in the correct anatomical location. The first prototypes, introduced in the early 1960s, most commonly consisted of a cloth-covered stainless steel ring that could be sewn in the aortic or mitral position after the affected leaflets had been removed. Curved struts from the ring formed a cage. Within the cage was a ball of Lucite or similar material that would rise from the ring as blood flowed around it, then seat firmly in place to prevent back bleeding. Although some of the evolving designs were effective, practical problems plagued others: clots formed on the struts and broke off as emboli; the synthetic balls disintegrated after months of use; the existing valves were often too bulky to be seated in the correct anatomical position. As time went on, however, improved models entered general use, making formal valve replacement increasingly possible.[17]

Despite technical advances, however, open-heart surgery remained relatively rudimentary. Each new type of heart-lung bypass apparatus seemed more unwieldy and complicated than the last. We residents had to fill out individual forms for eighteen units of blood the evening before operation: six to replace expected blood loss; twelve to prime the pump!

At the beginning of the procedure we connected the large artery and vein at the groin to the machine. Although the concept seemed straightforward, the actual tangle of plastic tubing was so complex that few of us understood the ever-changing circuitry. When the surgeon directed us to place the patient on bypass, we were supposed to unclamp one segment and clamp another. Not infrequently, we chose the wrong tube. After a pause, a connection would spring apart under pressure, and suddenly the floor would be covered in blood. Cries of outrage added to the confusion. Even when the patient was safely cooled and the heart had stopped its motion, these early operations were still hardly routine. With the left atrium open, we could, with judicious retraction, view the diseased mitral valve. We approached the aortic valve through the arterial wall close to the left ventricle. The surgeon then removed the diseased structure and sewed the prosthesis in place. These were tight areas, difficult to get at. We had to place multiple silk stitches through the heart wall and covered ring of the prosthesis, then tie them individually to seat the new valve in position. On occasion even the smallest device available would not fit into the designated site. Appreciable numbers of patients died despite our desperate efforts. Perhaps even more discouraging for all involved were the patients who awoke from anesthesia having suffered a stroke from an air bubble or fleck of clot that had formed in the tubing and had escaped into the brain. While it was not an easy time in those relatively early days, the promise of more effective technology and better results drove the field relentlessly forward.

Surgeons grew ever bolder and more skilled with operative approaches to the lungs, heart, and great vessels in both animals and humans. As the diseased heart became amenable to intervention or repair, they assumed new challenges. Some began to focus on the operative relief of angina pectoris, a subject not even mentioned in prewar surgical textbooks. William Heberden, the great English medical scholar, first described and named this condition in 1768, having confirmed the relationship between the chest pain that his friend and fellow physician, John Fothergill, experienced before his death and his severely diseased coronary arteries, discovered at autopsy. A century later, a practitioner in St. Louis,

Missouri, associated sudden clinical symptoms with acute closure of a coronary artery, an observation that physicians in Chicago subsequently clarified more precisely. The origins and importance of angina remained a mystery, however, as objective documentation was virtually impossible in the days before the stress test, coronary angiography, sophisticated imaging, and other diagnostic methods. Even Osler complained that "the opportunities to observe the paroxysm do not come often—and when they do the condition of the patient is such that our efforts are directed toward his relief than to the study of special points in the case."[18]

Long thought to occur primarily in older men, and associated with physical exertion, emotion, and excitement, angina pectoris is characterized by transient episodes of chest pain, breathlessness, and a feeling of impending doom. It took years before physicians realized that women were also at risk but that their symptoms are often more subtle. In late stages, all those with the condition may experience unremitting pain at rest. At the present time in the United States, 13 million people are affected, a substantial public health problem. Half a million die of heart attacks every year, by far the greatest cause of death.[19] Both angina and actual cardiac damage result from arteriosclerosis, the buildup of calcified and noncalcified plaque on the inside of the coronary arteries, like rust in a pipe. Arising at the base of the aorta where it joins the left ventricle and each about the size of the tip of a blunt pencil, the coronaries course over the surface of the heart. As in all other arterial systems of the body, their branches eventually form a network of capillaries that lie between each contracting muscle bundle. The capillaries, in turn, form coronary veins that carry deoxygenated blood to the right side of the heart. A strong family history of the disease, smoking, high levels of cholesterol, hypertension, obesity, and diabetes accelerate the progressive process. If an arterial segment becomes critically narrowed, insufficient blood gets to the area of cardiac muscle it supplies during periods of stress or bodily activity. This oxygen-starved portion reacts by evoking the symptoms of angina. This is a transient event; the circulation normalizes and the compromised heart muscle recovers after the patient relaxes. In contrast, a heart attack occurs if the narrowed segment of artery suddenly closes and blood flow ceases completely. The involved area of muscle then dies.

Before open-heart surgery provided the means to bypass the narrowed portions of the coronary vessels with lengths of peripheral vein, surgical investigators carried out vast numbers of experimental and clinical researches in attempts to ameliorate the problem. They pursued three different strategies. One was to prevent the pain of angina by cutting appropriate nerves in the neck and upper chest. Another was designed to reduce cardiac work. The third involved bringing blood supply to the heart muscle itself from other sources.

The sympathetic nerves influence the function of all organs and blood vessels throughout the body. Unlike the nerves to our muscles that we can control voluntarily, these act autonomously. They also may carry pain signals from tissues in distress. Surgical interruption of the nervous pathways to the heart was first suggested in 1889 as a means to relieve the symptoms of angina. Proponents in Europe, at the Mayo Clinic, and then in many other centers in the United States performed a variety of sometimes elaborate and extensive nerve-cutting operations on huge numbers of afflicted patients.[20] They continued this approach for several decades, encouraged by exuberant accounts of success. Unfortunately, although anginal pain was absent, the operated patients now had no warning of the onset of serious cardiac events such as heart attacks. At the same time skeptics became increasingly concerned that the intensity of the pain could not be gauged in objective physiological terms either in animals or humans, and that response to treatment could not be measured accurately. The subsequent discovery that removal of all nervous connections to the heart was not anatomically possible in cats also did much to dampen the ardor of the involved surgeons.[21]

During the 1920s and 1930s Cutler and colleagues in Boston introduced an alternative concept based on an extensive series of laboratory experiments in dogs that defined the relationship between the function of the heart and that of the thyroid gland. With the endocrine system gaining increasing attention, reports were arising that hyperactivity of the thyroid could masquerade as heart disease and produce the pain of angina.[22] Surgeons already involved with operative treatment of goiters became interested in the relationship, reasoning that if they decreased the metabolic rate of the body by removing most of the active gland, they could reduce the functional load of the diseased heart and relieve symptoms. However, as neither the experimental data nor objective effects in patients were convincing, those involved gradually abandoned the practice. Indeed, many individuals operated upon not only continued to experience angina but became lethargic and unable to carry out daily activities because of thyroid insufficiency.

Investigators then began to pursue other experimental strategies, particularly attempts to bring a new blood supply to the heart muscle itself. The concept was triggered by studies of pericarditis, inflammation of the membrane surrounding the heart. Claude Beck at Case Western Reserve University in Cleveland, Ohio, noted the presence of newly formed vessels in adhesions between the affected membrane and the organ beneath. These, he reasoned, could provide an external circulation that could revitalize cardiac muscle inadequately nourished by narrowed and diseased coronary arteries. He and others in North America and Britain demonstrated in animals that pedicle grafts of vessels from between the ribs or brought through the diaphragm from the abdomen would adhere to the heart surface and create a localized accessory blood supply.[23] Early in 1935 Beck carried out the first grafting procedure on a patient who did not experience angina again for seven months. Over the following decades, others reported at least subjective improvement. Beck was a renowned innovator and leader, and the first professor of cardiovascular surgery in the United States. His work in cardiac resuscitation and in revascularization of the heart was critical in the emerging field. Embellishing these observations, surgeons at McGill University dissected from beneath the breastbone a length of one of the paired internal mammary arteries that supply the front of the chest wall and breasts and buried its end into a tunnel made in the ventricular muscle. They performed this surgery first on animals and then on human patients, reasoning that the arteries' branches might ultimately connect with open segments of the compromised coronaries.[24] Others tested similar strategies during the 1960s using adjacent small arteries. Heart surgeons today not infrequently join the end of the internal mammary directly to a segment of normal coronary artery to bypass effectively an upstream blockage.

The enduring difficulty for the early investigators of the disease, as mentioned, was that angina pectoris involves pain, a subjective and nonmeasurable sensation. In reviewing the diverse approaches in the years before precise radiologic visualization of the coronary system was possible, physicians increasingly questioned whether some patients whose symptoms disappeared after operation actually had the condition to begin with. Were some patients' positive outcomes the result of a placebo effect? They quoted autopsy reports of persons with classical symptoms whose coronary arteries were uninvolved with arteriosclerosis. Some clinical researchers decried the lack of follow-up data in most of the studies and emphasized that the important psychic elements associated with the disorder made it difficult to clarify the end results of surgery. Others, more outspoken in their criticism, felt it unfortunate that those already convinced of the value of intervention should exploit any field where accurate diagnosis was undeveloped. Like the protracted but ill-conceived operative treatment of peptic ulcer disease and the overuse of appendectomy for less-than-compelling indications, these misgivings illustrate a pattern that arises intermittently throughout the entire field of medicine: widely heralded therapeutic claims are sometimes touted without adequate supporting clinical or experimental evidence. Another recent example of hope over experience has been the decline of hormone replacement therapy for the symptoms of menopause. A popular treatment for years, it lost favor with gynecologists and their patients because of the specter of increased heart disease, breast cancer, and other possible complications. In retrospect, many of the attempts at operative relief of angina, while based upon concepts popular at the time, were complex and unwieldy. The learning curve was long, and the results were unsatisfactory. Most of these substantial efforts later became obsolete with the introduction of coronary artery bypass grafting.

Occasional visionaries had considered the possibilities of direct repair of affected coronary vessels based, perhaps, on an unsuccessful attempt by Alexis Carrel in 1910 to bypass the mouth of a coronary artery of a dog with a segment of preserved artery.[25] A few investigators later widened the diameter of narrowed sections of the arteries with small vein patches in relatively small numbers of patients desperate for relief. Others removed localized areas of calcified plaque from inside the diseased vessel; still others joined vessels from other sources to the artery itself. Most attempts failed. It must be recalled that these pioneers had to operate on the beating heart, that sutures, needles, and the bulky surgical instruments then available were ill-suited for such fine work, and clotting often occurred at the operative site. Several decades would pass before improvements allowed new generations of surgeons to route a normal blood supply around localized obstructions of one or more of the small coronary vessels.

In the late 1960s René Favaloro first interposed portions of a normal superficial vein from the leg between the aorta of the patient and uninvolved segments of coronary artery below localized obstructions.[26] The venous channel he used was the one that forms varicosities in some people, as we remember from Mrs. Turner. Favaloro had trained for several years with pioneer heart surgeons at the Cleveland Clinic before returning to Argentina, his homeland, where he perfected his techniques and developed an important center for the study of cardiac surgery. A passionate spokesman for his people and often at odds with the repressive Argentine government, he became internationally recognized for his contributions. His coronary bypass operation was so successful that it quickly spread internationally, saving innumerable lives. Currently, about a half-million coronary artery bypasses are performed in the United States each year.

I have seen a number of these operations. They are choreographed like a ballet. The location and extent of the coronary disease is precisely documented in each patient with the most current functional and radiological diagnostic methods. Not only do sophisticated scans provide fine vascular detail, but ultrasound probes on the tips of tiny catheters can be snaked inside the vessels to transmit an even more accurate picture of the inside of the artery on a screen. Once the patient is asleep, draped and prepared in the operating room, the surgical teams go to work. One group removes a length of vein from the calf or thigh, dividing strands of constricting connective tissue on its surface and tying off all its branches. This is not a stripping operation as Cheever carried out on Mrs. Turner's varicosities but a careful dissection to preserve intact the normal thin-walled structure. Some use an evolving and less disruptive endoscopic approach for vein removal. The assistants then connect the patient to the heart-lung apparatus via tubes placed in the major artery and vein in the groin or high in the arm. If the operation takes place in a teaching institution, the senior cardiac trainee and a younger resident make a skin incision along the center of the breastbone from neck to abdomen; in community hospitals that carry out the procedure, staff members assist each other. Using a power saw, they divide the bone along its length in a single motion and retract the two sides of the chest wall widely apart. With the pericardial sac opened, the beating heart lies fully exposed, a sight that invariably moves me, perhaps due to a deep-seated consciousness of the psychic importance of the organ.

The team places the patient on bypass. I marvel at the compact and quiet machine, the lack of clutter of tubing and equipment, and the workmanlike motions of the pump technician, all so different from my own earlier experiences. With the device taking over the circulation and the body temperature cooled, the empty heart slows and stops. The surgeon carefully rechecks the scans and isolates segments of the coronary arteries below the site of narrowing. He clamps the aorta near its junction with the heart, punches holes through its wall and sews pieces of leg vein to it with tiny sutures. He then joins the other end of the grafts to the small incision he has made in the sides of the coronaries. When all grafts are in place (sometimes as many as five going to separate coronary branches) and the vessels carefully washed out to remove flecks of clot, debris, or air, the patient is warmed to a normal temperature. The heart, still and empty throughout the operation, gradually fills and resumes beating. With the pulsating vein grafts carrying blood into the open coronaries below the areas of blockage, the heart muscle regains normal color and tone. When the revascularized organ regains full function and is able to support the patient, who has been slowly rewarmed, the bypass is stopped. The team ensures there is no bleeding, closes the incisions, and takes the patient to intensive care for twenty-four hours.

The two or three open-heart operations we performed each week when I was a resident strained hospital personnel and physical resources. Current cardiac surgeons may perform a half-dozen a day. Indeed, surgeons in many hospitals throughout the world carry out millions of such procedures every year safely and effectively in patients of increasingly higher risk. Although the age at which the majority of the individuals accepted for the surgery has increased, and patients often carry the added risks of hypertension, smoking, generalized arteriosclerosis, and coexisting disease, the mortality rate is gratifyingly low (less than 2 percent for all comers).

Gibbon's introduction of the heart-lung machine, its refinement and perfection by others, the importance of hypothermia, and the development and routine use of the pacemaker and other mechanical adjuncts have been triumphs of surgical innovation. And innovation continues. Surgeons are able to perform more and more procedures through limited incisions or even without use of bypass. Clinical researchers are investigating the placement of heart valves via a distant vessel, rather like the "endovascular repair" of aortic aneurysms. Interventional radiologists widen areas of coronary narrowing with tiny metal coils, introduced through an artery in the groin of the awake patient. Pharmacological agents have become so effective that many individuals do well without surgery. Indeed, one of the reasons given for the present decline both in the incidence of coronary bypass operations and in deaths from heart disease is early control of high blood pressure. It remains a remarkable journey.

Early in 1969 at the Texas Heart Institute in Houston, acclaimed heart surgeon Denton Cooley removed Haskell Karp's failing heart and replaced it with an artificial device. The mechanical heart supported his circulation for sixty-four hours as Mrs. Karp spearheaded a nationwide search on television, radio, and the newspapers for an appropriate organ. With the numbers of potential donors having decreased significantly because of the highly publicized failures of the new procedure of heart transplantation, her desperation was palpable. "Someone, somewhere, please hear my plea. A plea for a heart for my husband. I see him lying there, breathing and knowing that within his chest is a man-made implement where there should be a God-given heart. How long he can survive one can only guess. I cry without tears. I wait hopefully. Our children wait hopefully, and we pray. Maybe somewhere there is a gift of a heart. Please."[27] Responding to Mrs. Karp's emotional appeals, doctors in Massachusetts identified a potential donor and transferred her to Texas by chartered air ambulance despite ongoing debate about her suitability. Although recognizing that she had sustained irreversible brain damage from a massive stroke, those caring for her had not yet pronounced her brain dead. On re-examination four hours later, however, Houston physicians felt that she had suffered a further episode on the airplane and finally gave her that status. Cooley performed the transplant. One day later Karp died.

A complex interplay of ideas, emerging technologies, false claims, self-aggrandizement, and institutional, professional, and personal competition suffused the development of the artificial heart. Feuds arose and careers were destroyed in parallel with important advances. I must stress, however, that a central theme of these often troubling events is of surgeons desperately trying all means possible to salvage a handful of dying patients using concepts and techniques still in their infancy. At such climactic moments, the individual responsible must be totally convinced of himself and his talents to make instantaneous and sometimes irrevocable decisions, cast aside philosophical, religious, or societal considerations, and leave debate about correctness, appropriateness, and even the ethics of the decision to the future.

The creation of a mechanical device to assist the failing left ventricle or to substitute for the entire organ is an intricate and difficult exercise that involves close collaboration between surgeons, physiologists, bio-engineers, instrument makers, and those studying the effect of synthetic materials on the circulation. The designers must prevent both the coagulation of blood within the artificial chambers and its failure to clot appropriately in the body with the coincident risk of bleeding. They must guard against the formation of small clots in the bloodstream that can cause strokes, protect the continuously circulating red blood cells from damage, and ensure that the power source is completely dependable. If the apparatus is to replace the entire heart, the investigators need to produce and test two conjoined pumps, one to propel the circulation at high pressure through the arteries, the other to ensure low-pressure venous flow through the lungs. They have to identify materials that will not degrade in the body over time and design valves that will stand up indefinitely. Research groups throughout the world have put strenuous efforts into these and related challenges.

Like most scientific innovations, the concept of an artificial heart was not new. Nineteenth-century German workers initially suggested the possibility. English physiologists built a pump in 1928 that simulated the native organ.[28] In the 1930s journalists introduced the term *mechanical heart* to describe the device that Carrel and Lindbergh had created to preserve tissues, extolled the design of the rotary valve that produced a pulse, acclaimed the efficacy of the pump driven by compressed air, and conjectured on its future potential.[29] Workers in France and elsewhere after World War II supported the compromised circulation of dogs and then patients with failing hearts by implanting a balloon in the aorta that inflated and deflated with each beat, augmenting the circulation into the coronaries, brain, and vital organs. Harken and others later refined this counterpulsation concept substantially. With coincidentally improving cardiopulmonary bypass prototypes, investigators designed ventricular assist devices to support inadequate function of one or both ventricles in a variety of large animals.

The placement of a total mechanical heart in Mr. Karp, the first such attempt, was particularly controversial. Not only was the exercise a contest between teams and institutions, but social and political pressures ongoing in the United States at the time seemed to encourage the race. The accelerating war in Southeast Asia was increasingly unpopular. Important political figures had been assassinated. There was racial strife and urban disruption. Upset, pessimistic, and disenchanted, the public clamored for answers and solutions. Craving something positive, they demanded and expected technology to solve many of the problems. Perhaps the artificial heart would fill the void.

In 1962 Michael DeBakey, an internationally recognized pioneer in cardiovascular surgery and president of Baylor College of Medicine in Houston, Texas, received a $4.5 million grant from the National Heart Institute to form an artificial heart program. He collected a team of experts that included Domingo Liotta, an experienced surgical researcher who had developed a prototype in Argentina. Supported by the federal funds, Liotta and engineers on the team designed and built a series of single pumps that could maintain a failing left ventricle until at least some of its muscle could recover adequate function. After trials in dogs, he used one of the devices to maintain the circulation of a patient for four days. A subsequent version functioned for ten days in a young woman with severe cardiovascular disease. She recovered and lived normally for several years thereafter. Production of a double ventricle pump to act as temporary support for the entire heart suddenly became more urgent, however, with the 1967 announcement from South Africa of the first heart transplant. Within two years Liotta implanted one of his newly produced mechanical models into a calf.[30] Curiously, however, he had submitted an abstract to a national conference the day before which claimed that his artificial heart had functioned successfully for many hours in ten calves. He acknowledged support by the National Heart Institute and listed DeBakey as one of the coauthors. DeBakey, annoyed and dismayed by his actions, had not learned of the abstract until a few days before the meeting. When the pumps were eventually placed in seven (not ten) animals, all but one died within a few hours; the remaining animal survived forty-four hours but was "virtually cadaver from the time of implantation."[31] The discrepancy between claims and reality was, at the least, disturbing.

Denton Cooley was a highly regarded and talented cardiac surgeon, head of the Texas Heart Institute and surgeon at its affiliated St. Luke's Hospital. He approached Liotta sometime during this period about working with him to develop an artificial heart for clinical use. No one asked or informed DeBakey, the Argentinian's sponsor and director of the separate and competing Baylor program. Enthused by the proposed collaboration, Liotta persuaded the engineer on the Baylor team who had designed the power source for the heart to build a duplicate apparatus—unofficially. Although receiving a salary from DeBakey's federal grant, this individual agreed because of the opportunity to work with Cooley and the incentive to perfect his machine. Unaware of any plans for its clinical use, he delivered the console to St. Luke's, but included a note stating that the untested device should be used only in experimental animals. Meanwhile, Liotta was producing additional units in the Baylor laboratory. He and Cooley later referred to nine animals with implanted artificial hearts, although they never published specific details. No one, including members of the St. Luke's Hospital pump team, was informed of plans to implant the mechanical heart into a human. While Karp and his wife were opposed

to a heart transplant, they had presumably given their permission sometime before surgery for the introduction, if necessary, of an artificial device
in preparation for such a step. Cooley placed the patient on cardiopulmonary bypass to salvage what he could. Seeing little normal ventricle
and unable to resuscitate Karp's heart or wean him from the machine,
he removed the barely functioning organ and substituted the mechanical
prosthesis.[32]

The line between placing such an apparatus in a dying patient as an
emergency last-stage endeavor and actually planning to do so was a fine
one. Many in the medical community felt that the extensive last-minute
preparations were prearranged. Priority for design and production of
the pump and the funds used for its development were also large issues,
particularly as the investigators who had built the device implanted at St.
Luke's were under federal contract at Baylor. Because of the increasing
national publicity and obvious controversy, both Baylor and the National
Heart Institute held inquiries. Liotta was suspended from the program
and his salary withdrawn. Although Cooley resigned his faculty position, he remained a formidable figure in cardiothoracic surgery, recognized
internationally for his intellect, technical expertise, and clinical productivity. His ambitions and hard-driving sense of achievement were widely
acknowledged. He did not lose patients lightly. But further activity on the
device ceased.

The second stage of the development of an artificial heart occurred during
the 1980s. In contrast to the prevailing mood a decade earlier, this was
a time of self-confidence, expansion, and optimism in the United States.
The Vietnam War was over. The economy was healthy. Industries sold
their products throughout the world. Technology was ascendant, driven
by new departures from the routine and a pervasive spirit of enthusiasm
and entrepreneurism. Commensurate with ongoing advances in medicine,
biology, and other sciences, the spirit of the times encouraged reconsideration of a mechanical device to fill a potential need for thousands of
patients with severe heart disease. The development of the second phase
was, like the first, primarily an American venture financed enthusiastically by federal monies. There was a mystique about it, as Robert Bellah,

professor of sociology at the University of California, Berkeley, noted: "It is a bit like a star on the 'American' flag, and stopping the artificial heart program would be like picking the star off the flag."[33] Despite previous misfortunes, the time appeared right to re-examine its clinical application.

Willem Kolff was a Dutch physician, inventor, and engineer who had developed the dialysis machine in Holland under the Nazi occupation. His father, also a doctor, was the director of a tuberculosis sanatorium, caring for patients terminally ill from that terrible disease. From his early observations and experience with his father, the underlying theme of Kolff's career became one of helping those to survive who were otherwise doomed. At the Cleveland Clinic in the 1950s, his increasing experience with the artificial kidney led to broader considerations of creating machines to substitute for other failing organs. This interest led him in 1967 to the University of Utah, an institution already interested in biomedical innovation, where he concentrated primarily on perfecting a mechanical heart. Within a few years, he and his colleagues produced pneumatically powered devices that could sustain calves over relatively long periods following removal of their native hearts. Although they extended and improved the existing designs, problems with engineering, materials, blood clotting, and infection persisted. It was a prolonged and taxing labor.

Two notable individuals had joined the project to work with Kolff. Robert Jarvik, a mechanical engineer then in medical school, was responsible for design of the device. A born entrepreneur, he was imaginative, flamboyant, and highly visible. Not only had he been featured in *Playboy*, but I later recall seeing his face plastered on the walls of the London Underground, wearing an eye patch and advertising shirts! When Kolff later formed a proprietary company with close (and controversial) ties to the University of Utah, the theatrical inventor became its president, ultimately supplanting his mentor in the process.[34] William DeVries was the other member of the team. A highly trained cardiac surgeon, he too had worked with Kolff as a student. He eventually became the only surgeon that the FDA authorized to test the artificial heart in humans.

The experimental results in calves that the group obtained were hardly ideal. Infection occurred commonly, initially at the skin site where the pneumatic tubes from the external power source entered the chest of the calves. Eventually, the infection burrowed inward to involve the apparatus itself. Regardless of this potentially devastating complication, pressures to embark upon clinical trials began to mount as the investigators perceived that the National Heart Institute, the primary source of support, was losing interest in the complete artificial heart and shifting its resources to less ambitious single ventricular assist devices. Concern grew among those in many disciplines that use of such a support system in humans would be premature and unwarranted.

In spite of these doubts, research on the subject was increasing throughout the world. In addition to the laboratory in Salt Lake City, groups in Berlin, Tokyo, and Hershey, Pennsylvania, reported that twelve goats and calves had survived total cardiac replacement with an artificial heart for more than six months. Initial tests were made in humans as well. DeVries tested the apparatus in recently deceased persons in Utah, Argentina, and East Germany. An investigator in Philadelphia implanted units into five persons with brain death, supporting the circulation of two for forty-one and seventy-two hours before elective termination; the other three became kidney donors after extended periods on the pump.[35] An attempt in a patient at the University of Tokyo increased the sense of urgency of the Utah team. Regardless of the unavoidable infections in their animals, the Utah team felt ready, approaching and receiving permission from both the University Human Subjects Committee and the FDA to proceed clinically. Carefully screening a group of candidates in end-stage heart failure, they chose Dr. Barney Clark, a 61-year-old retired dentist from Seattle, as the first subject. In December 1982, DeVries and a surgical colleague removed Clark's irreversibly diseased heart and implanted one of Jarvik's pumps. The patient lived for 112 complication-ridden days before dying of multiple organ failure and sepsis. It was a difficult period. At times he pleaded to be allowed to die. Unremitting media coverage compounded the misery surrounding his existence, even with strenuous efforts by his caregivers to protect him. Apparently immune to the stress of all involved and with surgical optimism consistently transcending common sense, DeVries later reported in the *New England Journal of Medicine* that "despite that relatively complicated postoperative course in our patient, the overall experience leads to an optimistic appraisal of the future potential for total artificial heart systems."[36]

Over the following months the young surgeon became increasingly frustrated with perceived obstacles to further trials. Arguments about priority of invention were arising. The gradual replacement of federal funding with private support intensified conflict-of-interest claims among Jarvik, the company, its stockholders, and the university. The institutional Human Subjects Committee objected to another attempt. But despite these local problems the FDA approved plans for a second implant in mid-1984. Within weeks DeVries joined the staff of a hospital run by the Humana Corporation in Louisville, Kentucky, one of the largest of the new for-profit health-care chains emerging in the United States. Although lacking university affiliation, their stated priorities included excellence in patient care, education, and applied research. They also announced plans to build an important center for cardiovascular disease, heart transplantation, and implantation of artificial hearts. For this venture, the company was prepared to spend a great deal of money.

DeVries moved ahead quickly, placing an artificial Jarvik heart into his second patient, William Schroeder, despite ongoing concerns voiced by leaders in American medicine, by members of the press, and from some in the FDA who expressed doubts about the rapidity and completeness of the review by the Humana Human Subjects Committee. Like Barney Clark before him, Schroeder's condition was reported, described, and discussed by the media in a stream of daily reports during the remaining 610 days of his complication-filled postoperative existence attached to a ponderous, refrigerator-sized power source. More operations followed. In February 1985 DeVries implanted a similar device into Murray Haydon. Like the others, Haydon endured sixteen months of strokes, pulmonary insufficiency, and a variety of serious and irreversible infections. The final procedure by DeVries occurred in April; Jack Burcham survived only ten disastrous days. About the same time, Professor Bjarne Semb in Stockholm implanted a Jarvik device in a 53-year-old patient, Leif Stenberg. Although the patient recovered, he died of multiple strokes seven months later.

Regardless of the brave talk from the principals and their respective institutions, it was clear that the patients fared no better in the second stage of development than had any of the calves studied nearly two decades before. Despite protestations of outrage by DeVries, the FDA withdrew support. In an issue devoted to the subject, the *Journal of the American Medical Association* allowed both the enthusiasts and the detractors to make their views known. The surgeon remained enthusiastic: "The total artificial heart is feasible, practical, and durable and offers life to those who would not otherwise be able to continue living. These patients have enjoyed their families, births of grandchildren, marriages of their children, fishing excursions, and even participated in parades, none of which would have been possible without the [device]. It is extremely rare—if ever—that clinical research has been so dramatically successful."[37] Others, however, including a surgeon who had himself implanted a mechanical heart as a bridge-to-transplant, felt differently. "The articles of DeVries define the serious problems that have cast a dark shadow on the currently available pneumatic heart. The suggested solutions seem unlikely to reduce substantially the incidence of complications. Adding patients to this [clinical] series would serve only to document further the magnitude of the complications rather than to demonstrate an acceptable lifestyle in the recipient."[38]

Those involved altered their careers. Kolff continued to invent and was widely acclaimed as the father of artificial organs until his death in 2009. Among his substantial contributions, the dialysis machine continues to sustain many patients throughout the world. Featured on the cover of *Time* magazine in 1984, De Vries settled into a quieter existence in private practice in Louisville. Jarvik went on to develop and refine a series of prototype ventricular assist devices in his company, a departure that was to find increasing application in patients with failing hearts. Until recently, we watched him advertising Lipitor on television.

The type of human experimentation exemplified by the development of the artificial heart opened a series of unresolved questions both within and outside the field. When, for instance, do attempts to salvage a patient slip from the usual, conventional, accepted, or even possible, to the extraordinary, heroic, or futile? When do efforts to prolong life merge with those prolonging death? Do the surgical pioneers involved in this and comparable undertakings throughout history ignore the need for painstaking science and laboratory studies before embarking on clinical attempts? Has enough work been carried out in animal models to justify human use? Moore discussed this situation eloquently a few years later:

> Desperate measures like the interim substitution of a machine heart, or the implantation of [an animal's] heart in man, call up for consideration a special ethical question: Does the presence of a dying patient justify the doctors taking *any* conceivable step regardless of its degree of hopelessness? The answer to this question must be negative. There is simply not evidence to suggest that it would be helpful. It raises false hope for the patient and his family, it calls into discredit all the biomedical science, and it gives the impression that physicians and surgeons are adventurers rather than circumspect persons seeking to help the suffering and dying by the use of hopeful measures. The dying person becomes the object of wildly speculative experiments when he is hopeless and helpless rather than the recipient of discriminating measures carried out in his behalf. It is only by work in the laboratory and cautious trial in the living animal that "hopeless desperate measures" can become ones that carry with them some promise of reasonable assistance to the patient. The interim substitution of a mechanical heart in the chest, in the location of the normal heart, had not reached this stage for the simple reason that animal survival had never been attained.[39]

But progress has continued and numbers have grown as over three hundred surgeons in several countries have attached over 850 single ventricular assist devices directly to the unhealthy heart for use either as a bridge for a cardiac transplant or as a means of allowing the failing organ to recover. Designs of pumps and power sources have improved. Such instruments are now wearable, compact, and powered by relatively small batteries. They function for prolonged periods with reasonable success.

A recent clinical series, for instance, describes the use of left ventricular-assist devices in 133 patients with refractory cardiac failure who would have died without further treatment.[40] One hundred of these eventually received a heart transplant after the device had supported cardiac activity for an average of 180 days. Most went home and lived relatively satisfactory lives while waiting. Although twenty-five of the remaining thirty-three died, function of the failing hearts of several others improved, precluding the need for a new heart. It seems clear that as technology improves, so do the results. A heart that recovers after support by the machine is not just a victory for the individual involved. It saves a transplantable organ for someone else in urgent need.

Whereas the ventricular assist devices have become an increasingly accepted part of the armentarium of many heart surgeons in large centers, the use of a complete artificial heart remains problematic. Like the original Kolff and Jarvik prototype, the current two-pound device replaces the entire diseased heart in an operation that may take seven hours. Unlike the action of the normal organ, where both ventricles contract together, a hydraulic pump directs blood in alternate sequence to the lungs and then to the body. The power source consists of an external battery pack worn around the patient's waist and an internal battery buried in the abdominal wall that can be used for short periods when the patient showers. While such devices have doubled the life expectancy of afflicted patients (about thirty days), their success remains relatively short in duration. At the time of this writing, twelve such artificial hearts have been implanted during an FDA trial that is limited to fifteen.[41] Although technology is always changing, the use of such devices seems limited, at least in the foreseeable future.

— nine —

The Transfer of Organs

Carmen Esperanza was a 17-year-old high school student when she first became ill. She had amassed good grades, played field hockey, was a cheerleader for the football team, and worked as a counselor at a children's camp during vacations. She lived with her parents and two sisters. Her future was bright. In the middle of her junior year, however, she developed increasing fatigue, loss of energy, and diminishing appetite. After some weeks she found that her ankles were swelling and that she couldn't button her skirt. Her urine became dark, and her mother noticed that her eyeballs seemed yellow. Her physician confirmed that she was jaundiced, her liver was enlarged, and fluid filled her abdomen. Liver function tests were highly elevated. Scans showed obstruction of the hepatic veins at the back of the structure, which normally drain blood into the systemic circulation, and a mass of abnormal collateral blood vessels carrying some of the flow around the blockage. The resultant and irreversible failure of the organ was from a relatively rare condition called the Budd-Chiari syndrome. This may present spontaneously at any time during life, but may also occur if abnormalities develop in the process of blood coagulation, when excess red cells produce vascular sludge or clots form to block venous drainage. Young women taking birth control pills are at some risk. As a result of the blockage, the liver becomes increasingly engorged from blood entering it but unable to leave.

With the exception of the skin, the normal liver is the largest organ in the body, filling the upper abdomen and carrying out a broad range of critical activities. It converts the products of digested food into simple sugars, storing and releasing these into the circulation on demand as energy for the body. It synthesizes new proteins, produces factors for normal coagulation of blood, makes cholesterol and bile, neutralizes metabolic wastes, alcohol, and other toxic substances, and destroys aged red cells. It is one of the few organs supplied by both arterial and venous blood. Arising from the aorta, the hepatic artery and its branches carry oxygen and nutrients to the liver cells. The portal vein, receiving the venous effluent from the intestines and other abdominal viscera, provides about three-quarters of the circulation to the organ. After entering the liver, this large channel divides repeatedly into vessels of ever-diminishing size, eventually forming sinusoids, capillary-like channels that run among and between hepatic cells. Their thin walls allow the ready transfer of digested nutrients from the bowel and products of metabolism from body cells out of the blood and into the liver, and efflux of energy-rich material and other intrinsic molecules produced by the organ back into it. The sinusoid network ultimately coalesces into several large hepatic veins that, in turn, empty into the inferior vena cava. Small biliary ductules arise near liver cells, run throughout the organ in parallel with the dense vasculature, and enlarge into channels that ultimately form the common bile duct. This hollow structure, normally as large as one's little finger in diameter and about four inches long, transports bile produced by the liver cells into the duodenum. Via a smaller conduit draining from the mid-portion of the common duct, the gallbladder collects, stores, and concentrates excess bile. When a person eats a hearty meal, the muscular bag contracts and releases its contents into the intestine to help break up and emulsify complex fats from ingested food into structurally simple component parts. After further digestion, these products eventually enter the portal circulation.

Carmen's hitherto pleasant, busy, and predictable life changed dramatically when the doctor told her and her parents that a liver transplant was the only recourse for her ultimately fatal disease. There are three operative choices if a deceased donor is to be considered. An entire liver would be used to replace the failed organ anatomically, a partial liver could be inserted as an auxiliary organ beneath the existing structure in a patient too ill for its removal, or a liver could be split for use in two small recipients, such as children. Alternatively, a segment of liver from a living donor like one of her parents could be transplanted. Carried out primarily in experienced centers, removal of a portion of a normal liver is an extensive and risky operation that is only possible because of the striking regenerative powers of the organ; the reduced mass eventually regrows to normal size in both donor and recipient. Many professionals in the field continue to express concern about the physical risks and ethical implications of performing life-threatening surgery on healthy donors, however. Taking all into consideration, Carmen's family opted for a whole organ from someone who had just died.

Carmen was placed on the national transplant list, a federally funded organization of involved professionals that ensures as even a distribution of available organs throughout the United States as possible. The criteria for optimal sharing have been carefully formulated. Time spent waiting by the potential recipients is carefully monitored in kidney transplantation, as most of the patients can be sustained on dialysis while they wait. In heart and liver transplantation, where there is no backup system, much depends on how sick the patient is. The more serious the threat to life, the higher the position on the list. Carmen's liver functions were declining at a frighteningly rapid pace. She was becoming increasingly incapacitated. Her skin color was deep yellow because the failing liver was unable to metabolize pigments from worn-out red blood cells that spilled into the circulation and were deposited throughout her body tissues. She vomited many of her meals. Her abdomen and legs became massively swollen with fluid. She developed large bruises from clotting deficiencies. She smelled of ammonia because of inadequate metabolism of proteins. Her mind wandered. She slept many hours of the day. Worsening progressively at home, she finally entered the hospital, near death with end-stage disease. The national computer network that ranks potential recipients throughout the country for available organs served Carmen well. Three days after her doctors had placed her at the top of the waiting list, she was matched with a donor of the same blood type. Within hours, she lay in the operating room, anesthetized, prepped, and draped.

The liver came from a young male in a nearby state who had skidded off the road on his motorcycle and hit a tree. He had not been wearing a helmet. He was rushed to a hospital, where the emergency room physicians and a neurologist declared him brain dead. The family granted permission for multiorgan and tissue donation after transplant coordinators from the local organ bank had carefully explained the horrific and irreversible circumstances. Procurement teams arrived to remove and perfuse the heart, lungs, liver, pancreas, intestines, and kidneys. The kidneys were used locally. A group placed the liver in cold solution and drove the one hundred miles to Carmen's hospital. Others flew the remaining organs to chosen recipients at various distant locations. In all, eight patients benefited from the sacrifice of that single donor. Additional persons received his corneas, skin, and bone.

The transplant team was highly experienced with the complex exercise to follow. The stored liver was brought into the operating room in a plastic cooler. The surgeon confirmed all details of both donor and organ, then made a long incision like an inverted V beneath Carmen's ribs, connecting this to a separate midline incision. Placement of retractors exposed widely the contents within. In normal persons, the pale pink colon, shaped like a series of fused pouches, drapes across the upper abdomen. The large, glistening, thick-walled stomach lies beneath. The omentum, a yellow, fatty apron attached to both organs, covers the small intestine. When lifted, one sees the smooth pink loops, rather like a delicate garden hose and half the diameter of the colon, filling the space. Unless enlarged by disease, the spleen, tucked high beneath the left ribs, is barely visible. Only the edge of the liver can be seen beneath the ribs on the right. A normal liver is smooth, firm, and a uniform nutmeg brown, with tiny lobules of cells fitting together like pieces of a mosaic beneath its cellophane-like capsule. In various disease states, in contrast, its color and quality varies markedly. A cirrhotic liver is irregular, shrunken, hard like the sole of a shoe, comprising obvious tan nodules separated by bands of scar. If the patient has severe hepatitis, the organ is flaccid and pale yellow. If there is fatty degeneration from diabetes, obesity, or other causes, it may be swollen and whitish, with collections of fat beneath the surface.

What the surgeons saw in Carmen's abdomen was quite different from the normal contents. All tissues, including the abdominal wall, were stained a deep yellow from bile. Because the venous outflow was blocked, the liver was hugely engorged, dark, and congested. Small collateral vessels, fragile and turgid from rerouting venous blood around the obstructed hepatic veins, were everywhere. Carefully and systematically, the team tied off as many of these delicate channels as possible as they slowly dissected the distended organ from its surroundings. They isolated and divided the portal vein, hepatic artery, and common bile duct, leaving adequate lengths to join to corresponding sites of the donor liver. They had to be particularly gentle dissecting the thin-walled portal vein with its easily torn branches entering it along its course. They then rolled the enlarged organ on its side to control the remaining collaterals and isolate the large affected veins on the back. Although these were completely clotted, the vena cava itself was uninvolved. Blood loss was substantial from cut surfaces and continuously oozing fine collaterals throughout the upper abdomen. In addition, the end-stage liver could not produce clotting factors to reduce bleeding. After they had removed the diseased structure, the size and extent of the resultant empty space in the upper abdomen was startling.

They placed the new liver in position after a separate team had cleared its vessels and bile duct of surrounding fat. Because it had been flushed with cold preservation solution during the ten hours since its removal from the donor, it was soft and pale yellow-brown in color. In sequence, the surgeons joined the donor hepatic veins to the recipient vena cava with fine stitches, then sewed the respective portal veins together. At this point, they released the clamps and allowed the venous blood to circulate. After they connected hepatic arteries of donor and host and restored arterial flow, the organ quickly regained its normal color and tone. It began to secrete bile as they joined the bile ducts. At the same time, the steady loss of blood from all raw surfaces slowed and stopped as the revascularized organ began to produce normal clotting factors. The entire operation took nine hours. After two days in intensive care, Carmen was taken to the surgical floor with the graft functioning nicely. All signs of organ failure had disappeared. Immunosuppressive drugs prevented her body from rejecting the new liver. Her large incision healed. She was discharged ten days later feeling well and returned to school after a further period of convalescence. It has now been eight years since her transplant. Although she remains permanently on low-dose immunosuppression, she lives a normal life, has finished college, and works full-time as a paralegal. She has just become engaged.

The astonishing advances that enabled surgeons to replace Carmen's liver serve as an excellent example of how the understanding and treatment of disease has benefited from laboratory investigations, and vice versa. Each evolved from relatively obscure origins; each has consistently cross-fertilized the other. Experience with animal models encouraged the substitution of healthy organs for failing ones and allowed the field to develop from occasional attempts by surgeons desperate to save their patients to routine practice with a high expectation of success. It has been one of the most remarkable surgical adventures of the twentieth century.

I became caught up in the new subject shortly after I arrived at the Brigham in 1964. This was only a decade after Joseph Murray and his team at that hospital had carried out the world's first kidney transplant between identical twins and only four years after they initially administered a chemical agent to inhibit the immune responses of a recipient of an organ from a genetically dissimilar donor. Despite hopes stemming from the success of subsequent identical twin operations, however, the few centers involved were struggling. In fact, a few months before I arrived, the handful of clinicians and scientists interested in the concept had met at the NIH in Bethesda, Maryland, to summarize existing knowledge. Twenty-five participants from France, Britain, Canada, and the United States attended. The clinical results were disheartening. The entire world experience included 216 nonidentical kidney transplants. By the end of twelve months, only occasional recipients remained alive, supported by their functioning graft.[1]

But when a transplant worked it seemed miraculous. I remember one of the early patients well. Bruce Campbell was forty years old. He was a large, heavily muscled ex-marine whose job as a telephone linesman had been to string heavy wires on poles high above the ground. He had developed kidney failure and required dialysis to survive, an imperfect treatment only sparingly available at the time. In fact, the existing prototype of the "artificial kidney" was unable to clear adequately the metabolic breakdown products from his blood. As a result Mr. Campbell became so weak he was almost completely paralyzed. The huge man lay in bed, helpless and unable even to raise his hands from the sheets. Lacking appropriate family members as potential donors, he was forced to depend upon the possible future death of a stranger who was relatively young and without infection, cancer, or other systemic disease. Such persons were usually victims of trauma. With the concept of brain death not yet a consideration, the team had to delay until the heart stopped before moving ahead with organ retrieval.

Watching someone die is never easy. Watching someone die, then rushing the body to the operating room to remove the kidneys is even more difficult. Eventually, a donor became available for Mr. Campbell. When as much as possible had been done for the patient and after everyone had given up hope, we waited until cardiac motion ceased and the electrocardiogram showed no electrical activity. We then immediately began the process of organ removal. This type of hurried donation, although startling, was leavened by the thought that we were helping someone else to live. Murray transplanted the kidney. I was a junior member of the team, retracting the incision and watching him use an approach he had previously developed in dogs and perfected on bodies in the morgue. The operation went smoothly. Within minutes after he connected the donor and recipient vessels and blood flowed through the organ, it regained its normal pink color and urine began to flow. Because such kidneys may be without circulation for hours, however, a substantial proportion do not function for days after operation. Some never recover. Such new recipients returned to dialysis. They hoped for the sight of urine, but realized that not all the grafts would work. Mr. Campbell was one of the fortunate ones. He improved dramatically as urine flow continued and function normalized over the next few days. His thinking cleared, and his energy and strength returned. To my amazement, he left his bed and began to walk around the ward. The change was so extraordinary that despite all the failures around me, I became a believer.

Like many advances, the concept of transplantation was not new. Indeed, the theme that one part of an individual could replace that of another had been a feature of lore and legend since ancient times. The Egyptians and Phoenicians worshipped gods bearing the heads of animals. In Greek mythology, creatures with attributes of both beasts and humans were plentiful. The horse, Pegasus, flew with bird's wings. Theseus fought and killed the fierce Minotaur with his bull's head and man's body. Satyrs with their goat's legs chased nymphs through classical landscapes. In ancient

Rome, Virgil described his own utopian Arcadia, that peaceful landscape inhabited by the half-boy, half-goat god Pan and other beast-gods. The tradition continues to flourish both in children's tales and in adult literature. A hippogriff, part eagle, part horse, is featured in one of the fictional Harry Potter's recent adventures. The chimera, a combination of goat, lion, and dragon, has become the modern symbol of transplantation.[2]

Early Christians reflected on the benefits of replacement of body parts, but only in the context of miraculous events. Christ restored the ear of a servant of the high priest after an angry Simon Peter had struck it off with his sword. Saint Peter, having witnessed this accomplishment, was later able to replant the breasts of Saint Agatha, pulled off with tongs during torture. Saint Mark replaced a soldier's hand lost in battle. Saints Cosmas and Damian, the fourth-century patron saints of transplantation, substituted the gangrenous leg of a bell-tower custodian with a healthy leg of an Ethiopian, the most famous instance of saintly surgery.[3] In the fifth century, Pope Leo I, tempted by a woman kissing his hand, cut it off. Appearing in a vision, the Virgin Mary restored the hand as a reward for his resisting further temptation. Two centuries later, Saint Anthony of Padua replanted the leg that a young boy had amputated in a fit of remorse after kicking his mother. These and other richly imaginative examples indicate the human psyche's longstanding yearning for the ability to replace diseased or missing parts with healthy ones.

Occasional surgeon-scientists considered transferring tissues from one site to another in the same or different living beings. The several early approaches ranged from the sensible to the absurd. I have discussed the restoration of noses in ancient India, in sixteenth-century Italy, and in World War I. John Hunter's novel observation that the spur of a rooster would grow normally after he had transposed it from its foot to its comb intrigued natural philosophers. He followed this initial experiment with the successful replacement of the first premolar of a patient several hours after it had been knocked from his jaw, then grafted a human tooth into a cock's comb. The ensuing rush by London dentists to transplant teeth in patients was a resultant misadventure that not only exploited the poor as donors but often ended in fatal infections among the recipients. A decade after Hunter's death in 1793, a Milanese surgeon and social activist,

Giuseppe Baronio, published an account of the grafting of skin between individual animals of both the same and different species, noting that those from the subject itself healed and grew hair but those from others did not.[4] These studies encouraged the transfer of healthy skin from an uninvolved site of a patient to cover a raw area too large to be closed primarily; in a well-known case, Sir Astley Cooper used skin from an amputated thumb to cover the open defect. By the end of the nineteenth century, surgeons frequently grafted normal skin from the patient's body to treat open ulcers and nonhealing wounds.

Evolving knowledge of the endocrine system and the success of treating deficient patients with glandular products such as thyroid extract and insulin opened another mercifully short-lived chapter in tissue grafting in the 1910s and 1920s. Over the centuries, interest in the functioning of sex glands has been enlivened by the enduring knowledge that growing old is associated with declining sexual prowess and vitality and the erroneous concept that tissues from youthful individuals might restore energy and slow the aging process. Much of the mystique involved the testis, long a symbol of bravery and vigor. The ancient Greeks and Romans drank extracts of the testis of the wolf as a rejuvenating tonic. The emperor Caligula allegedly sipped draughts of the material during his debaucheries. Seventeenth-century pharmacopoeias contained recipes of preparations from the gonads of a variety of species for similar human use. Even in modern times large animals such as the tiger, rhinoceros, and bear are at risk of extinction because of the reputed aphrodisiacal properties of their glands among some Asian cultures. In the West, cosmetics containing placental extracts are advertised as helping preserve youthfulness.

Toward the end of the nineteenth century an eminent but elderly French neurologist had the idea that individuals who were celibate experienced more intense physical and mental energy than those less sexually continent. Extending this hypothesis, he began to inject himself each day with a potion of gonadal tissues, seminal fluid, and testicular blood from dogs and rabbits, eventually reporting the apparently salubrious results at a professional conference. "Everything that I had not been able to do or had done badly on account of my advanced age I am now able to perform admirably."[5] "Everything" apparently included bladder control, enhanced strength, increased stamina, and improved potency. Although the audience remained appropriately dubious, within months hundreds of physicians throughout Europe were administering these materials to legions of males eager to receive them.

Blind optimism increasingly transcended common sense. The publicity reached the United States and encouraged a more exotic form of glandular restoration, the actual grafting of sex glands. This concept was as ill conceived as had been the transplantation of teeth. In 1916 a surgeon in Chicago reported the benefits of transplanting slices of testis from cadavers into the scrotums of large numbers of hopeful aspirants, including his own. Within a few years the doctor of San Quentin Prison touted the positive effects of implanting testicular tissue into 656 prisoners. The tissue came not only from executed prisoners but from goats, rams, boar, and deer.[6] The numbers swelled with reports from other prisons, particularly Indiana State Penitentiary. In Kansas a surgical quack and owner of a radio station named J. R. Brinkley attracted a huge clientele by grafting glands from goats, an animal known for its sexual proclivities. By 1930 he had reputedly made $12 million from 16,000 clients. Although eventually disbarred by the state medical society for not having an appropriate license, he narrowly lost a subsequent race for governor.

The Europeans were not to be left behind. Ten million soldiers had died in the carnage of World War I. The flu epidemic killed millions more. The loss of nearly a generation of young men and an already declining birth rate pressured older males to seek ways to regain their youthful energies and increase their sexual appetites in hopes of reversing the trend. A Russian surgeon working in Paris, Serge Voronoff, transplanted testes of young animals into prize dogs to improve the breeding stock, into racehorses to increase their speed, and into rams to enhance the production of wool.[7] Because of the apparently successful results, he shifted his emphasis to patients. The demand soon became so great that he opened a monkey colony in North Africa to ensure a ready supply of glands for the vast numbers of men clamoring for treatment. Anecdotal results were striking.

Medical skeptics from many countries, however, increasingly questioned the data. By the late 1920s scientifically objective information about the endocrine system, understanding of the importance of hormone replacement, and dispassionate expert assessment of both the experimental and clinical results of gland grafting put an end to such activities.[8] With the frenetic and irresponsible postwar gaiety of the Jazz Age ending precipitously with the stock market crash in 1929, the entire venture crumbled. Few of the gland grafters were heard from again. While some had considered themselves scientific visionaries, others were unscrupulous entrepreneurs who exploited the desires of aging males. Overall, in the hard light of unprejudiced scrutiny the entire approach was misguided.

Some surgical scientists had more pragmatic goals. As the twentieth century opened, a handful of Continental investigators began to explore the possibilities of organ transplantation in animals and in humans. The kidney seemed an obvious choice for such experiments. One of the pair can be removed without endangering the life of the donor. The blood supply is usually limited to a single artery and vein that can be joined to appropriate vessels at several sites in the recipient. Because the fist-sized, bean-shaped organ filters waste products from the blood and controls fluid balance, measuring the volume and concentration of the urine could determine its function with relative accuracy. The surgeons transferred dog and goat kidneys from their normal location in the flank to the neck using prosthetic tubes and rings to join the vessels. To their delight, they functioned well in their new location. Alexis Carrel used his precise suturing techniques not only to graft kidneys in dogs, but to graft hearts, lungs, and even legs. His mentor in Lyon performed the first two recorded kidney transplants in patients in 1906. Three years later, a surgeon in Berlin unsuccessfully engrafted both kidneys of a monkey to the groin vessels of a 21-year-old seamstress, an attempt stimulated by the emerging knowledge that monkeys and humans have a close genetic relationship.

The behavior of these early transplants confirmed Baronio's earlier impression that grafts from the same animal (*autografts*) or from identical twins (*isografts*) survive indefinitely, whereas those from members of the same species (*allografts*) fail within a week and tissues from other species (*xenografts*) undergo almost immediate destruction. The work of a young Oxford zoologist, Peter Medawar, triggered interest in the new biology with investigations he carried out during the later stages of World War II. Placing skin autografts and allografts on patients, he and a plastic surgeon in Glasgow confirmed that the former healed but the latter became inflamed and were inevitably destroyed after a few days. They subsequently observed that the tempo of destruction of a second graft from the same foreign donor was accelerated. It was this insight that led to the critical conclusion that host immunity mediated the event. After the conflict ended, Medawar refined and expanded his human investigations in beautifully controlled experiments in rabbits, defining *acute rejection*, as he christened the dramatic and powerful inflammatory phenomenon.[9] Medawar received the Nobel Prize in 1960 for findings that introduced the new subject of transplantation biology, an emerging science that led to an explosion of investigative activity into the meaning of the immune system and the function of the cells and tissues that compose it. As part of the bodily defense mechanisms that protect all living organisms from environmental challenges, its intricacies continue to fascinate subsequent generations of basic scientists and practicing physicians alike.

There was little clinical interest in the subject until after the war, when a few surgical investigators in Europe and the United States began to re-examine the possibilities of kidney transplantation. In 1947 three young surgeons at the Peter Bent Brigham Hospital were faced with a young woman dying of acute kidney shutdown following a septic abortion.[10] The professor of medicine suggested that if they could insert a kidney from someone else into her circulation, it might act as a bridge until her own organs could recover. Taking up the challenge, they located a patient who had just died and removed the organ in a side room off the ward, as the hospital administrator forbade them to use an operating room for such a bizarre purpose. Under a sixty-watt goose-necked lamp, they joined the vessels to those at the elbow of the recipient using local anesthesia. With resumption of the circulation, the transferred kidney produced urine and supported her until her own kidneys began to function two days later. They then removed the "bridge" graft and sent her home. She did well initially but died a few months later from hepatitis from a blood transfusion. Despite this patient's misfortune, a piece of the puzzle was in place; a kidney from a stranger could sustain one whose own organs were without function, at least over the short term. Other instances followed. In 1950, for the first and only time in his life, a surgeon in Chicago replaced a woman's failing kidney with one from a deceased donor.[11] To everyone's surprise, the graft functioned long enough to allow the remaining native organ to regain minimal activity. She lived for five more years. Emboldened by the report of this case, a group in Paris placed kidney allografts into eight patients, several from prisoners executed by the guillotine.[12] None excreted urine for more than a few days. About the same time, the Brigham surgeon involved with the original "bridge" graft, David Hume, transplanted cadaver kidneys into nine recipients. Surprisingly, one of these individuals survived for six months.[13] With the possibility that the coincidentally evolving "artificial kidney" machine could support terminally ill patients slowly becoming more realistic, interest in the treatment of end-stage kidney disease increased. In practical terms, however, enthusiasm was muted by the universal rejection of the transplants. At this point no one had considered depressing or inhibiting the patients' immune responses.

This was the state of transplant medicine when one of a set of genetically identical twins was transferred to the Peter Bent Brigham Hospital late in 1954. Richard Herrick was near death from kidney failure. He was convulsing and intermittently in a coma. His referring physician suggested the novel possibility of substituting a normal kidney from his healthy brother, Ronald, for one of Richard's nonfunctioning ones. Although earlier laboratory studies in dogs had implied that autografted kidneys transferred from one site to another failed over time, Murray's ongoing canine experiments provided more optimistic follow-up results. In addition, three times during the prior decade, surgeons had successfully grafted skin between human identical twins, confirming Medawar's findings in rabbits and mice. With these precedents, the stage seemed set. The Brigham team elected to proceed despite expressions of doubt by colleagues. The recipient was given a spinal anesthetic, an unusual approach in those days but used because he was considered too ill to be put to sleep. The donor was anesthetized with ether in an adjacent operating room. All went well until actual removal of the kidney. The surgeon for the donor had clamped and cut the kidney vessels. Suddenly the clamp slipped off the arterial stump at its junction with the aorta. Within moments, blood filled the deep incision. Fortunately, he was able to control the artery with his fingers and sew the open vessel shut once his assistant had suctioned out the blood so he could see. (He changed his technique for subsequent donor operations.) A colleague carried the organ across the hall into the next room. Murray flushed out clots from the artery and the vein and sutured them to the appropriate pelvic vessels of the recipient. Once he had re-established blood flow, he implanted the end of the ureter into the bladder. Except for the early moment of panic, all progressed smoothly. The graft functioned immediately and within days had completely reversed Richard's kidney failure. He returned to total normalcy, married his nurse, and fathered two children before dying nine years later of recurrent disease.[14] Ronald, the donor, pursued a long career as a high school math teacher in Massachusetts and Maine.

The success of this and subsequent transplants between identical twins answered lingering physiological questions. These included the influence of short periods without circulation on immediate urine output, and whether kidneys could behave normally after interruption of their nerve supply. Several female recipients later delivered healthy babies. Children whose growth had been stunted by organ failure grew rapidly after restoration of function. Anemia and defects in blood clotting corrected themselves. Although transplanted kidneys functioned well when no immunological barriers were present, a larger question remained. Faced with a growing number of patients seeking help, could the surgeons expand the benefits of this unique treatment to afflicted persons in the general population who lacked genetically similar donors? Investigators were also beginning to appreciate that a morphologically unprepossessing circulating white blood cell, the lymphocyte, was responsible for the immunological destruction of foreign tissue. The medical and scientific community became further excited by a report from London by Medawar and his colleagues about the indefinite survival of skin allografts in specially prepared mice. The problem was in translating such intriguing laboratory data to clinical applicability. Some type of modification of the host responses was obviously crucial for the successful engraftment of nonidentical donor kidneys. This involved inhibition of lymphocyte activity.

The devastating physical sequelae of the atomic bombs detonated in 1945 in Japan included destruction of all rapidly dividing cells in the body. The associated loss of intrinsic host defenses caused many of those surviving the initial blast to die of uncontrolled infection. Building on this information during the 1950s, investigators in several laboratories in Europe and the United States initiated experiments to study the influence of total body radiation on living cells and to determine the effects on host immunity. With refinements of equipment and techniques to control the dosage, they developed a variety of animal models that not only withstood the exposure but became unresponsive to foreign tissues. To the delight of the researchers, skin and even kidney graft survival could be prolonged. By the end of the decade, investigators in Boston and Paris were beginning to administer sublethal doses of radiation to patients in preparation for a transplant.[15] Despite never rejecting their grafts, however, eighteen of the twenty thus treated died quickly of infection. In contrast, the survival of two patients was unprecedented. One lived normally for twenty-five years supported by his brother's kidney; the other received an organ from his sister and lived for twenty-six years.[16] Similar instances occasionally followed.

The effects of total body X-radiation were so unpredictable and dangerous, however, that this approach was clearly not the answer. In 1959 two physicians from Tufts University in Boston reported that an anticancer drug could inhibit antibody formation in rabbits, the first suggestion that a chemical agent could influence the immune responses.[17] A handful of surgeons became interested, particularly a surgical resident from London who, on the advice of Medawar, arranged to spend a research year in Murray's laboratory. Arriving in New York on the *Queen Mary*, Roy Calne traveled to Boston, picking up some of the agent and several related compounds from chemists at the Burroughs Welcome Company on his way. Although Murray and his colleagues had tried to prolong graft function in dogs without success, one of the new derivatives changed the existing situation dramatically. Increasing numbers of the canine recipients that Calne transplanted survived, supported by their transplanted kidney. Although some of the dogs developed fatal infections, the grafts showed no signs of rejection. In addition, the presence of multitudes of lymphocytes throughout the substance of the foreign tissue, so much a microscopic feature of the rejection response in untreated animals, was minimal.[18] Murray summarized what had happened. "To try to put this breakthrough in perspective, consider our prior experience. For a decade in our laboratory several hundred renal transplants in dogs were performed using a variety of protocols. Our longest survival had been eighteen days. By 1961 we had reported dogs surviving over 150 days with normal function. [They] were not sick or debilitated. They ate well, maintained weight, and resisted kennel infections."[19] One named Mona even delivered a litter of healthy puppies.

It was also clear from the experimental data that the potential of immunosuppression with a chemical agent, in spite of significant toxicity, was superior to the poorly controllable X-radiation treatment. Indeed, the differences were so obvious that Murray and his team began to consider seriously the possibilities of testing the drugs in their patients. They treated the first early in 1961. He lived four weeks. The transplanted kidney supported the second for thirteen weeks. Despite several subsequent deaths, one patient lived over two years. By mid-decade, nine of twenty-seven kidney recipients had survived over a year.[20] About that time Thomas Starzl, a young surgeon from Denver who remained an important principal in the field for the rest of his career, reported substantial improvement in results by adding steroid hormones to the maintenance therapy, and reversing episodes of acute rejection with transient bursts of high doses of the agents.[21] With accruing interest in the possibilities of organ transplantation, additional transplant programs opened in North America, Europe, and Australia. At first half the patients died within a few months, but over time the results improved. For introducing a bold and unique approach to a fatal disease, Murray received the Nobel Prize in 1990.

Increasing understanding of organ failure and improvements in dialysis and postoperative care led to a significant decline in the mortality of transplant recipients during the 1970s. During this same period clinical investigators tested an evolving series of immunosuppressive adjuncts. While generally ineffective, the strategies allowed them to define more accurately the limitations, side effects, and toxicities of the available drugs. Tissue matching of potential donors and recipients became a major laboratory enterprise, as did methods to perfuse and store isolated organs for long-distance transport.

Although changing concepts of donor death and its relationship to organ donation drove the subject forward, it took time before clinicians and scientists began to reconsider the definition and criteria for the end of life. By the 1940s the long-accepted belief that death was synonymous with the absence of cardiac activity became progressively uncertain. The iron lung and subsequent generations of respirators allowed paralyzed patients to breathe, and the pacemaker and defibrillator kept the heart functioning. With these technological advances, the growing possibilities of transplantation and an increasing need for donors stimulated philosophical discussions about the actual meaning of death. Surgeons continued to wait for all cardiac movement to stop before removing the kidneys, but dialogue intensified about the morality of using organs from patients whose brains were irreversibly damaged but whose hearts continued to beat. Ethicists decried the idea. Jurists debated. Criticism about the motives of those involved in transplantation who accepted such donors was rife.

The concept of brain death emerged as a means to use organs from deceased individuals whose vital functions were supported by a machine. Indeed, dramatic news of the first heart transplant late in 1967 caused many to rethink their conception of death. Christiaan Barnard, a surgeon from Capetown, South Africa, had removed the heart from a young woman with massive head trauma and transplanted it into a patient dying of failure of his native organ.[22] Within a day after the operation Louis Washkansky was alert and talking. After two days fluid accumulation and other manifestations of terminal heart disease had disappeared. By eleven days he was out of bed. Although he died of pneumonia on the eighteenth day, the results were unprecedented. It seemed clear from this single experience that the use of brain-dead donors not only could increase the numbers of kidneys for transplantation but could encourage the grafting of other organs. In response to Barnard's operation and pressures by others in the field, the Dean of Harvard Medical School formed a committee in 1968 to examine the issue of "irreversible coma," a state following acute destruction of the brain that two French physiologists had described a decade before.[23] The group of physicians, ethicists, lawyers, and theologians concluded that if stringent criteria of brain death were satisfied and all cognition and central activity were absent, the patient could be considered dead even though circulation and respirations could be artificially maintained. They thought it inappropriate to continue extraordinary means of support without the possibility of donation, and felt that society could ill afford to dispose of healthy organs that might save those needing them.[24] The careful deliberations were convincing. Their guidelines continue to hold true throughout much of the world.

But regardless of the innovations and improvements, the results of transplantation remained relatively unsatisfactory. In 1977, a quarter-century after the first success with identical twins, pooled data from over 9,000 recipients of kidney grafts throughout North America were published. The rate of graft failure was dismal: by the end of the first year, one-third of recipients of living-related donor kidneys and over half those with organs from cadavers had rejected their transplants. Large numbers had died. After five years, the results were considerably worse.[25] Not only was the availability of dialysis inadequate to sustain those who had rejected their grafts, but over-immunosuppression produced serious and sometimes fatal consequences. Patients died of infections from rare organisms that did not affect the population with normal immunity. The side effects of chronic steroids to prevent rejection were difficult to bear, particularly facial changes, obesity, peptic ulcers, easily damaged skin, and a high incidence of bone loss and fractures. It was not an easy time, as few of the "successes" led normal lives.

Cancer was an unexpected complication. Joe Palazola provided the first clue. He received a transplant from a deceased donor in 1964 at the Brigham and was one of the relatively few to thrive. After sixteen months of excellent health and normal activity, he returned with a hard, immovable mass that encased the nicely functioning kidney graft in his lower abdomen. It could not be removed because it included the major vessels and nerves to his leg. To the shock and dismay of all, a biopsy showed lung cancer. Although the pathologists had registered the donor as dying from a primary brain tumor that only spreads locally, on re-examination of the tissues they found a tiny and previously overlooked cancer of the lung that had metastasized to the brain and caused his death. Presumably, the kidney carried a few cancer cells with it into its new host, whose depressed immune responses could not destroy them. The only thing Murray and his group could think to do was to stop the drugs in the hope that Palazola's defenses would recover and fight the tumor. Predictably, he rejected the kidney and returned to dialysis. But at the same time the mass began to shrink. Before the eyes of the incredulous team it became small enough for safe removal. They waited six months, until with trepidation and at the patient's insistence they transplanted a kidney from his mother. Again immunosuppressed, he lived for a further six years before dying from an unrelated cause. The donor cancer never recurred. As other cases were reported, it became clear that a variety of neoplasms develop more commonly in the compromised graft recipients than in the general population.[26]

The increased incidence of cancer and the occasional regression of a malignancy after withdrawal of suppressive treatment kindled basic questions about the function of the immune system. Populations of rapidly dividing cells reside in various sites throughout the body, replacing identical ones that age and die. Although the vast majority divide and proliferate normally, occasional genetic errors may occur. A single aberrant cell, for instance, may replicate or clone itself over and over, eventually forming a tumor. The intrinsic host defenses may have developed in part as a "surveillance" mechanism to identify and eliminate abnormal cells that may become cancerous. This intriguing possibility is supported by the relatively high incidence of cancer at the two extremes of life when these defenses are weakest; they are immature in infants and worn out in the elderly. Those in the middle years whose immunity is depressed by immunosuppressive medication, exposure to radiation, or other environmental factors are at similar risk. While the theory remains unproven, the argument seems reasonable.

The immune apparatus is an important part of the spectrum of host responses that have evolved to protect us from an alien environment beset with the potential for injury, infection, perhaps tumor formation, and other threats to life. The lymphoid tissues, primarily responsible for immune-system function, contain lymphocytes, small, round, nondescript white blood cells that circulate in the blood or reside predominantly in spleen, lymph nodes, and gut. In bulk, this "lymphoid organ" is of considerable size. The body's defenses developed early in evolution and have achieved considerable functional sophistication in higher animals. Even plants show some reaction to foreign stimuli. One can graft, for instance, various types of pears to a pear tree, but not apples. Primitive organisms such as worms can reject foreign substances slowly via the activity of a predominant blood cell. Lower marine vertebrates produce crude antibodies. Cartilaginous and bony fish, higher up the evolutionary scale, can reject skin grafts via discrete cell populations, and birds are the first vertebrates to produce distinct classes of antibody. Mammals can activate remarkably specific immunologic responses against foreign invaders, orchestrated by lymphocytes.

During the 1970s and 1980s transplant biologists made much progress in unraveling the complexities of host immunity. Having realized that lymphocytes are responsible for graft destruction, they found that two different classes of the cells were involved. A long-lived, continuously recirculating *T cell* population derived via the thymus gland mediates the actual destruction of foreign tissue. Sessile, noncirculating, antibody-producing B *cells* originate in the bone marrow and are found primarily in the spleen and lymph nodes. Having discovered the separate origins of these groups, investigators detected subpopulations with even more discrete functions and interactions, and identified a plethora of specific cell products orchestrating the rejection event. In more recent years they have defined the intricate molecular interactions arising between the lymphocyte and the allograft that lead to graft death, and devised how to block such interactions with highly selective cloned proteins. New understanding of this precise and intricate biology has burgeoned. It has been an exciting time.

Mediocre clinical results during the 1960s and 1970s proved no obstacle to the swelling roster of patients with end-stage kidney disease, who recognized the possibilities of help. A few pioneering surgeons also began to transplant hearts, livers, and lungs, first in large animals and then in patients. One research group in particular toiled diligently and carefully to place heart transplantation on a scientific footing. Norman Shumway and his colleagues at Stanford developed effective operative strategies and reported in 1965 that occasional animal recipients survived in satisfactory condition for months.[27] In contrast to the experimental advances, however, the initial forays into heart transplantation in humans were uniformly disastrous. Barnard had scooped the world with his first heart transplant. Within days he and two surgeons in the United States had performed four more. Another transplanted the heart of a chimpanzee into a human. With the exception of the South African's second case, no one survived more than a few days. Despite these generally appalling results, the enthusiasm of the surgeons, unrelenting hyperbole from the global media, and public excitement catapulted the subject to illusory heights.

A few clinician-scientists understood the intricacies of transplanting genetically foreign tissues and the virtual inevitability of rejection, but the majority of cardiac surgeons climbing on the bandwagon appreciated neither the power of the host responses nor the toxicities of the immunosuppressive drugs they had to use. They remained confident that technical expertise could transcend such theoretical matters. By 1969 over one hundred patients had received hearts; sixty-four new teams forming in twenty-two countries performed many more. Few recipients survived over six months. The situation became so difficult that the heads of several programs called for a moratorium on the procedure until the science had advanced.[28] Activity in heart transplantation halted nearly everywhere. Almost lost in the gloom were a handful of heart recipients who lived relatively satisfactory lives and stimulated occasional thoughtful enthusiasts like the Stanford investigators to continue their efforts.

Unexpectedly, compelling new information arose. The publication of a pair of short papers in November 1978 galvanized the attention of those struggling in the field. In one, a London group reported successful transplantation of bone marrow.[29] In the other, Calne and his colleagues at Cambridge University described the unprecedented survival of organ allografts in patients, including kidneys, pancreases, and livers.[30] Both

groups of investigators had treated the recipients with a unique immunosuppressive drug, Cyclosporin A. But as exciting as these findings
were, this agent had a difficult gestation. Field botanists from Sandoz
(now Novartis), a giant Swiss pharmaceutical house, had found a novel
strain of fungus on a highland plateau in Norway and in a valley in
Wisconsin. Company biologists isolated and tested a crude extract of
the primitive plant for antibiotic activity. The results were unexciting.
Because such compounds occasionally show characteristics different from
those expected, however, the laboratory supervisor assigned Jean Borel, a
young scientist who had joined the company three years before, to screen
the material for other pharmacological properties. He, in turn, noted that
one of the fractions of the extract was markedly immunosuppressive both
in the test tube and in mice. Indeed, its striking effectiveness soon piqued
the interest of colleagues interested in transplantation.[31]

Impressed by the potency and apparent lack of toxicity of the fungal
extract, Borel pushed ahead with his researches despite persistent executive doubts about their ultimate importance. As experimental data accumulated, he and others working with the compound found that it selectively
affected the T cells, the principal lymphocyte population responsible for
graft rejection, and that its specific inhibition of precise steps of cell acti-
vation and function contrasted with the few other available drugs that
indiscriminately destroyed all rapidly dividing cells. One of the research
fellows working in Calne's surgical laboratory in Cambridge heard Borel
present his data. Intrigued, he obtained a small amount of the fungal
extract to try in animal models. Learning to use it was tricky because
the powder would only dissolve in oil, not water, and was difficult to
administer. How much to give and for how long were other questions to
be answered. Within weeks, however, he and his fellow researchers noted
the unprecedented prolongation of skin and organ grafts in mice, rats,
and rabbits. With mounting excitement, they also found it to be effective in dogs, pigs, and primates. Investigators at Oxford, in our research
laboratory at Harvard, at the University of Minnesota, and then at other
institutions soon produced comparable data. The early results in the small
numbers of patients receiving the agent were equally compelling.

The news traveled rapidly throughout the international transplant community as growing experimental and clinical results confirmed the initial impressions. Only months after the first publications appeared, the halls of the major transplantation congress in Rome in 1978 were abuzz with conversation about the new agent. Lecture rooms overflowed during the few presentations on the subject. Other units in Europe, the United States, and Australia initiated clinical series. Two important controlled trials, one in Canada and one in Europe, enrolled hundreds of recipients.[32] By 1983, the data showed an increase in one-year kidney function compared to conventional therapy, from 50 percent to 70 percent.[33] The results of liver and heart transplantation also improved. Enthusiastic clinicians began to accept patients for transplantation whom they hitherto would not have considered, increasing both the number of organs grafted and persons demanding them. The discovery and introduction of Cyclosporin A were bellwether events for the emerging discipline.

But few drugs are without side effects, and this one was no exception. Calne quickly discovered what was to become a significant and unanticipated hurdle, the profound ability of the material to depress kidney function in humans but, curiously, not in animals. All of us testing it during that early period administered considerably higher amounts than are given today. Discovering the most advantageous treatment strategy took time. Eventually we improved the state of the recipients by dose reduction, standardization of serum concentrations, understanding the influence of other pharmaceuticals on its activity and toxicity, and conversion to different immunosuppressive medication. I remember two of our early patients vividly. One put out no urine for one hundred days after his transplant, the other for fifty-seven days. With repeat biopsies of the grafts showing no evidence of rejection, all of us waited helplessly. Finally, in desperation, we stopped Cyclosporin A and substituted the older drug we had used for years, a step far from standard practice at the time. Within twenty-four hours, both individuals began to excrete large amounts of urine. Kidney function returned to normal, and they were discharged. This unheard-of phenomenon gave us much to consider.

Thanks to the effectiveness of the new drug, transplantation became a routine treatment for patients with failure of a variety of organs. The introduction of a newer generation of immunosuppressive agents during the 1990s, each with a unique and selective activity on the immune responses, has improved the early success rates of most organ transplants to around 90 percent. Numbers of grafted patients have increased progressively in response. By the end of 2004, for instance, organ transplants were sustaining over 150,000 persons in the United States alone, many of whom live normal lives.[34] At present, about 20,000 organs are transplanted in the United States each year, a comparable number in Europe, and many thousands in other areas of the world. Considering the short history of the subject, its complexities, the still incompletely defined biology of the host responses, and the toxicities of ever-increasing choices of medications to sustain the grafts, the current record is striking.

The future of the field may be even more interesting than its past. It is likely that chemical immunosuppression will remain necessary for some time, although highly specific biological agents that interfere precisely with discrete steps of the host immune responses are increasing in number and effectiveness. Other innovative approaches are under continuing investigation. The concept of "immunologic tolerance," in which the recipient is manipulated in such a way that he cannot react against the specific foreign tissue but may respond normally to all other environmental stimuli, has been a subject of fascination for scientists since Medawar and his colleagues introduced it in the 1950s. Hints as to its possible clinical application continue to arise. It is unlikely that substantial advances are imminent in the use of organs from nonhuman species, although techniques to allow failing livers in patients to recover by transient periods of cross-circulation with a pig liver are being examined.

The inadequate number of donor organs available to meet increasing patient demands has provoked alternative strategies to salvaging failing organs. Because of its striking regenerative capacities and relatively homogeneous structure, the liver has received much attention. One intriguing experimental approach to limit this serious deficiency is to repopulate the diseased liver of a given patient with large numbers of healthy, functioning cells isolated from a biopsy specimen, then cultured in the test tube. Because these cells are from the individual herself, no immunosuppression is needed. Alternately, it may eventually be possible to remove from culture the most immunologically reactive cells from the liver of a deceased donor. After proliferation into large numbers, those remaining may evoke only a weak host response, decreasing the need for or dosage of maintenance medication. Not only could this inactive but well-functioning population help a single diseased organ to recover, it could be expanded for use in several patients, increasing the overall supply of donor livers for actual transplantation. Engineered tissues are also under investigation. Pieces of cultured cartilage and bone are already in use. Artificial skin increasingly covers large burns. Portions of liver, small bowel, bladder, and arteries have all been grown to significant size from appropriate cells on absorbable and biodegradable scaffolds. Engineered preparations of pancreatic islets have been transplanted into experimental models with some success, although inadequate numbers of these cells may limit their general use.

Despite its successes and a bright future, however, the field of transplantation is facing difficult and unexpected challenges. Like many other aspects of human endeavor, the results of a superficially simple idea, the desire for new knowledge, a substantive advance, or an encouraging early laboratory finding are almost invariably more complex than envisioned. With the clinical practice and its associated biologies spreading more widely over the globe and new scientific and medical knowledge perturbing established dogma and custom, theoretical, practical, and ethical issues are arising that are increasingly difficult to solve.

The patients are the most important consideration. Beset with a potentially fatal disease that they must deal with for the rest of their lives, they seek whatever help is available. Insufficient numbers of organs to meet the steadily rising demand, too much disappointment, sometimes inadequate health insurance, and the importance of the "bottom line" are all taking their toll. Although transplantation has become routine in the developed world regardless of these difficulties, engraftment of the kidney in particular remains a monumental challenge in developing countries, where failure of that organ is high, the medical and social infrastructures barely support such endeavors, laboratory facilities are inadequate, intensive care units do not exist, dialysis is rudimentary or unavailable, and expensive immunosuppressive drugs are not affordable. Many people die without relief.

Indeed, the possibilities of helping more than a relatively small percentage of patients seem overwhelming. That small percentage often includes the rich, important, and well connected who may exploit a widespread, clandestine, and underground commerce in organs sold by impoverished donors. There have been critical advances in encouraging altruistic donation and in making organ sales and transplant tourism illegal, but the problem is virtually impossible to eradicate. Individuals who can afford to buy an organ from someone desperate enough to sell find routes around accepted and acceptable behavior. Cynically abetted by commercial interests, by unscrupulous middlemen, and sometimes by the governments themselves, the rich continue to prey upon the destitute for their body parts.

Such irregularities have attracted international attention. Although denounced by the vast majority of practitioners, censured by public aversion, and forbidden by international law, this highly lucrative global traffic in human parts remains an unsolved problem. Simple necessity provides the driving force for individuals in desperate financial straits to sell parts of their bodies to those who can afford them. For instance, unscrupulous surgeons have performed thousands of kidney transplants using organs that the rich and powerful buy from the poor of countries such as India, Pakistan, Egypt, the Philippines, Turkey, less solvent nations in central Europe, and other areas.[35] While the brokers make large profits, the donors remain in financial and physical distress despite the transient infusion of cash. The removal and use of organs from the dead is a further extension of what has become a worldwide industry. The sale of body parts from executed prisoners in China is perhaps the most extreme example of this type of commerce.[36] It has been estimated that the majority of the ten thousand or more organs transplanted in that country each year were obtained from the four- to six-thousand prisoners executed for a variety of crimes. Foreigners from developed countries who can pay the high fees are the beneficiaries. Although the government officially denies the practice of "transplant tourism," these arrangements produce substantial financial rewards not only for hospitals and officials but for the state as well.

It should be noted, however, that professional societies, the World Health Organization, government bodies, international pressures, and recent reforms have curtailed at least some of this human trafficking, although it is doubtful whether it will ever stop completely. Perhaps we should not be surprised that the use of human organs as market commodities, a practice described as "neo-cannibalism," is little different from the activities carried out by the resurrectionists to supply the schools of anatomy nearly two centuries ago.[37]

Current transplant professionals are also enduring a variety of challenges. Numbers of surgical trainees entering the discipline may be declining. Some of those remaining are interested primarily in the complexities of grafting organs such as the liver. Others are frustrated by the difficulties of pursuing parallel academic clinical and research careers. The intellectual stimulation of the field, present since its inception, has for many been replaced by overwork, over-regulation, micromanagement, and the dullness of routine. Surgeons trying to solve difficult patient-related demands carry out long and complex operations, then confront unscheduled periods spent in organ retrieval, repair of dialysis access, acute changes in patient status, and the like. They may become drained by the exigencies of the extremely ill, the relative youth of many with organ failure, the inevitable complications, infections, and drug toxicities. Amidst all the optimism and progressive improvements, there are dark shadows.

As I will discuss in subsequent chapters, some of these shadows are endemic to surgery. It is also clear, however, that many talented individuals remain dedicated to their careers in transplantation and delighted to see their patients living relatively normal lives, sometimes many years later. The biology of the subject is fast moving and stimulating, with advances of potential relevance for patients appearing at an accelerating pace and results progressively improving. Overall, the successful replacement of failing organs with healthy ones has changed the purview of scientific research and clinical practice in one of the most remarkable advances in the history of medicine.

ten

Making a Surgeon, Then and Now

Young doctors entering a surgical career soon learn that they have become part of an evolving system in which much of the care they will deliver and many of the operations they will master were developed during their lifetimes, were in their infancy for their parents, and were nonexistent for their grandparents. Indeed, their grandchildren may one day express incredulity about the primitive nature of the strategies and approaches now regarded as state of the art. Less likely to change are both surgeons' and patients' expectations that any given procedure will enhance or prolong life. They expect excellent results, minimal complications, and fast, relatively painless convalescence. Despite the challenges facing the current field and those who practice in it, its appeal for committed individuals has remained substantial.

Mrs. Turner's granddaughter would have found me at the hospital in 1965 during an early phase of my training. The appointment to that highly regarded surgical program had not come easily. I still vividly remember my initial interview-examination three years earlier. I had traveled to Boston from Cornell University Medical College in New York City in an attempt to gain a place as a Brigham intern. If I was accepted and performed well, an invitation to become a resident might follow. The next morning I sat in the hospital amphitheater among a hundred or so fellow medical students from around the country competing for the six available spots. We gazed at the portraits of past professors lining the walls, considered their contributions, and began to sense the history of the place. After introductory talks about the institution and the department, members of the surgical staff passed out blue books for an hour-long written test. One of the essay questions, I recall, concerned a recent amendment to the Hill-Burton Act that authorized financial assistance to public and nonprofit medical facilities and provided free care to some patients. Although a lifeline for teaching hospitals in the days before Medicare, it was a complete mystery to me. Years later, I discovered that no one read our essays and that the examiners had organized the process to settle us all down for the oral sessions to follow. None of us, needless to say, appeared particularly settled.

In due course I sat at one end of a long table facing half a dozen of the faculty, some of whom looked as if they had stepped out of the portraits. Many of the questions put to me seemed appallingly obscure. One individual asked me to identify what clinical syndrome Henry James had described in his novella, *The Turn of the Screw*. Although I had majored in the humanities as an undergraduate, I was unfamiliar with the story, and thus with the malady–which turned out to be a form of epilepsy. It gradually occurred to me that the object of the exercise was to see how applicants such as myself would respond to stress. I did not realize it, but stress techniques were in vogue at the time. One admissions officer at Harvard Medical School, a psychiatrist, was well known for his methods. In the midst of the discussion, he would ask the interviewee to open the window. Struggle as he might (nearly everyone was a "he" in those days), the victim could not budge it; it was nailed shut. Requesting the subject to move his chair closer to the desk was another ploy. Again, the victim could not move it; it was fastened to the floor.

Fortunately, times have changed. When interviewing applicants for medical school and for residencies, we are now instructed to be nonconfrontational and to make the interaction a pleasant experience. From what we read in the letters we receive afterward, kindness is appreciated regardless of outcome. Back in 1962, however, nerves of steel would have been helpful. As the day progressed, those of us culled after the first round were thanked and invited to leave. Others endured a second, and some a third examination by other committees. The survivors eventually met with the chief of surgery, who picked the final six for the next class. Not having made even the first cut, I returned to New York unsurprised about my vanished prospects.

Until World War II three-quarters of those graduating from medical school served a year of internship and then entered general practice.[1]

Individuals wishing to pursue specialty practices assisted the few established experts for relatively short periods or took available postgraduate courses in their chosen subject. The relatively small numbers of new doctors who sought formal residencies in the programs modeled upon the plan instituted at the Johns Hopkins Hospital in the 1890s applied directly to the chiefs of individual departments. Halsted, for example, favored the best medical students from Hopkins. He accepted Harvey Cushing, a Harvard Medical School graduate and intern at the MGH, only after considerable procrastination and prolonged discussion.

For the first half of the twentieth century no applicant dared to present himself if burdened with qualities that Halsted, Cushing, and other early departmental chairmen felt were inconsistent with the conventional surgical image. Left-handedness was one such enduring bias. It reputedly (but incorrectly) precluded the effective use of standard instruments. Marriage was deemed incompatible with the total commitment to surgical training. A social life was certainly considered unimportant. My older brother walked through the doors of the Brigham as an intern on July 1, 1942, and did not leave the building until October. The regimen was worse at Johns Hopkins, where interns stayed on call throughout the entire year, never venturing outside the institutional walls. And they had to pay tuition for the privilege! Not surprisingly, many male residents married late and married nurses, the women they saw most often. The high divorce rate among doctors of both genders persists to this day.

With professional standards or certifications of competency being virtually nonexistent, one of the first tasks for the Hopkins faculty was to design and organize a residency system for individuals desirous of pursuing well-defined academic careers. These initial efforts to advance medical education and produce guiding principles in patient care were to become the fifth revolution in surgery. It was a long and competitive process. After completing eight years of training, for instance, one of Halsted's residents timidly asked the professor if the time was ripe for him to leave and enter practice. The chief quickly queried, what was his hurry?[2] Even among this small and select group of trainees, there was no guarantee of moving upward; they could serve indefinite periods as assistant to the professor until a satisfactory position became available.[3] Perhaps as a result, Halsted only graduated seventeen chief residents throughout his entire career.

While such a system still exists in European countries such as Germany, a "pyramid" system evolved in the United States in which the weaker individuals originally accepted into a given surgical program would not be invited to return the following year and would have to seek positions elsewhere. At the end of six or seven years the most favored would spend the final twelve months as chief resident and top of the list for a faculty appointment in either his own or another teaching institution. I remember the moment I discovered that of the sixteen interns beginning surgery at my teaching hospital, only one would eventually attain that exalted rank. During the 1980s most university-affiliated programs shifted to a more compact "rectangular" arrangement without such a built-in attrition rate.

The trend toward specialization accelerated in the years after World War II in parallel with the growth of biomedical research. Those entering general practice coincidentally declined in number, and the status and relative financial reward of careers in general practice declined as well.[4] In 1940 full-time specialists comprised only 24 percent of the total physician pool. By the mid-1960s, the number had increased to 69 percent.[5] In response to the influx of surgical trainees returning from military duty and seeking expertise in fields including orthopedics, urology, cardiac surgery, neurosurgery, or pediatric surgery, teaching hospitals throughout the United States increased substantially the number of residencies in all specialties. Between 1940 and 1947, for instance, these specialty positions grew from 5,000 to 12,000. By 1955, 25,000 slots had opened.[6] After professional societies formally assessed manpower requirements during the 1970s, however, numbers of available places leveled off, despite continuing pressure from both American and foreign medical graduates. One result of producing too many well-qualified and highly skilled young professionals during those years was that a significant proportion entered community hospitals and competed directly with their teachers in university settings.

Even with its stringent commitments and challenges, the medical profession was a favorite career choice of undergraduates for nearly four decades after the end of World War II because of its prestige, autonomy, job satisfaction, and associated scientific knowledge. One-third of my college classmates in the late 1950s pursued a premedical curriculum. The demographics were predictable. Students, the residents in training ahead of us, and the professors themselves were almost invariably white and male. Although some medical schools accepted the occasional outstanding female student and a handful of establishments were dedicated to that gender, the mindset prevailed that medicine wasn't proper for a young woman and that investment in her education would be wasted when she married and started a family. The few African Americans who became doctors attended the few institutions created exclusively for them, formed in the late nineteenth century. The College of Medicine at Howard University and Meharry Medical College were the first. Surgery may have been the most resistant of the medical disciplines to societal shifts. Although there was no explicitly stated barrier, the Brigham's department of surgery did not accept its first black or woman resident until the early 1970s.

Jews, Catholics, and some other groups also faced rigid quotas. Medical schools in the 1940s accepted only one in thirteen Jewish applicants compared to three of every four non-Jews.[7] Jewish and Catholic private hospitals rarely affiliated with local medical schools. Mount Sinai Hospital in New York, for instance, opened in 1852 to care for the Jewish community. Of distinguished clinical reputation, it did not form its own medical school for a century. St. Elizabeth's Hospital opened in 1868 to serve Irish and Italian domestic servants from Boston's South End but did not become a teaching hospital for Tufts University Medical School for over fifty years. Not atypical of other established centers, no Catholics served on the MGH's surgical faculty until after World War II.

Medical students initially applied to teaching hospitals within a reasonable train ride of their institutions. But as air travel became more ubiquitous and convenient, the possibilities of seeking residencies in distant regions broadened. However, logistical problems sometimes emerged. Each hospital had its own schedule of interviews and of sending out acceptances and rejections. The Boston programs, for instance, haughtily delayed their appointments until all others in the country had committed themselves, putting aspirants seeking a place in hospitals in that city in a precarious position. Finally, between 1951 and 1952 an association of medical schools and hospitals organized a uniform national scheme to match hospitals and applicants.

Programs still vary in quality. Just as the admissions committees of the most prestigious medical schools accept the bulk of their applicants from a spectrum of top-tier colleges, faculties in the most desirable teaching hospitals primarily fill their residencies with those from highly rated medical schools. Other academic institutions remain more regional in their scope and expectations, turning out practitioners who usually remain in the local area. Among the hundreds of teaching programs in the United States that accept residents, many are large community hospitals unaffiliated with a medical school.

The first steps in applying for postgraduate training have changed little since my classmates and I experienced them and since teaching hospitals first organized themselves on the Hopkins model. Medical students complete a standard application that includes their academic records, letters of recommendation, and personal statements of intent, and send it to the residency programs they favor. Each department invites those applicants it considers most promising for scheduled interviews. These remain relatively formal affairs, although virtually all training programs dropped actual examinations in the 1970s. Both students and program directors then rank their choices in order and submit them to a national computer center that as closely as possible synchronizes the aspirations of the applicant with the selections of each department. The results of "the match" on "Match Day" are revealed simultaneously across the country in mid-March. Medical schools have ritualized the event. Envelopes are laid out in the dean's conference room, and with varying degrees of apprehension, students open theirs to learn where they will spend the next several years and what their career paths may be. Pandemonium ensues. When I opened my envelope in 1962, I learned, hardly to my surprise, that I had not won one of the coveted six training positions at the Brigham. My next choice was a large teaching hospital in Chicago that had chosen me as well. I had applied to medical school in New York to experience a new city after receiving the bulk of my education in

Massachusetts, and here was a chance to familiarize myself with a city in the Midwest.

In 1964 I applied again for surgical training at the Brigham. With many of the more senior residents throughout the country being called into the military, spaces in the various programs were in flux. I had assistance this time from the longstanding Old Boy network. An elderly ex-Harvard oarsman, knowing of the accomplishments of the varsity crew I had captained in college, put in a good word to his doctor, Francis Moore, the chief of surgery. "The boy," he puffed, "is all right." It worked.

Like everyone else training in surgery during much of the twentieth century I entered a structure that Halsted had introduced seven decades before: at a minimum, it entailed a year of internship, two years as a junior resident, then two more years as a senior resident. One or two outstanding individuals in the senior group would be invited to spend their final year as chief resident or spend time in a research laboratory. Increasingly, residents spend additional years in specialist training. As an example of the enduring nature of this form of educational apprenticeship, Moore recalled that when he began in the 1930s, the new interns were called "pups."[8] Their primary responsibility was to test the urine and feces of the patients for any abnormalities each morning at six o'clock. The senior residents would occasionally put a drop of blood on a stool sample or a pinch of sugar, bile, or protein in a tube of urine. Those who missed the decoy would hear of it! During rounds, a tour of the patients led by the chief resident or an attending surgeon, the pups had to walk three paces behind the junior residents, who in turn trailed the seniors. Both Mrs. Turner and Mr. Costello would have recognized the hierarchy instantly.

Perhaps more structured and tightly organized than training programs in community hospitals, the system of graded responsibility in teaching institutions remains firmly in place. As did their predecessors, current interns spend two-month rotations on the general surgical services, anesthesia, the intensive care unit, and a variety of subspecialties. They remain responsible for all details of individual patients from admission through operation and discharge, supervised and instructed by the senior residents assigned to each unit. They assist in simple procedures with the staff surgeons, where they attain basic skills. They master their surgical craft in a well-established manner, opening and closing incisions, dissecting along anatomical planes, tying knots, and joining structures together. Learning and maturing as they climb, the junior residents care for sicker patients than the interns and act as second assistants on more complex heart and lung operations, extensive cancer resections, and organ transplants. By their fourth and fifth years, the senior residents have become relatively autonomous in patient care. As their technical skills advance and with growing expertise in minimally invasive techniques, they are allowed to perform increasingly intricate maneuvers commensurate with their level of experience and always under the gaze and assistance of the responsible faculty member. Competent to perform a range of operations and qualified to take their Surgical Boards by the end of their residency, their five- to eight-year apprenticeship is complete.

The surgeons on the hospital faculty admitted the majority of the private patients, having seen them in their offices usually via referrals from other doctors within the institution or in the community. Having given a tentative diagnosis, they would book an individual into the hospital, where the interns or junior residents would carry out the workup. Patients with simpler conditions came in the day before their operation. Those with more complicated problems needing additional assessment, such as cardiac evaluation or arteriography, arrived several days ahead. Those of us on the house staff, the interns and the residents, learned well both the natural history of disease and the indications for operative intervention. Early each morning we wrote orders for medication, infusions, diet, and activity for the twenty or so individuals for whom we were responsible. The nurses carried out these orders during the day. We drew blood for testing and started intravenous drips. We checked our few charges in the intensive care unit where, in addition to standard management, we were expected to understand all the monitoring devices, adjust mechanical ventilators (breathing machines), and take and interpret electrocardiograms. We then retrieved the X-rays for the day's operations and met the first patient in the operating room before eight o'clock. After assisting with the surgeries and writing the operative notes and postoperative orders, we returned to the wards, where we collected and transcribed individual laboratory results into the patient records and memorized the details in time for afternoon rounds, often with the attending surgeon present. If the fluid balance or electrolyte concentrations of a given patient were not perfect, those in senior positions demanded prompt explanations. The constant exchange of information up and down the chain of command kept mistakes to a minimum. Today, transparency of practice has increased even from those high standards, with results made available to third-party payers and to the public. Gradually, the physical and physiologic mysteries that many patients posed became clear.

At the end of the afternoon, the residents and medical students assigned to a particular rotation made "work rounds," tending to unresolved problems and planning for the next day. Those who were "off" went home, usually well into the evening. Those "on call" every other night and every other weekend worked up the new patients, discussed the operation with them, received written consent to proceed, and ordered laboratory tests and X-rays. We learned the most at night, when we were nominally in charge. Our tasks included isolating arteries and veins and inserting lines, placing catheters in bladders and stomachs, and introducing breathing tubes into the windpipe of patients in extremis. Not infrequently we assisted on or were assisted on emergency operations. We stayed up all night with the ill, then, without a break, reported for morning rounds and spent the next day assisting in surgery.

Chief residents in many teaching hospitals throughout the United States were assigned as junior staff members in charge of the "Ward Service," care for indigent patients who came from the emergency room and from the resident-run surgical clinic. Chief residents and their teams ran their own services, orchestrated the workup, performed the operations, and assumed full responsibility for patients long after discharge. If the team had a problem it couldn't solve, they called an appropriate attending surgeon for help. The patients and the house staff liked and respected each other. The quality of care was excellent. The follow-up was thorough. The trainees experienced a broad spectrum of surgical disease among those in the open wards awaiting their procedures or recuperating from them. An individual recovering from ulcer surgery or excision of a portion of large intestine lay in the next bed to one operated on for thyroid disease. In an adjacent room an individual with jaundice awaited removal of gallstones. Nearby might have been a person in traction for a broken leg. Bottles sat on the floor under many of the beds, collecting urine, bile, or bloody fluid. Persons of different ethnic groups, races, and religions were thrown together in their desire to get well. Outside societal discord was forgotten. The experience for everyone involved—the ill, the doctors, and the nurses—was unique. The clinical and administrative responsibility afforded to the chief resident and his group put the final polish on years of training. Changes in health-care delivery that evolved during the 1980s gradually eliminated chief residents' service in this capacity, however.

Nurses were integral to the success of the house staff, particularly in our early years. Trained primarily at the hospital's nursing school, they were an experienced and capable group who delivered hands-on attention, comfort, food, and pain relief to their patients. Many spent their careers in specialized units. This was a halcyon time for the nursing profession, before their responsibilities shifted from traditional patient care to the completion of forms, interpretation of computer screens, and relegation of their clinical roles to aides. Intimidating to the neophyte house officer, nurses were a source of important advice in the support and treatment of complicated cases. Residents who acted in a haughty or superior fashion learned to regret it.

In addition to gaining practical experience on the wards and in the operating room, the head of the department and his surgical faculty made sure residents received formal education. On a weekly basis we attended Grand Rounds, where experts reviewed clinical subjects in detail, and various specialty rounds, where less general topics were discussed. The Morbidity/Mortality Conference was a particularly important aspect of our learning process, a tradition of the academic curriculum for a century and now required in all hospitals by credentialing bodies since the 1980s. As nonpunitive peer reviews of surgical failures, deaths, and errors, they were an unforgettable means of improving patient care, sometimes leading to important changes in overall policy. We residents would listen, sometimes with glee, as the chief interrogated the individual responsible for the patient, going through the case and discussing what had gone wrong and what could be learned. As part of the process, the pathologist would bring in the diseased organ or show relevant slides. As diagnosis was not as certain before the advent of modern imaging techniques, we picked up many hints concerning disease presentation and recognition of symptoms and signs. These important closed sessions for the faculty and the house staff remain a dynamic form of self-regulation.

The individual officiating at the hour-long Chief's Rounds, usually the department chair, chose residents in turn to present interesting summaries of certain patients. With the group standing around the bedside, he would listen, examine the patient, then spend what seemed like an eternity questioning the presenter closely about various aspects of the disease, its complications, and its treatment. The range of subjects was wide. If a person was recovering from an open-heart operation, a still relatively infrequent procedure, the chief would ask about details of the heart-lung bypass machine. If another had sustained a large burn, the resident had to know the intricacies of water and salt metabolism, the significance of fluid shifts after acute injury, and plans for future care. If the patient was on a respirator, queries about the design of the device, pulmonary management, and oxygen concentrations would tumble out. Woe unto those who were uninformed! These sustained efforts instilled enduring medical precepts and required total responsibility for all aspects of patient care. They were lifelong lessons.

Although Boston was a relatively quiet city, we saw all of society's problems when we were called to the emergency room. We set simple fractures and applied casts, sutured lacerations and cared for minor burns. We learned to identify and treat gynecological infections and to diagnose acute appendicitis. At that time only a few patients used the facilities as a clinic. Many of those we treated were often in real distress. Some had been injured in an automobile accident, a stabbing, or rarely, a shooting. There were victims of rape. We worked up patients with acute abdomens: some had perforated a hollow organ like the stomach or bowel, whereas others had bleeding ulcers. Young women seeking help after an illegal abortion sometimes died, despite our best efforts. When we needed additional help, we called our senior resident or the attending surgeon. If emergency removal of an appendix or relief of a bowel obstruction was indicated, they not infrequently allowed us to perform the operation.

There were times, certainly, when we wanted to give up. Hours and sometimes days on call took their toll. We were often exhausted. I remember sitting in relative somnolence in Grand Rounds, seeing those around me asleep and wondering how the faculty in the front row could be so alert. Sometimes, while retracting for several hours during a long, complex operation, a sense of futility dampened any remaining embers of altruism or empathy. On rotations in the emergency room, I treated a seemingly endless stream of individuals with venereal disease (often for the third time that month), sewed up lacerations in drunken patients whom I had sewn up only a few days before, and dealt with a variety of other irreversible social ills. At times I doubted the sanity of my career choice. My children were growing up at home and I was missing the entire process.

If we knew that surgery was so demanding, why did any of us consider it? An enduring speculation among all medical students involves which classmates will enter which specialty. We soon learned that particular personality types gravitate toward particular fields. Those choosing internal medicine tended to be thoughtful, enjoying the discussion of complex problems and formulating means to solve them. They expected to follow their patients for years. We surmised that individuals entering radiology were less interested in direct contact. Budding pathologists were scientifically curious puzzle solvers, willing to spend long hours at the microscope or in the library seeking answers to clinical problems. The individuals entering psychiatry were particularly interested in human interactions and relationships. A few seemed to have their own demons.

For decades, surgery was the chosen path for about one-quarter of the graduating fourth-year class of many medical schools. These were usually optimists who were comfortable taking charge and leading a team. They were energetic and directed, and they had often been athletes in college or had become expert in playing a musical instrument. They enjoyed anatomy and the types of diseases, abnormalities, and conditions they could see and touch, the challenge of pressing and dramatic problems, and the possibilities of controlling them. Admiring the no-nonsense pragmatism of their surgical professors, they envisioned themselves staunching hemorrhage, closing a perforation, repairing damaged hearts, or reconstructing disfigured faces. There were even intriguing clues in the early 1960s that organs could be transplanted. To cure a patient of an important disease or relieve an acute condition with one's hands was the ideal for those entering the field. As emergency medicine hadn't yet become a discipline, surgeons also expected to cover the urgent problems that arose intermittently.

Most residents were thrilled to be part of a competitive training program, and few resented those years. Quitting was unheard of. Although we worked every day until the work was finished, we learned constantly through operating on and caring for patients. We experienced nearly every human drama and dealt with situations we had never envisaged. We were part of a close-knit alliance to do what we could for those needing help. No one questioned the overwhelming commitment that we and our families accepted as the norm. Many of the faculty acted as mentors, teaching us the nuances of treatment, and indications for and intricacies of operation. They advised us about which research projects we should pursue. As we became immersed in the spirit of the place, we felt part of a rapidly moving, innovative, and dynamic whole. The years passed quickly.

By the time we had completed our training and were individually responsible for our patients, we felt ready for almost any eventuality. It seems a dictum that the reason one puts all the effort and commitment into such a career is not only to treat effectively routine surgical disease but to get oneself out of the untoward circumstances that may arise during an operation. Our experience served us well when we faced a new situation for which we needed to make instant and occasionally irreversible decisions. Pride of endurance was cultivated. We knew we needed to develop the capacity to work for long stretches without rest. The time we were on duty in the hospital matched the needs of the patients and fulfilled our desire to follow them during the critical hours and days until their discharge. But in my case the years of training, a period in research, and service in the military in the middle of training made for a long apprenticeship. I did not get my first staff appointment until I was thirty-seven years old. In addition, this deliberate rite of passage offered but modest compensation. I earned $7,500 during my first year of residency, $15,000 in my last, and $27,000 the first year I joined the staff.

One feature shared by all successful surgeons is the ability to stand confidently beside a trusting, helpless, and anesthetized patient, make a deliberate incision in unblemished skin, and carry out often complex and sometimes life-threatening maneuvers inside a body cavity. Although this act violates the body itself, the identity of the subject as a fellow human being must always be consciously maintained. The individual on the operating table must never become a "specimen" or "just another case of colon cancer." Retaining one's humanity may be difficult at times when cool objectivity and detachment must preclude emotional involvement. I tried to resolve this complex challenge by attending to the physical and emotional needs of the individual as best I could before and after the operation but concentrating completely on treating the disease process during the procedure itself. Although the usual depiction of the surgeon includes the word *ego*, the term *hubris* may perhaps be more accurate. *Hubris* encompasses the surgeon's desire to help someone with hands and mind, accompanied by the unswerving conviction that such surgical treatment is the patient's best recourse. It has been stated, perhaps with some hyperbole, that it takes fifteen years to mature as a surgeon: to learn to operate takes five; to learn when to operate takes another five; to learn when not to operate takes the remainder. The time to develop good judgment and experience is long, and it takes faith in oneself to carry out what is necessary for the welfare of the patient. But the stereotype endures; one author, with reason, described Cushing as representing one of "the least humble members of one of the world's least humble professions."[9]

Along with the dialogue and dynamics of health-care delivery, medical education, applied biology, and increasing information and communication among disciplines have evolved progressively. As a result, professionals and trainees alike are adopting new concepts, forming new habits, accruing new knowledge, and accepting unfamiliar cultures. Surgical practices are an integral part of these changes. When a careful clinical history and complete physical examination were the traditional means of assessing disease, for instance, the clinician could often only guess the identity and extent of tumor, location of vascular involvement, or the presence of pus. Emerging technologies have altered these practices substantially. Clinicians still take a history to assess symptoms, but sophisticated imaging techniques detect existing abnormalities more accurately than physical examination alone. Collaboration among specialties is critical. Except in some emergency situations, there are relatively few diagnostic surprises.

Although surgeons performed a relatively standard series of operations for predictable disorders for a century, changing patterns in the incidence and patterns of surgical conditions have modified their practices. Peptic ulcers and cancer of the stomach have declined in frequency in the West. Tumors of the pancreas, in contrast, have increased. Diverticulosis, an illness in which tiny out-pouchings of the wall of the large bowel may become infected, perforate, or cause obstruction, was relatively unknown in the nineteenth century but is now relatively common. Cancers of breast and prostate have become almost endemic, possibly because one is detectable at an early stage by mammogram and the other with a blood test. Their surgical removal is only one of several current treatment options. Indeed, a new field, surgical oncology, has arisen that combines radiation and chemotherapy with appropriate operative control of the tumor. With such a team approach, the control and cure of a variety of cancers have improved in a gratifying way.

Many of the operations that we and our teachers learned laboriously and carried out routinely have virtually disappeared. Several examples come to mind. Stripping of varicose veins, as Cheever performed on Mrs. Turner, was long an integral part of the surgical armamentarium. In recent years, the pendulum has swung toward less invasive approaches. An interventional radiologist slides a fine catheter along the inside of the enlarged vein. A laser or radiofrequency pulse emanating from the catheter tip destroys the inner surface of the vessel, causing it to seal, scar, and in time, virtually disappear. Sclerosing injections, heat, or laser treatments can eliminate smaller veins for cosmetic purposes. Performed during an office visit, these minimalist methods have gained broad appeal.

Generations of surgeons spent much time and effort removing gallstones. As mentioned, the contracting gallbladder ejects its supply of bile into the bowel via the common duct to digest the load of ingested fats from a large and rich meal. If a stone suddenly blocks the egress of the stored bile, the patient may experience severe abdominal pain and tenderness from the distended and inflamed gallbladder. If stones form within the common duct itself and obstruct normal flow from the liver, the patient develops jaundice, a serious complication. To correct the first, the operator traditionally removed the gallbladder through an upper abdominal incision. For the second, he had to explore the common duct and extract the stones. Excision of the gallbladder is a relatively straightforward procedure. Like an appendectomy, it was one of the first operations younger trainees learned.

If the common duct is obstructed, however, the problem became more difficult. The staff surgeon and the senior resident had to dissect a portion of the duct free from the adjacent portal vein and hepatic artery, open it, and attempt to wash out the concretions by saline irrigation, or take them out with a spoon-shaped instrument or forceps. In later years short catheters with inflatable balloons on their tips became available. If these maneuvers failed or a stone was impacted tightly in the muscular end of the duct as it entered the duodenum, they dilated the area with probes to allow the stone to pass. As this was essentially a blind procedure carried out by feel alone, they intermittently filled the duct with dye and took one or more X-rays to monitor progress. If the obstruction remained, they had to enter the bowel, find the tiny site of entrance of the duct, and open it. They could then remove the stone directly. These operations could be tedious and frustrating, often taking several hours. In contrast, surgeons now remove the gallbladder via a laparoscope, or capture a common duct stone by passing a flexible endoscope through the mouth and stomach, guiding its end into the duodenum, localizing and dilating the opening of the duct using tiny instruments, and extracting the stones with balloons. For this latter maneuver, no invasive surgery is necessary. Never having seen the open procedures that we performed in such quantities, our current residents consider them dated and rather quaint. Patients have undoubtedly benefited from the noninvasive approaches, despite minimal but sometimes significant complications.

The treatment of breast cancer is another example of the changes evolving in surgery. Traditionally, if a woman found a mass in her breast, she visited a surgeon. If cancer was suspected, radical mastectomy was usually the next step, a procedure that Joseph Lister in Britain and William Stewart Halsted in the United States popularized late in the nineteenth century as a means of removing large breast masses. Their disciples and trainees in turn considered the intricate dissection, based on strict anatomical principles, to be the ultimate treatment. We carried out many of these operations during my residency, learning much about anatomy, surgical technique, and how to handle tissues. What we didn't consider enough, however, was the brutal progression of events to which the women were subjected. Major disfigurement was often only the first step. If the tumor recurred, as many of them did, more operations followed.

One patient in particular comes to mind. I assisted on her original operation and knew her for years afterward. Mrs. Townsend lived in a suburb of Boston with her husband and her three children. Handsome and athletic at 42 years, she was proud of her appearance, active in the community, and popular with her friends. Her life was happy and fulfilled. One morning, however, while taking a shower, she discovered a thickening in her left breast. Panicked, she called a neighbor, a surgeon, who quickly arranged an appointment. On examining her, he confirmed the presence of a mass deep in the breast. He also felt a firm lymph node under her arm, a sinister finding that implied tumor spread. The news fell like a dark curtain across her pleasant life. She soon entered the hospital to face a battery of tests to detect metastases. All were negative. Operation was arranged. Mrs. Townsend was anesthetized, not knowing if she would awaken with her breast intact or with a permanent deformity. As had been routine for decades, the lump was excised through a small incision and sent to a pathologist, who made a frozen section for diagnosis under the microscope. If negative for cancer, the patient would be sent back to the wards to awaken, rejoicing. If positive, the mastectomy would continue. In her case, the news was bad. The surgeon opened a large ellipse of skin well beyond the margins of the tumor and elevated thin skin flaps that encompassed the entire circumference of the breast tissue. He isolated the major artery and vein of the arm in the armpit, identified and spared important nerves, then removed the breast, its underlying muscles, and the chain of draining lymph nodes and surrounding tissue in a single specimen. He finally tailored the skin flaps to cover the exposed ribs. As cancer surgery became more extensive in the 1950s and 1960s, some operators even opened the chest to extract lymph nodes lying within. The whole exercise resembled an anatomical drawing.

The overall result was that the patients were mutilated. Not only did the lack of tissue on the chest wall preclude their ability to wear anything but high-necked garments, their arms and hands on the affected side often became chronically swollen because of interruption of normal lymphatic drainage. To reduce the swelling, they had to wear a long elastic glove and endure a compression machine at night to squeeze fluid back into the circulation. Many experienced a lasting loss of body image, sexuality, and self-worth. Despite support from her husband and family, Mrs. Townsend took much time to regain the happiness of her former life.

Regardless of the extensive removal of tissue, recurrence was relatively common, sometimes after years, because the masses were often initially detected at a relatively late stage. Because many breast cancers are dependant on female hormones for growth, the next treatment strategy was to change the hormonal environment of the body, based on the discoveries of Charles Huggins and others years before. This implied removal of the ovaries, a step that sent young women precipitously into menopause and accentuated the condition in older ones. It also involved an abdominal incision, as minimally invasive techniques did not exist. If the tumor did not regress or recurred later, the final step to reduce female hormone production further was the elimination of the adrenal glands from their location above the kidneys or the pituitary gland from deep in the brain. These extreme operations produced their own complications. Four years after her mastectomy, Mrs. Townsend developed a shadow in her lung. By that time I had joined the surgical staff and was asked to eliminate her ovaries. Even though her chest X-ray improved, she died five years later with spreading cancer. These events were all too common.

Although radical mastectomy was long the treatment of choice in the United States, local excision of the mass and radiation to the area became relatively standard in Britain after World War II. Even though the results were comparable, enthusiastic American surgeons remained convinced that extensive removal of the site and its surroundings was the optimal treatment. One can only conjecture whether this striking geographical difference in approach to a common disease was due to skepticism about data from other countries, cultural variance, or divergent economic philosophies.

How different and more merciful is the strategy pursued since mammography became widely used in the 1970s. If there is a suspicious shadow, the radiologist performs a needle biopsy under ultrasound. If the specimen is positive, the surgeon usually removes the local area, then refers the patient for adjunctive chemotherapy and/or radiation. When the mass is large, the breast itself may be sacrificed but the chest muscles and most lymph nodes are left intact, a substantially less extreme procedure than a radical mastectomy. In this situation, the defect can be reconstructed at the same or a subsequent operation using flaps of adjacent muscle and fat or by inserting a silicone implant to produce a new breast of satisfactory bulk and shape. For the current treatment of many cancers, including breast, the surgeon has become part of a multidisciplined team of individual experts working toward a common goal. Therapy may be increasingly tailored to the molecular or hormonal responsiveness of a given tumor and the genetic makeup of a given patient. In addition to radiation and chemotherapy, alternatives to operation may include laser pulses, localized freezing, radio waves, and placement of radioactive seeds. The improving results provide optimism for those with malignancies.

The changes in health care during the 1980s and 1990s produced critical changes in many medical practices. They were particularly obvious in teaching hospitals that adapted to increasing patient loads, complexity of care, and inter-institutional competition. Mrs. Turner or Mr. Costello would find the new Brigham and Women's Hospital unrecognizable, for example. The vast complex of high modern buildings houses a collection of world-renowned institutions with their specialty units, clinics, and research laboratories, so different from the original small wooden structures. More buildings are rising and still others are being planned. Like many other such university-affiliated academic centers in the United States, the Longwood site has become a medical city. Patients like Mrs.

Laverne flood through the doors for treatments and approaches to disease inconceivable even a decade ago. The four departments of the Peter Bent Brigham–Medicine, Surgery, Pathology, and Radiology–have expanded to fourteen, each with their own divisions staffed by scores of specialists.

Surgery remains amply represented. In 2006 the departmental staff numbered more than 130, performing or assisting at over 20,000 operations each year. Its specialty education programs included 120 trainees. Research funds totaled $19 million, half from federal sources. The patients include an ever-increasing proportion of older individuals with significant co-morbid conditions. Despite the high potential risk, diagnostic evaluations, invasive procedures, and frequent multidisciplinary treatments are, in the main, efficient, safe, and effective. Although those admitted are often discharged before they consider themselves ready, as demanded by their insurance plans and administrators desirous of ever-shortened hospital stays, most achieve satisfactory results.

With the transformation of the small Peter Bent Brigham and older university hospitals like it into large, full-service aggregates, care of the ill has shifted from relatively leisurely treatment strategies and directly applied investigations involving comparatively few patients to corporate-driven care plans for "clients" by "providers" (business terms introduced during the beginnings of "managed care," a general title that implies cost control of medical services).[10] With the faculty required to increase its clinical output to combat declining reimbursements, reductions in traditional academic activities such as student and resident instruction have become important sources of concern. Burgeoning regulations, attendant paperwork, and the ever-present possibilities of litigation have increased progressively, while the numbers of individuals committed to basic and applied laboratory investigations have declined as funding opportunities narrowed. These and other forces have transformed the traditional "triple threat" image of teaching, patient care, and research that the faculties of academic hospitals had prized for a century to one based on more obvious budgetary goals and demands. The structure of medical education long accepted by the entire profession has particularly changed.

A watershed moment occurred at 11:30 PM on March 5, 1984, when the enduring foundations of medical training came under intense and highly publicized scrutiny. This involved a patient named Libby Zion.[11] She was an 18-year-old woman admitted to the emergency room of a prestigious teaching hospital in New York City with fever, chills, and body aches. A junior resident examined her and discussed her case over the telephone with the referring staff physician. They formulated a treatment plan with the intern who admitted her for workup. Adhering to the tenets of the discussion, he and the resident ordered appropriate laboratory tests and prescribed medication to relax her muscles and decrease her fever. Becoming increasingly unresponsive, however, she died eight hours later. The cause of her death was never determined, although information later emerged that she had taken large amounts of medication for stress plus illicit drugs.

Her father, a prominent lawyer and newspaper columnist, "claimed that his daughter had received inadequate care in the hands of overworked and under-supervised medical house officers," and arranged that the district attorney convene a grand jury to investigate the case. Although their 1986 report did not indict the physicians, it condemned graduate medical education in New York and, by inference, throughout the entire United States.[12] Events accelerated. The New York State Commissioner of Health called a committee that eventually endorsed the grand jury's findings. Relevant professional organizations were informed. In response, they formulated new rules that limited the number of hours that all residents could work each week. Stimulated by additional reports in the media about sleep-deprived house officers, the highly publicized road-traffic death of an exhausted cardiology resident driving from the hospital to take his board examinations in January 1999, and swelling public outrage, the laws toughened. The contrary opinion of a high official in the American College of Surgeons that "constrained work hours do not prepare residents for the real world of surgical practice" garnered little sympathy.[13] Senior surgical educators, however, quickly echoed these sentiments, while attendees at the subsequent annual meeting of program directors described the atmosphere as "funereal."[14] One surgeon was quoted: "We have to act as cops and chase [trainees] out of the hospital. It is antithetical to everything being a doctor is about." A distinguished professor summarized the general feeling of those in teaching hospitals.

"The [limited] work week is seen as damaging to the essence of surgery's being. It is the denial of the foundation of continuity of care."[15]

Although it seems inevitable that young doctors in training who toil under conditions of fatigue and stress make occasional errors of observation, judgment, and ministration, these occur remarkably infrequently in the strict hierarchical structure of graded team responsibility. But some instances inevitably arise. In response to Zion's death and other incidents, national credentialing committees and the United States Congress mandated in 2001 the number of hours residents could carry out their hospital duties without a break. At least one subsequent study found, not surprisingly, that there are fewer errors when residents are more rested.[16] The congressional mandate altered the entire construct of medical education. The discussion has continued abroad. The work week for German residents has been pared to forty-eight hours, and British trainees spend even less time at the hospital. In the United States, the current rules limit periods spent in hospital by the house staff, at least during their first four years, to eighty hours per week, plus eight additional hours for education. They are scheduled on a twelve-hour "shift" system, with at least ten hours off between sessions. During their time on duty, they are involved with about fifty patients on two or even three services, but inevitably on a fragmented basis. Communication is stressed by necessity. The residents obtain current patient information through the ubiquitous hospital computers and write orders electronically. Email and text messages flood the ether.

A perhaps inevitable result of these dynamics is that current surgical education may lack cohesiveness. Face-to-face contact between the house officers and the patient is relatively minimal. Instead of staying for the entire operation, the resident may have to leave in the middle, when her shift is up. They are no longer directly responsible for patients in intensive care at whose operations they have assisted but rotate for relatively short periods as junior members of permanent and autonomous anesthesiologist-run teams. Although some residents violate the work-hours regulations and stay until all tasks are completed, they must defend themselves to the program director if caught. If infractions occur too frequently, accreditation bodies may place the entire program on probation. In response, and to buttress deficiencies in the handoffs between shifts, department chairs have hired physician's assistants to provide routine and continuing care. The surgical faculty work harder, taking on direct patient responsibilities previously performed by the residents and physically covering all operations and emergencies.

The Morbidity/Mortality Conference, traditionally so important to teaching by correlating a disease state with operative findings and pathology and replete with lively faculty and resident interchange and constructive criticism, has become a victim of the new changes. The current system generally involves discussion of two or three patients chosen by an attending surgeon. The resident who carried out the surgery describes the case and answers relevant questions. Following this, he makes a ten-minute slide presentation on some general aspects of the history. Unfortunately, this often dry and boring format, without any consideration of pathologic findings, lacks spontaneity. No one but the presenter is expected to speak. As a learning experience, deficient in debate or dialogue, it suffers.

Trainees today face a plethora of additional challenges. Conrad Jacobson had become as familiar with Mary Agnes Turner as I was with Mr. Costello throughout their stay in the hospital. With nurse practitioners and physician's assistants responsible for orchestrating outpatient work-ups as in Mrs. Laverne's case, the house staff now rarely meets patients admitted for elective procedures until immediately before the operation. These increasingly standardized outpatient exercises, often adhering to strict protocols, presumably provide fewer opportunities for mistakes or omissions on the part of doctors and nurses. Unfortunately, the strategy provides little opportunity for the younger doctors to equate the symptoms and signs of the patient with the full rationale for surgery or associated therapies. Compounding this problem has been both a substantial increase in outpatient surgery and an appreciable shortening of in-house stay that precludes full consideration of postoperative changes and complications. Indeed, periodic institutional publications disseminated to all personnel are replete with the gleeful announcements of administrators that patient stay has, once again, been reduced and money saved. The most recent information I received was that thirty minutes had been shaved from the average time in hospital! My perception of such advances, correct or not, is that the comfort and well-being of the "clients" have fallen far down the list of "cost-effective" priorities. It should be stressed, however, that the quality of care, despite these exigencies, generally remains at a high level.

In contrast to residents of an earlier era, who were products of the traditional system in which they bore full responsibility for all aspects of care, medical students and even some currently in training appear to view surgery as just another career choice like investment banking; perhaps the more "heroic" persona of the surgeon of prior generations has been diminished and the discipline's image has moved toward one of technician. The coincident expectation that work hours must balance with the lifestyle and personal interests of the trainees and their families has become potentially problematic for optimal patient care.[17] Even with reduced hours and other lifestyle changes, a troubling proportion of surgical residents leave in the midst of their training to enter other fields. The current national attrition rate of those in surgical programs in the United States is between 20 and 30 percent, although this may be leveling off.[18]

Like the high official of the American College of Surgeons, many program directors are concerned that the residents may not assimilate an adequate repository of experience, information, and participation in clinical decision making, and that the new shift system may both diminish continuity of patient care and increase the number of mistakes and near misses. Indeed, a primary feature of the Libby Zion case was concern about patient safety, a fear intensified in an age of rush-through hospitalizations and mass-produced treatment. While the data are widely debated, medical recklessness, incompetence, or negligence are relatively rare. More common is the inevitable human error, inadequate communication, and inadvertent deviations from the routine. Although the figures vary widely, it has been thought that about 3 percent of patients are injured during their hospitalization; 7 percent of this cohort die from adverse circumstances and 9 percent from negligent events. About 40 percent of the injuries occur after surgery, and many of the others stem from medication-related problems.[19] The incidence remains low even as the patient population ages and develops coincident risk factors. Nevertheless, this ongoing problem is attracting well-deserved attention both in organized medicine and in the corridors of political power.[20] But despite satisfactory training, compulsory continuing education, and

intermittent mandatory recertification examinations throughout a professional career, mistakes are made and patients suffer.[21] An atmosphere
that couples often unrealistic patient expectations with the specter of
medical mistakes not only challenges the traditional doctor-patient relationship but contributes substantially to professional dissatisfaction and
disillusionment.[22] Some of the problems are unavoidable. Others stem
from stress and fatigue. Some difficulties arise from substance abuse;
doctors are notorious for protecting their friends and colleagues who
may drink too much or take easily available drugs. The rate of physician
suicide is appreciable, a generally unrecognized aspect of high achievement and a demanding life. One study notes that the equivalent of an
entire medical school class is lost through suicide each year, about 400
physicians.[23]

The residents have noted another change in medical convention. This
involves the interaction between doctor and patient. The relationship
between Dr. Cheever and Mrs. Turner, and between Dr. Warren and Mr.
Costello, was undeniably paternalistic. Although each patient had to give
written consent for the operation, neither would have thought to question
the surgeon's judgment, nor probably would the surgeon have accepted
skeptical questions without reflex indignation. The times were such that
the subject would never have arisen. Neither the relationship with their
doctors nor the prevailing customs encouraged a patient to promote his or
her rights beyond accepted limits. With relatively few certainties available, they were grateful for the care and relief they received. If either Mrs.
Turner or Mr. Costello felt the outcome of surgery was less than expected
or their condition had worsened, there was little recourse for help or
compensation. Both would have been incredulous and possibly appalled
if they could have seen into the future and learned about the Patient's Bill
of Rights, an atmosphere of questioning medical opinions, dissatisfaction
with results, and a general breakdown in mutual trust. Current patients
are increasingly involved in decision making regarding their treatment.
They may gain extensive and sometimes conflicting knowledge from the
Internet and other public sources, but they must still depend on professional advice, a potential source of frustration and conflict.

Physicians and graduates entering high-risk specialties appreciate how different the atmosphere has become. Perhaps in part because of the current emphasis on rapid patient turnover, the transient relationship between provider and client may never develop beyond artificial familiarity, impersonality, or detachment. Always under potential threat of lawsuit, many in the profession are forced to practice defensive medicine by ordering a spectrum of sometimes unnecessary and inevitably expensive tests that may not always be in the best interests of the patient. They may spend tens of thousands of dollars each year for malpractice insurance. Some cease practicing or retire early. Although many doctors feel pressured by these societal forces, we should appreciate that the situation appeared considerably more problematic 4,000 years ago. The Code of King Hammurabi of Mesopotamia is carved into a huge stone now in the Louvre Museum in Paris. Among these remarkable series of laws that govern human behavior are statements concerning both the benefits of successful surgery and punishment for failure. For instance, "If a physician makes a large incision with an operating knife and cures [the problem], or if he opens a tumor [over the eye] with an operating knife and saves the eye, he shall receive ten shekels in money." However, "If the physician makes a large incision with an operating knife, and kills him, or opens a tumor with the operating knife, and cuts out the eye, his hands shall be cut off." Perhaps modern litigators are preferable!

In this regard, I should mention the human subjects who were pioneers in many of the advances in surgery that we have discussed. Why would a patient agree to an unproven and dangerous cardiac procedure during the early days, or receive an organ transplant when there was little chance of a favorable outcome? The ill, as Giles Mullins, victim of bladder stone, exemplified so long ago, are desperate; there is often little choice but to continue to endure unbearable symptoms or to die. Without such legions of selfless individuals, realizing the odds against them but perhaps looking for miracles, there would have been fewer improvements, fewer successes, and fewer cures. Subsequent generations of patients and surgeons alike owe them a great debt.

Despite the challenges buffeting the surgical profession, the unremitting satisfaction of improving the lot of a patient in need with one's knowledge, experience, and hands remains a privilege. Full responsibility for his welfare is a critical facet of this satisfaction. Francis Moore encapsulated this theme in his statement:

> The fundamental act of medical care is assumption of responsibility. Surgery has assumed responsibility for the care of the entire range of injuries and wounds, local infections, benign and malignant tumors, as well as a large fraction of those various pathologic processes and anomalies that are localized in the organs of the body. The study of surgery is the study of these diseases, the condition and details of their care. The practice of surgery is the assumption of complete responsibility for the welfare of the patient suffering from these diseases. The focus is entirely on the care of the patient.[24]

Regardless of the present maelstrom concerning how patient care is conducted, these tenets remain the basis of the profession.

eleven

Shifting Foundations

I recently attended the goodbye ceremony for the graduating senior surgical residents, a yearly event well in keeping with the enduring rituals of academic medicine and its educational precepts. It was held in the hospital amphitheater, the same large, portrait-filled hall I first entered fifty years before and where I had sat through untold numbers of rounds and lectures during my career. Faculty and trainees filled many of the seats in front; spouses and a scattering of parents beamed from the upper rows. An occasional baby made itself heard. The programs were printed on crisp paper. The colored shields of hospital and medical school headed the list of honorees and the awards for teaching and mentoring. On a table in front lay an array of framed diplomas and book prizes. The mood of the audience was expectant and good humored, with the buzz of conversation conveying a sense of achievement, pleasure, and pride in those about to finish. The ceremony was no different, perhaps, from any other graduation except that the individuals involved were few, in their thirties, and embarking on lifelong responsibilities after years of preparation.

The seven honorees were diverse in origin, background, and culture. Most were married with children. Three were women. I was struck by how different they were from the virtually uniform population of white males from comfortable Protestant backgrounds that made up the majority of surgeons of my generation and those before. Like their peers throughout the country, they had spent five or more years in surgical training after medical school. Additionally, four had worked extensively in laboratory research. Two had doctorates. One was an engineer. Four were planning to take supplemental specialty fellowships. They all knew each other well, having cared for patients, struggled with difficult clinical or investigative problems, and experienced many hours together in the operating room. It had been a long apprenticeship.

The chief of surgery introduced each in turn, noting their future plans and asking them to summarize their surgical experience. With well-prepared presentations, they enumerated the types and numbers of operations they had performed at the Brigham and at its affiliated hospitals during their years of training, information critical in fulfilling the credentialing requirements of the American Board of Surgery. Several enlivened their talks with amusing pictures and stories about colleagues, faculty, and the foibles of the institution itself. Some became emotional as they extolled the sacrifices of their families and of those who had influenced and supported them along the way. They emphasized their indebtedness to their mentors and role models, particularly important because of the intensity and stresses of residency, time commitment, challenges, and extended periods spent as part of a team. The group noted that their teachers had ensured exposure to an array of surgical disease, overseen their developing technical expertise and experience, and insisted that they learn how, why, when, and when not to operate. The awards, named after distinguished figures in the department, came last. Individual residents at each level were recognized by their peers for their enthusiasm in instructing those below them. Members of the staff collected teaching awards as well, a tribute to their time and efforts. It was a pleasant and satisfying occasion.

Listening to the proceedings, I reflected on those currently entering the profession. Each autumn, applications from college seniors hoping to become doctors flood the admissions offices of the 126 medical schools in the United States. The number of students peaked in 1994 when nearly 47,000 applied.[1] It declined by 25 percent in the following years as many bright young people, especially males, chose careers in finance, technology, and other lucrative areas; in 2004 the total number of applicants had decreased to about 38,000. During the current recession, in contrast, the numbers are again rising.

About 15,500 medical students in their fourth and final year compete for over 23,500 first-year residency positions available nationwide, a number that has remained relatively stable since the 1970s.[2] Foreign medical graduates fill many of the remaining 8,000 slots.[3] In years past the majority of these came from Europe, although now increasing numbers from other global regions apply. For those intending a surgical career, about 90 percent are accepted in the 1,050 openings offered by the 251 accredited programs in the 120 university-based teaching hospitals and many nonaffiliated institutions; the remainder do not match or withdraw before entering. Less prestigious programs may remain unfilled or accept those less well suited.[4]

As a representative example of changing admission patterns at a post-graduate level, the Brigham department of surgery received 965 applications for internship in 2010. From these, 120 aspirants were granted interviews. Eight were taken. Only 532 of the 965 applied from schools accredited in the United States; the remainder, unsolicited and not considered, were from a variety of developing countries that included the Ukraine, Jordan, Iraq, India, the Sudan, and others. Of those granted interviews, about 90 percent were from the Brigham list of nineteen "top tier" schools. On occasion, an impressive individual from another school was accepted.

Although some medical schools and hospitals do not require interviews with prospective candidates, many believe these to be an important part of the admissions process. Selection is difficult because the applicants have generally amassed exemplary records, top national test scores, and highly supportive letters of recommendation. Experienced admissions officers invite those with the best apparent potential to visit. I have interviewed such individuals for medical school and for residency for many years, and consider the interaction to be crucial in gaining impressions and information that the written records do not provide. We converse for about an hour in a free-ranging discussion as I assess motivation, experience, leadership skills, and interests. Some of the young people are more impressive personally than their application would suggest. Others discuss interests and challenges they emphasized in their essays in a surprisingly unenthusiastic and disinterested manner. The following is a not-uncommon example of a dilemma we commonly face; an excellent candidate who I did not recommend to enter the incoming medical school class.

David Cross was from a large town in New Jersey. His father was an executive, his mother a lawyer. Always academically gifted, he developed an obvious interest in science in high school. He performed brilliantly at an elite university, majoring in biology with a minor in chemistry. His grades were mostly A's, his test scores were in the highest percentile, and he had received several awards and scholarships. He worked for two summers in a basic science laboratory, examining a gene involved in diabetes. The project led to a presentation at a national conference and authorship on a paper in a professional journal. He accrued some clinical experience volunteering at a local hospital, spending time with patients in a nursing home and shadowing a physician. In addition, he was the film editor of the school newspaper and was active in a church group. The university letter of recommendation was laudatory, noting him to be "one of our most outstanding" applicants. Other letters described him as "extremely intelligent and highly motivated." All placed him in the top 5 percent of the class. During the interview, he articulated well his desires for his future career. Although his knowledge about his research project was appropriate, his comments about patients he had met and his other experiences were conveyed with a curious sense of apathy. Indeed, as much as I tried and as many topics as I introduced, I couldn't get beyond rather superficial generalities. I felt that all had come rather easily for him and that his premedical activities and interests seemed rather pedestrian.

We see many highly qualified applicants like David. All have impressive qualifications and spotless records. He will certainly be accepted by a medical school and will pursue a successful professional career. I was, however, looking for more. I wished he had spent more time and energy traveling, working in another culture, learning a language, playing in an orchestra, or taking a leadership role in some community activity. I was not convinced that he pursued his commitments and achieved his successes out of real passion for a career as a doctor, or merely to pad his résumé. Overall, even with his obvious talents and intelligence, he just didn't seem very interesting. The other interviewer felt the same way and discussion by the entire admissions committee was unfavorable, so he was not offered a place.

The interview process is subjective by nature, but it is difficult to envisage designing anything more deliberate and considered. Despite all the care and effort put into selecting candidates with energy, passion, intelligence, and skill, our choices sometimes fail. Occasional promising medical students do not live up to expectations, opt out, transfer to other medical fields, or move to industry. We have admitted academic "superstars" to the residency who dealt poorly with the practical day-to-day issues of patient care. Perhaps the current system with its emphasis on grades, test scores, and highly polished applications tends to disregard those who are somewhat different—the free thinkers, the eccentrics, and the innovative spirits who may later become generous, concerned, and giving physicians or mature into productive clinician-scientists. Indeed, the apparently less accomplished but more personally compelling individuals on whom we have taken a chance have often turned out to be the best. It is interesting to consider some in this latter category who were not initially accepted either to their medical school choice or to their desired residency. Two examples from the Brigham come to mind. In the 1950s Harvard Medical School turned down David Hume because of a relatively mediocre academic record in college. He later applied to the Brigham surgical program and was admitted with the less-than-enthusiastic comment that he "talked fast but made sense." He went on to carry out highly regarded original research on the endocrine response to injury and to become one of the principal figures in the new field of transplantation. Outspoken, creative, and iconoclastic, he was a towering figure in American surgery. Robert Gross attended Harvard Medical School but was accepted grudgingly and only after a long delay into the residency program at Boston's Children's Hospital. His lukewarm recommendation read: "Mr. Gross is an interested, eager, and active student somewhere above the average, and has a pleasant personality and a good appearance. He should make a satisfactory house officer."[5] He became, as discussed, one of the greatest contributors to pediatric surgery.

Perhaps the most obvious change over recent decades has been the diversity of the applicants. A striking demographic shift has encompassed the entire spectrum of education and achievement, from college through medical school, residency, and the attending staffs of hospitals themselves. Although the majority of applicants are Caucasian, there are increasing numbers of second-generation students of both genders from the developing world. Many of their parents, often Asian and professionals in their own countries, immigrated to the United States and took menial positions to give their children a chance. Other talented individuals obtain a green card for university and postgraduate education in the United States. In both instances, children have often repaid their parents for their assistance by excelling in excellent colleges, involving themselves in community service, and assuming leadership roles in a variety of activities. Family pressures, however, sometimes appear intense.

Some outstanding candidates have succeeded despite a lack of support from parents, peers, or community. Parents' goals for their children may differ, or parents may be entirely absent. Educational opportunities, particularly for some African American and Hispanic applicants from urban communities, may have been few and far between compared with their suburban counterparts, making their achievements even more impressive. Alonzo Hollis, now a medical student, grew up in difficult circumstances in East Los Angeles. His father had disappeared years before. His mother worked long hours as a maid to support him and his sister. The large high school he attended was, unfortunately, typical of many urban public institutions. Academic excellence was low on the list of desirable attributes. Drug use and violence were rife. Many of the girls became pregnant and dropped out, and a significant proportion of the boys joined gangs. Only six of the two hundred seniors went on to college. Highly motivated and industrious despite intense and distracting peer pressures, Alonzo was one of them. He entered a local community college, where he showed unexpected talent in the sciences. After a year an enthusiastic teacher helped him transfer to one of California's excellent universities. He did well academically while working part time to aid his mother and sister. Somehow he found the energy to form a successful after-school mentoring program that protected local children from the influence of the gangs. Again, a professor thought so highly of Alonzo's potential that he encouraged him to apply to prestigious medical schools. He was accepted at Harvard and has thrived, earning the respect of faculty and colleagues for his intellect, work ethic, and unflappable personality. Following residency he wishes to return to an inner-city hospital in Los Angeles to help the indigent. Interested and sympathetic teachers have consistently opened doors. He has taken full advantage of what they offered.

Who attends medical school has changed, and so have the particulars of what students are expected to learn. Technical advances over the past three decades have produced important differences in the curriculum of medical students and residents. New imaging devices, for instance, have reached such sophistication in visualizing contents and abnormalities of body cavities that they have altered substantially long-accepted means of diagnosis, allowing diseases to be discovered at earlier stages and remedied appropriately. The traditional "exploratory" operation, for instance, in which a surgeon opens the patient with only a tentative diagnosis or guess as to what he will find, has become a thing of the past. Some scans discriminate between individual structures; others detect functional differences. Body parts stand out in textbook detail and clarity, often in color. The exactness of the pictures allows radiographers to place catheters precisely into remote places of the body to instill drugs, to dilate narrowed vessels of the heart with a tiny balloon and insert a mesh cylinder to keep the site open, or to clot off a discrete area of bleeding deep in the brain.

At the same time, the teaching of surgical skills is undergoing a massive transformation. Expecting perfect results always, the public assumes their surgeons to be highly experienced in the treatment of their conditions, even though the newer generations of graduating trainees may lack full exposure to a potential spectrum of ills. Part of this lack has to do with the curtailed work hours, part due to less actual time in the operating room, and part to concentration on minimally invasive techniques such as laparoscopy. In response, the technical training of young surgeons is increasingly benefiting from the use of simulation technology. In growing numbers of academic departments, program directors are exploiting the availability of incredibly realistic (and expensive) human models and mannequins with relatively lifelike tissues and organs to help the neophyte resident gain expertise in the manipulation of instruments, stapling, suturing, knot tying, and other basic skills. This departure is based on simulation training of airline pilots, in which the students learn to cope with all eventualities, routine and emergent, while sitting in an exact mockup of the cockpit of a commercial or military plane. Similarly, the model patient lies in an operating room, exact in every detail. Sitting in an adjacent room and viewing the proceedings through a window, a technician can control all facets of a given operation electronically. He can make the blood pressure decline as with rapid loss of blood. The patient may stop breathing and need to have a tube inserted into his windpipe. He can create cardiac arrhythmias. He can make red dye squirt from a fresh incision in plasticized skin. All surgical instruments are real. Practicing on rubberized tissues, joining ends of simulated bowel, and sometimes dissecting and manipulating animal organs, the fledgling interns learn one-on-one from instructors how to suture, what material to use, which stapler to choose, and so on. Nearby, residents hone their laparoscopic skills on organs viewed on a screen. Established trauma surgeons take refresher courses, currently offered in thirty centers around the world, in which they repair specific injuries in anesthetized pigs, enhanced with visual aids and close instruction. Although no models can simulate real situations, much can be learned. In particular, the intern will have developed rudimentary skills before he or she approaches the first patient.

Actual surgical operations are evolving in parallel. As we have seen with Mrs. Laverne, minimally invasive methods allow precise dissections with decreased postoperative pain, lessened inflammation, reduced length of stay, and improved convalescence. Indeed, laparoscopy is undergoing continuous refinement, with some surgeons now carrying out abdominal operations by inserting a specialized instrument through the umbilicus that combines viewing and manipulation of internal structures in a single unit. The advent of robotics is another example of surgical evolution, a futuristic innovation that is slowly gaining popularity. Military strategists in the 1980s first proposed that a surgeon, miles away from the action, might carry out a lifesaving procedure on a severely wounded soldier by telesurgery using a robot.[6] To accomplish this, they designed and programmed a computer-controlled manipulator with artificial sensing to perform a variety of intricate tasks. A decade later, visionaries in the National Aeronautics and Space Administration suggested that a surgeon on Earth might use a robot to excise the inflamed appendix of an astronaut in space. With the imaginative instrumentation and three-dimensional viewing of this technology spreading into specialized institutions, correction of abnormalities in a variety of relatively inaccessible anatomic locations is becoming possible. Increasingly, urologists remove prostate glands with more exactness and less disruption than under direct vision with an open approach. Indeed, they performed 62,000 robotic prostatectomies between 2000 and 2007, with the frequency increasing substantially since.[7] Experts in well-equipped centers will eventually use robotic surgery to operate on patients miles away in underserved or remote areas.[8] For some complex procedures on the central nervous system, the entire neurosurgical team—surgeon, assistant, nurse, and anesthetist—are enclosed in huge scanning devices with the patient lying on the operating table. This futuristic arrangement allows them to visualize specific areas of the brain continuously and with astonishing clarity for accurate removal of spreading tumors invisible to the naked eye. Heart surgeons not only are beginning to replace diseased valves with substitutes introduced through the vascular tree but are precluding the necessity for the artificial structures themselves by clipping together the edges of the leaflets of incompetent valves with tiny instruments, monitored on a television screen. If the early benefits of ongoing clinical trials hold, these minimally invasive techniques may save many patients from a formal open-heart operation.

An increasingly popular innovation that combines both surgery and radiology is the "endovascular repair" of aortic aneurysms, working from inside the abnormal vessel rather than outside.[9] With appropriate imaging devices positioned directly over the operating table, the size, shape, and extent of the sac can be clearly defined. The surgeon can then choose a graft of appropriate size with flexible rings incorporated into each end. Sharp metal teeth protrude from the rings. He inserts a catheter with a large, deflated balloon at its tip into the artery at the patient's groin. Under continuous imaging, he threads the catheter up through the aneurysm and into the normal aorta at the level of the diaphragm. Inflating the balloon to block incoming blood flow, he insinuates the graft over the catheter through the diseased segment and localizes the ring precisely in the uninvolved aneurysm neck. To anchor it, he positions another balloon within the flexible ring. Inflation of this balloon forces the metal teeth deeply into the arterial wall. He repeats the process at the lower end. The new arterial conduit, now seated firmly in place, runs through the intact but empty aneurysm. Deflation and removal of the balloons allows blood to flow normally to the legs. Instead of awakening in the intensive care unit and staying in hospital for ten days in pain from a large abdominal incision, as Mr. Costello experienced, the patient endures only one small groin incision, recovers quickly, and leaves the hospital in two days. If the relatively satisfactory early results continue, this imaginative innovation may change substantially the traditional open repair of aortic aneurysms.

Completely noninvasive possibilities to moderate this disease also lie on the horizon. Aneurysms form because of degradation of structural molecules responsible for the thickness, elasticity, and strength of the normal artery. One of the features of arteriosclerosis, the underlying cause of the condition, is inflammation, a normal protective bodily response to injury or insult. Among the many activities associated with this complex process, however, is the release of destructive chemical products by white blood cells that may weaken the aortic wall. Selective pharmacological inhibition of these inflammatory factors is under investigation and may eventually prevent the development of this serious and potentially fatal disease. In theory, at least, surgical intervention would become a thing of the past.

The "hybrid operating room" is a recent innovation in the care of fragile, high-risk patients with severe and generalized arteriosclerosis. It exploits the dictum that older individuals can withstand one operation well, but tolerate poorly either more than one or an untoward complication. Present in a few specialized cardiovascular centers, the large room contains all equipment needed for the combined repair of diseased hearts and abnormal vessels, allowing the correction of several serious conditions in a single session. State-of-the-art fluoroscopy and other imaging devices guide stent placement in coronary arteries plus coincident endovascular correction of aortic aneurysms, for example. If heart-lung bypass is necessary, coronary artery revascularization can be performed along with reconstruction of the arteries of the neck or legs. Perhaps it may seem grandiose in concept, but this approach is saving lives.

Surgeons are devising other unique approaches, particularly the use of a natural body orifice to access or remove internal organs. Only mild sedation is necessary because manipulation or dissection of the intestines and other viscera does not elicit pain. The operator inserts an endoscope through the mouth into the stomach. He passes the device through a small hole he has cut in the stomach wall, and with excellent visualization of the adjacent viscera, maneuvers the instruments to take out the gallbladder or spleen. On completing the procedure, he closes the gastric defect from the inside with staples. He may remove the appendix or even a portion of colon via the anus, and can reach the ovaries and other pelvic organs via the vagina. Surgeons in France have removed a patient's gallbladder trans-vaginally, while in America they have extracted donor kidneys for transplantation and performed gastric bypass operations using this route. For all these procedures there is minimal discomfort, no external incisions, and little time needed for recovery. Threats to the body's homeostasis and defenses diminish. Risks of infection or respiratory compromise are reduced. Although much remains to be tested before the strategy becomes routine, it is an intriguing concept. A potential difficulty with this approach, however, is that if the patient returns to the hospital at a future date with another disease process, lack of scars on the abdomen may complicate the reconstruction of a complete medical history.

Perhaps the most spectacular interplay of the new methods involves the repair of debilitating or ultimately fatal abnormalities of the developing fetus. A well-timed intervention may cure a given condition or allow the baby to be born and grow large enough for later definitive intervention. Several methods have been used. With precise imaging, specialists can make a small incision through the muscular wall of the mother's uterus and move the abnormal area of the developing infant into direct view. After repair, they close the maternal tissues. If prenatal scans identify a congenital obstruction of the airway, the operator may correct the problem before the child breathes and while oxygen still comes from the mother via the placenta. In instances where the developing vertebral bodies fail to fuse, as in spina bifida, the specialist can cover the open defects of the spinal cord with skin to promote healing and reduce subsequent disability. To decrease the risk of premature birth after direct fetal manipulation, surgeons may insert tiny laparoscopes or catheters through the uterine wall and into affected areas in the body of the infant. If an embryonic tumor has been detected, for instance, they can place ultrasound-guided radiofrequency probes near or in the mass and activate sound waves to destroy its blood supply. This prevents further growth and facilitates its complete removal during infancy.

A successful operation on a five-month-old fetus with a severe congenital heart defect was a dramatic example of these techniques, attempted only a few times before. A resident in pediatrics involved in the baby's care told the story.[10] In the autumn of 2003 a young woman, five months pregnant with her first baby, was undergoing a routine ultrasound near her home in Los Angeles. Suddenly the obstetrician performing the examination stopped his cheerful conversation as he noticed that the tiny heart looked abnormal. After careful examination of multiple films and consultation with the pediatricians, he broke the news to the patient and her husband that the fetus had "hypoplastic left heart syndrome" and that the chances of survival were remote. Although most of his colleagues confirmed the diagnosis and suggested termination of the pregnancy, one told the couple about a team at Children's Hospital in Boston experienced in fetal surgery. They soon learned what was known about their child's condition. The primary defect is a congenital constriction and partial fusion of the leaflets of the aortic valve that prevents the left ventricle from developing to a normal size and ejecting normal amounts of arterial blood. To compensate, the right ventricle sustains the entire fetal circulation by pumping blood through the open ductus arteriosus. Even though the 1,000 children born each year in the United States with this anomaly appear normal at birth, they die quickly when the ductus closes. During the 1980s a handful of surgeons attempted to correct the condition with three separate, staged, and individually serious heart operations. A few of the survivors received heart transplants, although long-term complications were frequent and often severe.

The doctors at Children's Hospital proposed to open the fused valve of the fetus by positioning and inflating a tiny balloon. Several teams had attempted this approach a dozen times during the 1990s, but only two babies lived. In their previous single successful attempt, the Children's group had opened the valve at an earlier stage of fetal life than the others to allow more time for the underdeveloped ventricle to grow during subsequent development in the mother. In the present case, they felt that five months' gestation was still early enough to give the baby a chance. Everyone involved, including the parents, the doctors, and the hospital ethics committee, agreed with the plan. But like Gross's first closure of a patent ductus and Blalock's "blue baby" operation, this was essentially new territory. Like so many innovations throughout the history of surgery, the risks were large and the benefits relatively unproven. In fact, success was probably remote.

Specialists from different disciplines stood around the mother as she lay asleep on the operating table. Under ultrasound monitoring the radiologist pushed a long, thin needle through her abdominal wall and into the uterus lying directly beneath. After the anesthesiologist had temporarily paralyzed the fetus to prevent movement, the obstetrician carefully guided the tip of the needle between its ribs and into the tiny left ventricle of the grape-sized heart. A pediatric cardiologist then threaded a hairlike wire down the needle and passed it through the narrowed valve. Over the wire he ran a fine catheter with a deflated balloon on its tip. Once in exact position, he inflated the balloon to the size of a small pea, opening the site of obstruction by forcing the valve leaflets apart. Three months later, a healthy baby, William, was born.

As remarkable as these advances are, however, they are creating an array of logistical, ethical, financial, and societal difficulties. The technologies and their continuing refinements are used increasingly, not only for routine health care but as powerful marketing tools for individual physician practices, for competing hospitals, and for patients who consider that the most advanced tests, procedures, and medications define good health care. The traditional means of diagnosing an illness by history and physical examination—and confirming and often curing it with an open surgical exploration—have been transformed into a battery of investigations and treatments that progress from simple X-rays through a variety of scans to interventional radiology, and perhaps finally, to minimally invasive operative interventions. There is no question that definition of a given problem is accurate, time spent in hospital is reduced, and the patients suffer less. But the techniques are time consuming and extremely expensive. In addition, the results are not always superior.

The use of robots in surgery is an example of the problematic use of such methods. A robot may cost between $1 million and $2.5 million, with additional yearly outlay of many thousands for maintenance and ancillary equipment.[11] While many surgeons agree that they can carry out an open procedure as effectively and in considerably less time than with a robot, they often feel that they must use the new device to satisfy consumer demand and to uphold the "cutting edge" image of the institution. Indeed, in some instances, robotic technology may replace equally effective nonsurgical or conventional surgical approaches, driving up overall costs further. Experience is also a problem because the learning curve is long; it has been thought that a surgeon must carry out 150–250 operations with the robot to become fully proficient, although most operators currently take only a short course of instruction and use the equipment a few times a year. Although the approach diminishes immediate postoperative complications and shortens length of stay in the hospital, recent data analyzing robotics in prostate surgery, for instance, have suggested that long-term complications may be substantially increased.[12] But like other minimally invasive methods, such operations hold much promise in the future as overall results improve, expertise broadens, and methodology develops. Some expenses of the technology may be offset by reduced postoperative charges. Patients may recover more rapidly and be able to return to work sooner. Judging the ultimate effectiveness of robotic surgery versus its costs and general availability remains an unsolved problem for health-care providers.

The high quality of those graduating from surgical programs and exciting advances in surgical technology provide much hope for the future of medicine. Yet less-optimistic developments threaten the foundations of the surgical profession. We live in an era in which a broad array of medical and scientific advances can salvage patients with conditions hitherto regarded as hopeless. Many, however, feel uneasy that increasing technology and an emphasis on pharmaceuticals has replaced clinically structured, humanitarian, and individualized care. How many times, while watching the news each night, are you encouraged to "Ask your doctor" about some incessantly advertised nostrum? Others perceive that the well-publicized efforts of third-party payers to hold down costs are paradoxically transforming the physician-patient relationship and the art of healing into an impersonal and commercial interaction between "provider" and "client," forcing the medical profession to adopt the less socially conscious and more opportunistic ethics of business.

Individuals with vision and imagination have emphasized that the benefits of computerized data gathering, the rapidity of global communication, and other innovative departures from long-accepted norms may provide unprecedented opportunities in the practice of medicine. Others remain skeptical, pointing out that the gap between rich and poor, educated and undereducated, skilled and unskilled, and those who receive adequate health care and those who do not is greater than ever, and that sophisticated technologies, as effective as they are, have contributed to health-care funding woes. Indeed, the high cost of these technologies is a major factor influencing the continuing and still relatively unresolved debates regarding affordable quality health care for all citizens. The ethical implications—that huge financial outlay and much professional effort are limited to relatively few, complex patients—conflict directly with the need for general care for many. On one side rest the demands of well-insured individuals seeking the most advanced treatments in the most experienced institutions; on the other, primary care for the underinsured, adequate prenatal evaluation and child health, screening for cancer, prevention of hypertension and heart disease, health education, and public health measures. With both sides at least partly correct, true reform will take effort, altruism, money, political skill, and diplomacy. Such reform is essential to resolve the differences and allow the benevolent side of the profession to transcend the all-pervasive power of the market and regain its traditional profile. Whether doctors, their organizations, politicians, and the skeptical public could ever agree on such measures remains moot. Meanwhile, active practitioners often struggle to keep the opposing forces in balance. The residents and their education are caught in the middle, and their newly graduated peers are stepping into an uncertain future.

I recently discussed these and related matters with two of our current trainees. Their opinions are broadly representative of those of their colleagues. Damanpreet Bedi is in his third year of residency. A devout Sikh, he is already an experienced laboratory researcher desirous of an academic career. His father came to the United States from India to earn a degree in biochemistry and is now a professor at a state university. His mother owns her own business. Their son has taken full advantage of the opportunities granted him. Among the several subjects we considered were the effects of the federally mandated changes in work hours on his surgical training. He commented, "Like many of my colleagues, I fully understand that the face of surgical training has changed significantly, and we worry whether the current scheme will provide the necessary tools to equip us to fill the shoes of previous generations of surgeons. Residents and faculty alike are holding their breath apprehensively as we go through our education, hoping that it will be 'good enough' to give us the appropriate tools to forge us into confident, competent, and strong surgical practitioners." We discussed the current emphasis on lifestyle, noting that all generations of young doctors felt crushed by busy work, although its character has changed over time. Bedi observed,

> Surgical residents now feel that somehow life outside *and* inside the hospital can be balanced. Residents worked hard back then, but we still do now, and I often wonder if we're trying to do in the eighty-hour work-week what previous generations did in 120 hours. Physician's assistants provide some help, but the work placed on the house staff has increased correspondingly: patients are sicker, operative volume is higher, consult notes are generally expected to be typewritten and emailed, computer-generated medication lists must be compiled by residents, discharge summaries must be complete, notes in charts must be thorough, and serial vital signs must be collected.

We noted that the improving technology, particularly in imaging, has sharpened and simplified hitherto lengthy diagnostic workups.

Next we considered morale and expectations. Bedi commented,

> I fear that morale is low amongst the residents, particularly the juniors. We see our anesthesia colleagues in the operating room being relieved by staff personnel every two hours for lunch and coffee breaks, then leaving at 4 PM. We hear of the "miserable" night float system when the medical residents work four or five ten-hour shifts, compared to

our six thirteen-hour stints. Yet we tell ourselves, over and over again, that it is OK. Why? Because we are surgeons. We have elected to live this way. And living this way gives us the privilege of caring for patients, opening their body cavities, and being trusted to work on the vital structures within. What we do is incredible, and thus, the sacrifices we make must, too, be incredible. Surgical residency is similar to religion. One must believe, almost blindly, that there is a higher purpose to all of this, and that a select few must endure hardships and make sacrifices to taste the ultimate fruits.

To gain additional perspective I spoke of some of the current dynamics with Caprice Greenberg, a newly appointed member of the department who had been a resident just before the conversion to the eighty-hour work week in 2001. She spent six years in general surgery plus a specialist fellowship, then an additional two years earning a Master of Public Health degree, examining the statistical outcomes of various treatment protocols for breast cancer. She recently joined the Brigham staff as a breast surgeon and clinical investigator. She has published several papers and is on the medical school faculty. I inquired about her perceptions of the current design of surgical education.

> Today's residents are caught in a transition period and are unfortunately not getting adequate training. I would predict that general surgery residency will be reduced to three to four years with earlier specialization. Given the limited work week and the incredible increase in surgical knowledge, there is simply no way to be an expert in everything anymore. Early specialization will allow trainees to learn what will be practical in their eventual careers. For example, as a breast surgeon, I learned most of what I use in my daily activities during my fellowship. I will never again use the skills that I acquired during my residency.

I questioned her regarding the widespread professional anxiety about the disappearance of the general surgeon and the threat that surgeons are losing their broad professionalism and are turning into technicians.

> I think the biggest concern right now relates to increased specialization. Almost everyone completes a specialist fellowship following residency, as few people completing general training feel adequately prepared to go out and practice at the end of it. Another reason that many do not feel general surgery to be a viable career, at least in academic centers, is that there seems to be little control over the schedule, and fellowship-trained specialists are taking most cases—colorectal, breast, laparoscopy—what is left? In addition, most who are fellowship-trained do not want to take general surgery call, nor do they necessarily feel competent to do so. This is leading to many problems related to emergency room coverage.

What a contrast this answer was to the situation in earlier years, when surgical trainees completed their residency feeling competent to care for the majority of problems they would encounter throughout their careers.

Educational debt also looms high in the consciousness of all entering the medical profession in general and surgery in particular. This underlying concern was illustrated during a recent conversation with a distinguished chairman of surgery at a major medical school who came to our hospital for a few days as a visiting professor. He is an enthusiastic educator, highly successful investigator, and an experienced clinician. He is the editor of a major surgical journal and sits in leadership positions of prestigious professional societies. He had trained at the Brigham years before, so I knew him well. During his visit he joined the residents on rounds and in the operating room, gave several lectures, and met with many of the staff. I happened to see him shortly after he had spent a couple of hours with the dozen third-year medical students going through their surgical rotation. All were interested in the subject, intrigued with the patients, impressed with the residents, and enthusiastic about witnessing the operations. They were enthralled with the types of diseases and the ability of the surgeon to care for them. They were excited about seeing the anatomy, the new technologies, and the intricacies of the intensive care unit. Many valued the experience as practical exercises in physiology and pathology they had only read about. But when my friend asked who of the group was considering a career in the field, there was a deafening silence. When he pressed them for the reason behind their reticence, several expressed concerns about the length of training, limited lifestyle, and still-apparent gender barriers. The majority mentioned educational debt.

The financial burden that many students and young residents face is a serious consideration in their career plans. Unlike Cheever and many of the earlier surgeons, few of the current residents are independently wealthy. Even for those few, the increasing cost of eight years of higher education can be overwhelming. When my Harvard undergraduate tuition increased from $750 per year to $1,000 in 1956, my father gasped. When our youngest daughter matriculated in 1998, the cost had risen to $40,000. In 2010 many colleges have announced that the yearly rate will be over $50,000. Acceptance to medical school adds a frighteningly comparable outlay. As a result, many students enter their residency over $200,000 in debt from their medical education alone. If they marry a classmate, the couple has accumulated a deficit of half a million dollars, with up to a decade of relatively low-paid training still ahead of them. With many practices no longer particularly profitable, these individuals face many years of repaying their educational loans. This burden may prevent talented and motivated individuals from following careers they find captivating but which involve prolonged training.

Greenberg addressed this all-too-common concern in the context of our conversation:

> In general, residents have either huge amounts of debt or no
> debt depending on their family's financial situation. I was
> terrified about my ability to clear my loans and support
> my family following my training. Luckily, I was accepted
> to the NIH Loan Repayment Program, which is paying
> back substantial amounts. Without this help, we would

be struggling to make our mortgage and pay for childcare
and other expenses while my husband is still in residency.
That's pretty pathetic after nine years of training [follow-
ing medical school]. Despite it all, I don't think most people
make career decisions based on educational debt. I didn't.

I am not so sure about this last point, particularly as one views the
increasing popularity of specialties with a more satisfactory lifestyle
and relatively good pay. I probed her feelings about a medical career
in general and her future financial hopes. "Residents seem surprisingly
unconcerned about declining reimbursements for work done, although
many are discouraged when they look at the career paths of many of our
peers. Most of our college friends had starting salaries in business or after
law school that are the same as we have at the end of residency. They
are now a decade older and still make at least twice what I am currently
paid and expect to be paid." We both mentioned, however, that many
well-compensated young businessmen and lawyers become bored and
disenchanted with their careers within a few years. Finally, I contrasted
her present modest financial realities based primarily upon an unrelenting
patient and procedure load with those of us in academic medicine during
prior decades. Although we too had started well behind our nonmedi-
cal peers, we received reasonable salaries for our clinical work as faculty
members and still had time to teach, run a laboratory, and pursue other
scholarly endeavors.

The subject of medical manpower has become an urgent issue and one
with which graduating seniors must wrestle. A quarter-century ago the
Accreditation Council for Graduate Education, a nonprofit group that
evaluates and accredits residencies in the United States, predicted that
by the year 2000 there would be a 15–30 percent surplus of physicians.
In a remarkable turnabout, a study only four years later concluded that
a deficit of 200,000, about 20 percent of the needed workforce, would
arise by 2020 or 2025.[13] Indeed, the decline has already begun, although
physician's assistants with specialty training, nurse practitioners who
have earned doctorates, and foreign medical graduates are taking up part

of the slack. Some of the existing 126 medical schools are responding to a recent recommendation by the American Association of Medical Colleges to enlarge their class sizes by 30 percent. Despite plans for the creation of twenty-five new schools in several states, one wonders whether adequate numbers of experienced faculty will be available to fill needed positions. Of course, plans to increase the number of physicians will take time and could eventually produce an unwarranted physician surplus.[14]

Evolving societal issues are complicating the decreasing numbers of medical personnel. The population of the United States will allegedly increase by 27 percent by 2050, up from the recent census number of 307 million.[15] The public is also aging. The United States Census Bureau predicts that the numbers of those over 65 will rise from the present 13 percent to 20 percent during the next twenty-five years; individuals older than 85 years are the fastest-growing group. In addition, recent passage of the health-care reform bill will purportedly provide medical coverage for over 30 million previously uninsured people plus millions more with inadequate coverage. Health problems of the underserved are expanding in parallel, with obesity, hypertension, and diabetes taking a particular toll. In partial response, remotely monitored systems have been introduced in areas where staffing for intensive care units is in short supply. The outsourcing of X-rays to distant readers is becoming common. "Concierge practices," in which primary care physicians take exclusive responsibility for relatively small groups of affluent subscribers, are gaining attention. The expanding pool of potential patients will also require considerable surgical involvement as hearts need repair, joints require replacement, cancers must be removed, and complications of arteriosclerosis and diabetes treated. At the same time the demographics and practices of doctors are changing. With lifestyle an obvious and important consideration, many recently graduated professionals are involving themselves in less-demanding specialties or in disciplines not directly concerned with patient care.

The surgical workforce (over 63,000 current members of the American College of Surgeons, about ten general surgeons per 100,000 population) has been especially affected. The 25 percent of the senior classes of medical students entering the field in the decades after World War II declined to 10 percent by the late 1980s and to 6 percent in 2001.[16] The average age of general surgeons is now over 50 years. It has been calculated that 10–15 percent are retiring early, burned out and depressed by the restrictions imposed by health plans, administrative overload, and litigation. That the health-care system is losing such highly experienced individuals at the height of their skills has profound implications regarding manpower.[17] For years the numbers of committed trainees were adequate to replenish the ranks of those retiring. As discussed, 70 percent of the approximately one thousand new surgeons produced every year in the United States pursue specialty fellowships. This trend is creating difficulties in coverage by existing general surgical practitioners, particularly in rural areas or in small urban hospitals on which 54 million people depend for their acute care; such institutions require an annual recruitment of about three- or four-hundred trained personnel to cover their professional attrition rate.[18] Indeed, when a staff member of a critical access hospital retires, it may take fourteen to sixteen months to find a replacement. Recent data projected a potential shortage of 13,000 general surgeons by 2010.[19]

Some previously sought-after specialties are in difficulty as well. Cardiac surgery is an example. Traditionally, entrance into this field was highly competitive, with about ten applicants for every available position. The trainees would become board certified in general surgery after a five- to six-year residency, then spend two additional years in a cardiac fellowship, and often extra time in the laboratory. As members of an elite and high-profile profession, they expected to live comfortable and productive lives pursuing a challenging and interesting career. But enthusiasm has declined significantly in recent years through reduction in prestige, diminished professional satisfaction, the threat of litigation, and concerns about financial shortfall. In 2007 only ninety-seven residents applied for the 130 slots available nationally; twenty-nine of these had come from other countries.[20] With interventional radiologists treating successfully many individuals with less advanced heart disease, operative cases have become increasingly complex and difficult. Although formerly an especially lucrative specialty (some may say over-lucrative), reimbursement in real dollars has decreased by 30 percent since the 1990s, while the annual costs of malpractice insurance are considerably over $100,000 in some states. Many existing cardiac surgeons (about two-thousand currently board certified in the United States) are, in fact, discouraging medical students from considering the specialty despite the growing need for their services as the population ages. Indeed, by 2025 the demand for cardio-thoracic surgeons has been projected to increase by 46 percent, whereas the number of those in active practice is expected to decline by 21 percent.[21] Whether existing units will be able to compensate by consolidating into fewer and larger centers and by collaborating more closely with related specialties is unknown.

Another compelling problem directly related to the decline in surgical manpower is the impending crisis in the staffing of emergency rooms and trauma centers. For decades, the uninsured gravitated to city hospitals or to teaching institutions, where the residents treated every patient seeking urgent help, regardless of financial status. The facilities were used relatively appropriately; people came only when they were ill. Dedicated hospital funds or monies from cities, states, or federal programs covered the expenses of those unable to pay. Insured patients with acute conditions more usually went to private hospitals, where the nurse in charge would assess the situation and contact the staff physician on call or seek help directly from an in-house resident moonlighting for extra funds. Young staff doctors often began their private practices by caring for those with emergent problems. This relatively stable situation began to shift in the 1980s, when hospitals increasingly competed to attract a broader clientele by upgrading their facilities, providing specialists expert in the handling of discrete problems, and marketing the most current diagnostic and therapeutic technology. Greater numbers of patients lacking a personal physician or unable or unwilling to make a timely appointment began to use emergency rooms as walk-in clinics, expecting care for often trivial complaints at any time of the day or night. Costs accelerated and waiting times lengthened. Overall, an astonishing 116.9 million visits to emergency rooms were recorded in 2010. Nearly 40 million were injury-related, implying at least some surgical involvement.[22]

Street violence, road traffic accidents, an aging population, poverty, and other societal problems have sharpened the demand for acute services.

Overcrowding of existing space has become an everyday event. We not infrequently hear of sick patients filling the halls outside the emergency rooms of large centers, waiting for beds to open so that they may be admitted. Others sit for untold hours before being seen. With many of the ill lacking adequate medical coverage, institutional costs have soared. Remuneration for professional services by third-party insurers and by Medicare has also declined progressively; the already low payment for emergency room physicians will decrease by an additional 40 percent over the next eight years in the face of a 20 percent increase in practice costs.[23] In consequence, some hospitals are limiting those they accept. A disturbing result of these dynamics is that about 425 emergency departments closed between 1993 and 2003 in the United States, even with a 26 percent increase in overall number of visits. A distressingly prevalent corollary to this situation, despite laws against such activities, is the pattern of ambulances rerouting the uninsured from local facilities to already overextended city or university hospitals.[24] In 2003 alone, ambulances were redirected 501,000 times.[25] The unfortunate patients involved are placed at risk. Some have died unnecessarily. Experts warn of an impending national crisis.

As my colleague Caprice Greenberg intimated, many general surgeons no longer participate in emergency rotations. Indeed, specialists willing to do this work have become so scarce in some areas that affected hospitals are offering generous financial enticements for time on call, and are even hiring "headhunters" to locate appropriate staff. Some newly graduated surgeons feel that they are asked to provide acute care beyond the scope of their expertise. Many balk at declining standards, feeling that inadequate medical coverage may adversely affect outcome. Appallingly, one recent study noted that the rate of perforation of the appendix varied in proportion to the insurance status of those afflicted.[26] Litigation is also a constant specter. The relatively high incidence of lawsuits against the first emergency room doctor to see a given patient is presumably fed both by the frustrations of those who have already waited long hours and an often hurried and impersonal interchange during treatment of acute conditions. Indeed, liability insurance premiums have risen 12 percent per year since 1975 for those covering emergency rooms in general. The premiums are considerably higher for those in high-risk specialties.[27] Some insurers are offering discounts on their malpractice coverage if surgeons *do not* take emergency call.

Medical educators and leaders of university hospitals have become less sanguine about the future of their customary commitments to academic medicine since the dynamics of health care began to change in the 1980s. The area of applied laboratory investigations, an established part of the "triple threat" role of the faculty, has come under particular pressure and has virtually disappeared from many departments. In addition, with research funding shifting toward new areas such as subcellular and molecular biology, gene therapy, proteomics, and associated esoterica, new generations of full-time scientists are replacing laboratory-oriented clinicians, filling postdoctoral positions, and accruing appropriate financial support.[28] The process of gaining adequate funding for research remains difficult for everyone, particularly as congressional appropriations for science vary from year to year and from political administration to administration. Residents aspiring toward an academic career but starting out without a recognized reputation not infrequently become discouraged and do not pursue avenues for monetary support.[29] Indeed, more than a few experienced figures have warned that M.D. scientists are an "endangered species" in the United States and note that research publications come increasingly from foreign laboratories.[30]

Surgical careers in university hospitals have been particularly affected. With faculty promotion traditionally grounded on scholarly output in addition to patient-based activities and teaching, current academic surgeons feel less competitive than their laboratory-centered colleagues. Unrelenting pressure to increase clinical output is accentuating this issue by precluding the time for scholarly reflection so necessary for innovative minds.[31] Indeed, a subject not infrequently discussed in university departments is whether traditional applied surgical research has become obsolete. Opinions vary. Skeptics may consider such activities to be irrelevant in an age of sophisticated biology. Cost-cutting and profit-oriented medical managers may doubt that such efforts will fit into their budgetary planning. This mindset, often promoted by necessity and accepted grudgingly by at least some departmental chairs, directly impacts those desiring academic careers.

In response to these and other pressures, prescient surgical chiefs are promoting new areas of investigation for their residents. Outcomes research, the collection and statistical analysis of particular medical practices and treatments, has become an important area of concentration. With more objective information about benefits, risks, and effects of treatment and medical practices, clinicians can improve their performance and make better decisions for and with their patients. For instance, by assessing the outcomes of elderly individuals with pneumonia, a common disease, investigators have developed guidelines with which practitioners can determine who can be treated safely at home and who should go to a hospital. Not only do those afflicted prefer this approach but Medicare costs are reduced substantially. Practices in the operating room have received comparable attention as it has become clear that complications of the 234 million operations performed yearly around the world are not uncommon but often preventable. To improve safety and reduce error, surgical investigators have introduced a tool that mirrors the preparations of commercial airline pilots before takeoff. The result is a nineteen-item checklist used by the entire surgical team before each major procedure to confirm that no operational detail, no matter how small, has been forgotten or omitted, and that all preventative measures potentially harmful to the patient are in place. The product of a few surgical researchers, the World Health Organization's Surgical Safety Checklist is now in place in a variety of operating rooms throughout the world. Its implementation has reduced overall surgical deaths and complications by more than one-third in both low- and high-income countries.[32]

But despite such novel measures, mistakes still happen. One category of misadventures, wrong-site surgery (wrong side, an incorrect site, wrong procedure, wrong patient) is especially prevalent in orthopedics and neurosurgery; 68 percent of claims against orthopedic surgeons, although comprising only 5.6 percent of overall reported medical errors, involve this subject.[33] The response to such misadventures includes rapid disclosure and transparency to patients and their families, to peers, to the institution itself, and to professional organizations. Ever-increasing attention to the education of all operating-room personnel is improving the problem. Regaining the trust of the injured party, supporting both the injured and the doctor, waiving hospital charges, and decreasing the threat of lawsuit are obvious priorities.

The role of the chairs of surgical departments, the program directors, and those in other positions of responsibility reflects ongoing societal changes and differs substantially from that of the often larger-than-life figures of prior generations. These latter individuals acted with virtually complete autonomy, limited little by institutional, state, or federal oversight. As such, they encouraged clinical investigations, often without rudimentary knowledge and adequate supportive data. Funding was relatively easy to obtain. As we have seen, some laboratory projects had no import. Others were remarkably successful. The often-disastrous early attempts at organ transplantation, heart surgery, and other departures from routine practices eventually produced unprecedented advances. The new leaders, in contrast, face a spectrum of challenges unknown in years past. One current surgical chief summarizes the dynamics with which he and his colleagues must deal.[34]

> Reductions in reimbursement for clinical services rendered, cutbacks in medical education funding for academic medical centers, rising malpractice costs that have now reached crisis proportions in more than a dozen states, and a national nursing shortage are just some of the blows that have been doled out. Their net effect? Make no mistake about it, the business of medicine is no longer medicine, it is business governed by market forces and escalating competition. Few would disagree that these changes have led to an increase in institutional bureaucracy, complexity, anxiety, stress, and physician disenchantment.

The changes he alludes to certainly have influenced surgical education and its related activities.

Unfortunately, many young academic surgeons brought up in the current atmosphere and deprived of relevant scientific nourishment in their daily activities are forced to become business-oriented technicians, investing their creative energies overseeing clinical trials sponsored by pharmaceutical companies and involving themselves in management training–subjects foreign to their traditional role as clinicians, teachers, and investigators. These issues may also be influencing the declining numbers of medical students committing themselves to a surgical career. For continued progress, chairmen and faculties of departments in teaching hospitals realize fully that they must cultivate and protect the energetic and imaginative trainees and young colleagues desirous of an academic position. They must encourage them to apply scientific knowledge toward specific problems posed by the ill. It is heartening that some of these talented and inquisitive individuals continue to investigate the fascinating scientific possibilities that are continually emerging. Indeed, professional meetings remain packed with enthusiastic researchers presenting their data. Science and its application to clinical use have rarely been more exciting.

The challenges buffeting the surgical profession have altered significantly the way in which much surgery is currently practiced. This changing context, however, relating particularly to over-regulation, economic worries, and high costs, may not be too different from events occurring in other fields that entail years of training and a prolonged commitment. Airline pilots, schoolteachers, university faculties, those in the arts, and even those in the sciences have felt the effects of cost containment and new regulation. It may be that all these disciplines are suffering from an increase in national pessimism regarding our ability to produce satisfactory solutions to the problems of a complex world.

twelve

Unsolved Challenges

When the Peter Bent Brigham Hospital opened in 1913, the staff performed relatively few operations. These were always under the threat of infection. Diagnostic tools consisted of little more than a determination of numbers of blood cells and chest and abdominal X-rays. Ether was the only anesthetic agent available. Drugs were few. Intravenous support of the ill patient with water and electrolytes was neither used nor understood. Monitoring methods and intensive care did not yet exist. Most cancers could not be cured. Some common procedures were based on false physiological premises. Manipulation of the heart was never considered. The successful removal of Agnes Turner's varicose veins was considered a relative tour de force. Resident education and research efforts, however, moved along effectively.

I have discussed the development, breadth, and success of the modern field in previous chapters. Among many other improvements, precise imaging methods that leave few surprises for the operating surgeon have evolved in parallel with operative and peri-operative advances. Minimally invasive technologies have revolutionized patient care and rehabilitation. Whereas childhood cancers were almost uniformly fatal in past decades, a significant proportion of afflicted children now survive with a combination of surgery, radiation, and chemotherapy. In similar fashion, such conjunctive measures can cure or turn many adult cancers into chronic diseases. Those previously debilitated with the pain of angina regain full activity after an open-heart procedure or arterial dilation with balloons. Joint replacements rejuvenate individuals previously crippled with arthritis of hip, knee, or shoulder. Those with failure of a vital organ are resurrected with a transplant. Patients with morbid obesity can return to normal lives.

The future holds even more promise as necessity propels new areas of knowledge inexorably forward. Several examples come to mind. Increasing the tempo of the healing of wounds has been an enduring dream of surgeons throughout history, stimulated further by the production and propagation of sheets of skin in the laboratory to cover burned areas, restore extensive tissue loss from war wounds, and heal the ulcers that may develop on the legs of the ever-increasing numbers of diabetics. In one important subject of ongoing investigation, cells from a small biopsy of normal skin are dispersed and cultured under sterile conditions with a variety of recently defined growth factors. The resultant "artificial" skin originates from the patient, so there is no difficulty with rejection. The newly generated substitute, sometimes grafted in combination with a biodegradable matrix for reconstitution of deep defects, is increasingly becoming a realistic alternative to taking skin grafts from uninvolved donor sites. Some surgical scientists are developing strategies for faster wound repair by altering the local temperature or tension of skin edges and flaps.

Teams of surgeons, computer experts, and biomedical engineers are currently pursuing the use of embedded micro-apparatuses to restore activity to poorly functioning body parts, investigations driven in large part by the needs of soldiers disabled in combat. In preliminary studies, for instance, minute transmitters activate the nerves of hearing to relieve deafness. Electrodes implanted behind the eye may energize tiny cameras, producing an "artificial retina" that can record some visual images for the brains of blind patients to process into at least some sight. "Neural prostheses," implanted on spinal nerves, are designed to stimulate hand and arm muscles of individuals with quadriplegia. Computer chips placed in the spinal cord or on individual nerves near sites of limb amputations direct sophisticated bionic prostheses to obey commands sent from the brain. Already, first-generation prototypes for upper-extremity amputations activated by such electronic nerve impulses allow a mechanical arm to move appropriately and an artificial hand to pick up a glass or guide a pencil. Leg prostheses stimulated in a similar manner govern a bionic knee to bend and an ankle to push the body forward for normal walking.

The possibility that transplanted stem cells may populate deficient tissues or even form new organs has generated excitement among both researchers and clinicians. Arising early in embryonic life, these progenitor cells are potentially capable of differentiating into any developing tissue or organ in the body. However, the selection of an aborted embryo as a source or the use of cells from frozen embryos produced by in-vitro fertilization and otherwise discarded has engendered considerable public debate, media exposure, and political posturing. Because of social and emotional issues surrounding the use of fetal cells, the potential application of adult stem cells is gaining attention. In general, these differentiate in a narrower range than embryonic cells and have been less satisfactory in experimental systems. But these observations are tempered by recent reports from laboratories in Japan and the United States that have introduced nuclear material into adult skin cells to produce functioning and differentiating stem cells, and the reprogramming of mature cells from various tissue sources into fully immature forms or intermediate steps of differentiation. Indeed, practical advances from such researches are evolving further as scientists develop techniques to transform one type of the patient's own cells into an entirely different population, obviating the need for immunosuppression for similar cells from genetic strangers. If the results of such experiments hold, many of the problems associated with fetal cell use may be avoided, removing ethical barriers and accelerating research. Although stem cells have long been visualized as progressing inexorably from an undifferentiated population to those in a highly specialized state, it is becoming increasingly clear that their full capacities have been unappreciated. Means to improve repair of damaged sites in the brain and spinal cord with their use, for instance, is an exciting prospect for the large numbers of patients with stroke, paralysis, or other central nervous system deficiencies. As mentioned, surgeons may substitute all or some of failed or failing solid organs such as liver or heart muscle with appropriate primitive cells produced in culture.

Finally, knowledge about the human genome and the genomes of cancer that has been collected during the past decade will eventually allow individualized treatments of maximum effectiveness and minimal toxicity in persons of known genetic makeup. On the horizon are the possibilities of defining and introducing specific genes into patients to cure diseases that occur because a single gene is omitted during embryonic development. Biologists are also increasingly using the techniques to combat the emergence of bacterial and viral variants resistant to current antimicrobial agents.

———

Although new and evolving approaches for the control and cure of disease give much hope for the future, it is less easy to be sanguine about health-care delivery, a subject that is of increasing concern not only to the medical profession but to every citizen. This subject and its immediate outlook fuels much national discussion and debate. The inadequacies and inequities in the existing system seem to obviate or trivialize many of the ongoing medical and scientific advances. Conflicting forces include political enthusiasts both desirous of and opposed to rendering adequate care to as much of the population as possible, commercial ventures interested in improving their bottom line, and a public that expects the best services without increased costs. The consequences for academic institutions, medical education, research, and the effectiveness of patient care itself range from fear, to uncertainty, and to myopic satisfaction with the status quo. In this final chapter I stray from a discussion of surgery and surgeons to wider issues that concern all of us, speaking not as a policy expert but as a long-term and bemused participant in an academic hospital trying to provide optimal care to those who require it.

"To say that the current US health-care 'system' is a dysfunctional and costly patchwork of employer-based insurance, private markets, public programs, and special initiatives is, by any measure, an understatement," note two researchers in an article in the *New England Journal of Medicine*.[1] All physicians, whether in training, in private practice, staff members of a health maintenance organization (HMO), or on the faculties of teaching hospitals, are currently caught in a maelstrom of review and reform of an increasingly fragile and uncertain system. On a daily basis practitioners face patients who vary in their medical coverage. Some have health insurance that safeguards any eventuality, some have inadequate protection despite employment, and some lack any safety net whatsoever. Coverage may suddenly disappear depending upon job loss, unforeseen life changes, or merely the whim of the company providing it. Some insurance companies facing medical bankruptcy may suddenly discontinue coverage. Although the role of doctors and their institutions is to treat each patient to the best of their collective abilities, the ever-shifting foundations of health-care delivery constantly challenge the ingenuity of all involved.

My own awareness of problems of medical coverage stems from my early experience with patients who had developed kidney failure in the 1960s. Their plight posed, in microcosm, a crisis that currently faces us all and certainly influences national policies. Relatively young and with young families, these unfortunate persons were struck down indiscriminately by an ultimately fatal disease. They had to choose among three options: to go on dialysis, which was scarce, expensive, relatively ineffectual, and often organized on a commercial, pay-as-you-go basis; to receive a transplant, which was of high risk and usually unsuccessful; or to do nothing and die. Financial considerations were paramount; existing insurance plans rarely covered their care. Only the wealthy could afford treatment, although occasional minimal support from the NIH and emergency monies from a few states carried a portion of the hospital expenses for some of the less financially endowed. With such persons and their families paying out of pocket to remain alive, patient groups formed to raise money to provide necessary medicines, rent, clothing, even food. Bake sales, auctions, and church activities all contributed. "Death committees" of doctors, priests, businessmen, and other members of the public were established during the 1960s to decide who should receive dialysis—who should live and who should die. The problem became unanswerable. "Should machines or organs go to the sickest, or to the ones with the most promise of recovery; on a first come, first serve basis; to the most valuable (based on wealth, education, position, what?); to the one with the most dependants; to women and children first; to those who could pay; to whom? Or should lots be cast, impersonally and uncritically?"[2] Is a bank president more valuable to society than a housewife, a car mechanic of more worth than a student? How could one choose? It is interesting that during the vituperative debate on national health-care reform in 2010, opponents once again deliberately evoked the erroneous possibilities of "death committees" to frighten the public.

In 1973, the United States Congress debated the fate of thousands of such patients dying each year because of lack of facilities (24,000 died in the following year). Patients and their caregivers lobbied for change. In response, Congress passed HR1, an act that provided support under Medicare for patients with end-stage kidney disease, the only disease so provided for and a departure from the federal coverage that, since its inception in 1965, had included only those over 65 years and on Social Security. The expense of this venture has grown exponentially and now supports 355,000 patients in the United States currently on dialysis and an additional 10,000 who receive a kidney transplant each year. Unfortunately, the expenses for this population have been unremitting. In 2007 Medicare paid $8.6 billion for dialysis support alone, over $43,000 per patient per year.[3] Such funding for a specific disease is merciful and necessary on the one hand and highly costly on the other. It seems clear why its translation into general policy for the nation remains unsolved.

Full realization of the problems with the cost of health care and its coverage evolved slowly. Most medical professionals were relatively unaffected until the issues became increasingly obvious in the 1980s. Through the earlier decades of the twentieth century the majority of doctors treated the ill in solo practices. Hospitals cared for all those who came to their doors. As noted, surgeons earned reasonable salaries, operating on the indigent for free and charging the more affluent whatever both parties agreed was fair. The field of medicine gradually broadened in scope, initially with the formation of Blue Cross and other prepaid health insurance plans in the 1930s, followed by Medicare and Medicaid three decades later. As a result, practitioners flourished with an ensuing increase in clinical income. Private and public hospitals increased their net worth and endowment as more patients emerged to take advantage of the improving care. Teaching institutions enjoyed additional subsidies for resident education and support for research, much from public funds.

This "Golden Age" could not last, however, as the need for services continued to expand. With medicine becoming big business, the profiles, profits, and administrative presence of insurance companies and emerging health plans grew. Costs rose and insurers attempted to decrease their financial outlay by controlling professional practices and diminishing physician autonomy. A new type of market-driven strategy, "managed care" and its most common manifestation, the HMO, arose in the 1980s to regulate coverage for subscribers and their families through contracts with clinics, hospitals, physician groups, and salaried staff. Both private and university-based medical institutions joined such plans to retain their referral base and their fiscal solvency.

Although a significant proportion of the population is relatively satisfied with their medical coverage, the existing system is unraveling. Many legislators and much of the public are vocally in favor of reducing taxes, yet demand a wide array of social programs. This obvious dichotomy is difficult to resolve, particularly when the sophisticated advances of modern health care inevitably engender both high expectations and high costs. Combining these benefits with a comprehensive, affordable, and equitable system is an enduring challenge for policy planners, politicians, and professionals alike. Demands for the most current treatments compete with the often more basic needs of the uninsured and underinsured, at the same time that existing services such as primary care and emergency room coverage are near the breaking point and numbers of practicing obstetricians and general surgeons are declining significantly. Battered by excessive insurance costs, the public additionally perceives that the pocketbooks of executives, stockholders of profitable medical plans, and the executives of nonprofit hospitals take precedence over their coverage and services. The public may decry the unrestrained influence of powerful lobbies against meaningful reform, yet oppose a single-payer system. While the quality of care is excellent for many people, distribution remains inconsistent and often dependent upon economic status, employer responsibility, position in the social hierarchy, and geographic location.

Even though organized by the allegedly more efficient rules of business, the vast medical bureaucracy has become an imposing part of our diverse market-driven health-care scheme. Administrative costs constitute an important proportion of the annual expenditure, accounting for over 27 percent of the total health-care budget in the United States as compared to 3 percent in Canada and less than 10 percent in France, Britain, and other countries with universal coverage. Indeed, a 2003 study concluded that about one million "middlemen" were involved in activities inherent in the system, and that $375 billion could be saved with a single-payer scheme.[4] Those of us who have changed health plans can appreciate this point all too well while trying to fathom the rules, limitations, and fine print of their policies and ensuring that coverage is available for pre-existing conditions. The ever-shifting variables of the insurance industry and pharmacy assistance programs are confusing to all. The patients are particularly frustrated by the often-unintelligible torrent of bills, statements, and directives that flood their mailboxes after an illness or change in coverage. The numbers of doctors, social workers, financial officers, pharmacists, and bill coders in private practices, clinics, and hospitals of every variety spend untold hours navigating an ever-changing labyrinth to collect payment for services rendered; as a small example, 1,300 billing clerks currently labor in the 800-bed Duke University Medical Center just to keep the books.[5] The collective efforts of these and others in all medical facilities throughout the country must be added to those of the thousands of workers in the insurance plans who decide the costs, receive the bills, and organize the payments. A veritable army is involved. And despite all the manpower and all their efforts, nearly 30 percent of expenditures for health care are thought to be wasted on activities that do not benefit the patient directly.[6]

I discussed this subject with a long-term Brigham admissions officer and a group of social workers working with her. She is among the first persons the patients meet to ensure permission by their health plan for a surgical intervention; her colleagues will advocate further for their clients if there are undue difficulties. She notes,

> I have been a manager in Inpatient Accounts for years and have seen many changes in the insurance industry. It has become increasingly difficult getting permission for many procedures, with vast documentation required for every step. Even with complete information, cases commonly approved in the past now require individual physician peer-to-peer review, and are often approved for [less expensive] outpatient day surgery and denied at the in-patient level. In our present economy when patients not infrequently lose their insurance because their jobs are terminated, we often assist them with the complexities of both state and out-of-state coverage. Some may be approved for Medicaid but only after a prolonged waiting period or after any remaining insurance funding is exhausted. Tragically in many

cases they have to deplete their assets to pay the bills or to qualify for federal help.

She gave recent examples. The first was

> an urgent transfer of a highly problematic patient from a community hospital in a neighboring state. Although the insurer denied authorization, the transfer was eventually approved after several calls between the transferring physician, the Brigham physician, and company spokesmen. Because of the serious and prolonged nature of her illness, however, her private policy exceeded its maximum and coverage ceased while she was here. With much difficulty, we eventually received Medicaid approval. Unfortunately, the family had to meet the high interim expenses and had to sell her house.

The second involved an individual "who had a policy that denied treatment at our hospital. I had to give a self-pay estimate and the family came together to raise money for a deposit at a considerable sacrifice."

The social workers recounted comparable situations in a sobering conversation. They noted that the rules and guidelines of many of the private plans are not only bewilderingly Byzantine but vary depending upon individual circumstance. Like the variables influencing the diagnosis and treatment of a medical problem, compensation formulas may shift for a variety of factors, including but not limited to age, locale, marital status, pre-existing conditions, income, employer contributions, layoff or job change, and existing disabilities. Patients, accounts managers, and the social workers themselves may spend hours on the phone with little immediate satisfaction from the private insurer, often inadequate resolution of the problem, and the possibilities of the sick person going into debt to pay for necessary treatments.

In contrast, they stressed that while Medicare and Medicaid eligibility is sometimes equally difficult to comprehend, a single call by a patient advocate will often suffice to resolve the sticking point. Multiple plans produce additional difficulties. If an elderly patient protected by Medicaid plus private insurance fails to complete the paperwork for reauthorization of coverage, if return to work with a resultant increase in income forces the person off Medicaid, or if a younger individual develops a disability and has too much income for Medicare coverage but not enough to afford private insurance, what then? If he or she cannot afford it, a person who has developed a new condition may go without care during their two-year wait for Medicare benefits to be activated. Coverage for medications may be equally complex and may depend on brand, generics availability, co-pay, and deductibles; older people may have to choose between drugs or other necessities of life. These and related dynamics add confusion and administrative costs to the heavily bureaucratized and overburdened system.

What happens if the uninsured or underinsured cannot pay the inflated hospital bill? In many instances, the hospital will lower the overall costs, although the final figure may amount to tens or even hundreds of thousands of dollars due within thirty days. Alternatively, property and even the house may be taken. If the family still cannot afford it, a credit card may be issued, allowing incremental payment over forty years at 17 percent interest. I strongly believe that all citizens need insurance coverage to avoid becoming impoverished as a result of a health issue, like the original patients with kidney failure. That a judge in Virginia, and apparently judges in a few other states, have recently ruled such a matter unconstitutional seems not only counterproductive but cruel.

Inconsistencies also abound throughout the system despite efforts at standardization. Costs of treatment and practice patterns may vary widely depending on social groups, geographical areas, and the choice of hospital. Insurance costs, regardless of source, may be substantially higher in some regions than others without delivering better-quality care or increasing the satisfaction of those receiving it. The incidence of amputation for diabetes or peripheral vascular disease, for example, is four times higher among blacks than among whites, possibly because removal of the leg is a less expensive alternative to a lengthy and expensive vascular reconstruction.[7] One study determined that 63 percent of children under 16 years of age from a town in Vermont had their tonsils removed, but only 16 percent in another town seventy miles away received similar treatment. The incidence of knee replacements among Medicare patients living in Nebraska is twice that for individuals living in Rhode Island.[8] Women covered by Medicare in South Dakota undergo mastectomies for breast cancer seven times more frequently than women in Vermont. The numbers of operations for some types of back pain carried out each year in a city in Idaho are five times the national average and twenty times those performed in a city of similar size in Maine.[9] Significantly, these and similar analyses show that the spending profile of the available medical facilities influences the number of doctor visits, hospitalizations, and tests. As one staff member put it: "In a payment system that rewards everybody for staying busy, every bit of capacity you have, whether it's the number of specialists or the number of intensive care beds or the M.R.I. scanner, has to stay fully occupied because they bought them already and they have to keep paying for them."[10] It may be that in the future, the results of relevant outcome studies may reduce some of these discrepancies and standardize both treatments and costs.

In collaboration with Medicare, the HMOs reduced costs in a variety of ways. They hired primary care doctors to work for them exclusively, exhorted them to increase their daily clinical load, act as gatekeepers in referring patients to specialists only as they (the gatekeepers) deemed necessary, and limit laboratory tests, drug prescriptions, and hospital admissions. For a time the companies implemented a system of "capitation" whereby they rewarded their staff members for staying within stated financial boundaries and imposed penalties for those who exceeded them. The plans promoted rapid discharge from the hospital, encouraged the performance of operations in less expensive outpatient settings, and set restrictions on some treatments.[11] When faced with an emergent clinical problem, professionals responsible for an ill patient not infrequently had to call the relevant insurance company to convince the sometimes recalcitrant authorities to allow them to proceed, to argue about appropriate medications, and to discuss the expected length of stay in the hospital. Contacting HMOs was particularly difficult at night and on weekends. Meanwhile, those seeking care were often becoming sicker. How different were these arrangements from traditional practices, when the doctor diagnosed a given condition, treated it as necessary, orchestrated specialist consultation if appropriate, and attended throughout the recovery period.

I remember well one such interchange with a third-party payer. One of my patients, Mary Burrows, was a 42-year-old woman who had developed kidney failure secondary to uncontrolled urinary tract infections. I had transplanted an organ from a deceased donor some days before. To our mutual delight, the graft functioned well. However, about a week later she developed fever and a severe cough. A chest X-ray showed diffuse pneumonia in both lungs. No bacteria grew on culture. With a lack of diagnosis, we didn't know what to treat. In desperation, we biopsied her lung. Characteristic signs of a serious virus were present on microscopic section. Fortunately, an antiviral agent had recently been introduced. As Mrs. Burrows belonged to a large HMO, I called their headquarters in a distant city for permission to administer the new agent. I explained to the nurse who answered that the patient was a transplant recipient taking powerful immunosuppressive drugs, that she had a rapidly worsening lung infection, and that we had identified the virus. I also expressed fears that without the special treatment, her life was in danger. The conversation was disappointing. The person on the other end of the phone was not only unfamiliar with transplantation and the effects of immunosuppression, but totally unfamiliar with the new drug—except its high price and the fact that it was not on the plan's list of authorized medications. She refused my request. I did my best, stressing the severity of the infection and arguing that if the patient survived, we expected her to live normally for many years. Increasingly frustrated, I asked to speak to the senior company physician. The results were the same. I finally went to the administrator of our hospital, who eventually agreed to bear the not-inconsequential costs of administering the agent. Mrs. Burrows was treated, improved dramatically, and was discharged. I last saw her a decade later, doing well and enjoying her life. This initial experience, however, one of several, still bothers me, although I can well understand the ongoing and as yet irreconcilable debate concerning the expedient use of available resources and insurers' inability to fund costly and nonroutine, albeit potentially promising, treatments.

Additional cost-saving measures have arisen in sequence. Both private and government insurers are consistently reducing reimbursements for care. Recently rescinded, the Medicare sustainable growth rate formula planned to cut the rate of physician payment for its subscribers by 22 percent in mid-2010. The federal division in charge of Medicare payments has recently announced that it will cease reimbursing hospitals for care made necessary by "preventable complications" from presumed inadequate treatment or medical error.[12] However, complications may inevitably develop that no one can predict, much less "prevent." Untoward events occasionally occurring after surgical operations in a small proportion of patients are particularly prone to administrative scrutiny. University-affiliated hospitals may be especially liable from these measures, as many of the patients entering such institutions are uninsured or underinsured, are of high risk with coexisting conditions, and often require complex care.

Some of the financial strategies the HMOs and their associated hospitals have introduced are sensible. Contracts with pharmacological companies allow exclusive purchase of their products at lower prices. Smaller institutions employ commercial laboratories to perform their diagnostic tests, as bulk determinations are less expensive than assays performed in-house. The computerization of records for all subscribers of a given plan is showing promise. Although software programs between member institutions are not always compatible and confidentiality issues problematic, computer technology increasingly allows accurate and rapid transmission of information anywhere. A consulting specialist at a teaching hospital a considerable distance away from a given patient and his or her doctor in a remote or rural area, for instance, can review records online and deliver opinions and advice about diagnosis and treatment. Such an arrangement is often cheaper for the local hospital than employing full-time staff specialists, particularly for night and weekend call. Similarly, outsourcing of X-rays, mammograms, and scans to outside readers is becoming relatively common. The talents of "teleradiologists" in India are often used–their readings are accurate and the turnaround time rapid. This practice may be threatening to those in practice locally, however, as one such individual noted rather poignantly: "Who needs to pay us $350,000 a year if they can get a cheap Indian radiologist for $25,000 a year?"[13] Certainly, individuals in many other lines of work in the United States have been experiencing the difficulties of outsourcing for years.

"Medical tourism" is a related but perhaps unexpected phenomenon. Each year increasing numbers of patients travel long distances abroad for surgery that is, in most cases, significantly less expensive than they can get at home. In 2007, 750,000 Americans received medical care abroad, a figure rising to 6 million by 2010.[14] In many instances, third-party payers or employers footing the insurance bill encourage such offshore activities and arrange specialty care. Some plans provide attractive tourist package tours as added incentives. The Joint Commission International, a section of the major accrediting organization in the United States, has sanctioned many of the institutions involved. These state-of-the-art hospitals, staffed by well-trained surgeons, are on nearly every continent. Patients desiring a facelift, for instance, fly to Argentina, a country known for excellence in plastic surgery. There, the procedure costs less than half that in the United States.[15] They arrive in Mexico, Costa Rica, or South Africa for cosmetic operations and for dental implants. Thailand is a popular location for hip replacements, vascular procedures, and sex-change operations. One beautifully maintained hospital near Bangkok, for instance, has served over a million foreign patients from 190 countries, 64,000 from the United States alone. Individuals with heart disease are sent to India, Singapore, or Malaysia for coronary bypass operations; the cost varies between $10,000 and $19,000 versus $130,000 in the United States.

Although the surgery carried out in some countries is usually excellent, some of the nursing and ancillary services may not meet expected Western standards. Individual patients may also find follow-up care to be a problem upon their return, as some American surgeons do not feel much obligation to treat postoperative complications that have developed half a world away. The field of transplantation has not been exempt from these challenges. Jonathan Marston was a 43-year-old patient I became peripherally familiar with. A successful stockbroker, he lived the high life in New York until struck down by progressive kidney disease. He had to go on dialysis. No family or friends were available to donate an organ. Growing increasingly distraught and feeling that his life was slipping away while waiting on the national transplant list, he found information on the Internet about traveling to other countries to obtain an organ. One glossy advertisement described a clinic in India that stated: "If you are in desperate need of a transplant we might be able to help [with] hospitals located where organs are readily available."[16] Another from China extolled their program; the complete transplant package, excluding travel expenses, cost $55,000.[17] Against the advice of his physician, he pursued the latter avenue. Payment was arranged. Arrangements were surprisingly easy. A date and time for the operation was set. The hospital was modern, the amenities apparently excellent. The operation was carried out successfully on schedule. Immunosuppressive drugs were given. Within ten days he was ready for the long trip home. Feeling so well upon his return, he delayed contacting his doctors. When he eventually presented himself, however, the local transplant team was appalled and frustrated with what they were suddenly asked to deal with. The patient was obviously ill. His incision was poorly healed. The grafted kidney was swollen and tender. He had finished the medication he had been given and had brought no records or reports from China. His situation became increasingly problematic after the kidney was lost despite strenuous attempts to save it. Having put himself outside accepted tenets of care, he learned that neither Medicare nor his private insurance would cover the extensive hospitalization. He had to return to dialysis, but he had lost his place on the national transplant list. Not until later did he discover that the organ had come from a prisoner who the Chinese government had executed on schedule for his operation.

I should emphasize, however, that medical tourism is not limited to patients from developed countries traveling abroad to specialty clinics in less economically fortunate areas. Many large teaching hospitals and major private clinics in the United States improve their financial structure by treating the very rich from other lands, offering "boutique" floors to care for the needs of the patient, their families, and their entire entourage. I know of one important clinic that caters almost exclusively to important individuals from the Middle East. Like other areas such as airlines, hotels, and resorts that prioritize their services for the wealthy, the hospital surroundings are luxurious, special food is served, and a local television station broadcasts in Arabic.

Policy experts from both industry and government predicted that the emerging managed care plans and their "providers" would control costs and provide comprehensive medical delivery. However, the desire of private payers to maximize their profits relegated much medical coverage to a business model of competition, outsourcing, and sometimes appropriate and sometimes draconian limitations. Unfortunately, despite full-page advertisements in the newspapers and optimistic reports on radio and television, the strategies generally failed to reduce expenditures, caused the ranks of the uninsured to swell, and arguably diminished overall quality of care. Public confidence eroded, with dissatisfied voices clamoring ever more loudly about perceived shortcuts in treatment, accelerated and hasty appointments, and an inadequate and impersonal relationship with their physicians. Primary care doctors complained that the controls and bureaucracy imposed by the system curtailed the time they could dedicate to the ill.

Rushed and over-regulated specialists felt equally frustrated as patients occasionally developed unnecessary complications and even threats to their lives from cursory attention to conditions that should have been diagnosed promptly and treated readily. Indeed, some of the corporate pronouncements required a culture shift from the ideals with which doctors entered their profession to those based on monetary gain and the application of business principles to their practices. Productivity and performance were at risk, with every aspect of physician activity apparently having a price tag, a stultifying awareness of expenses and reimbursements permeating daily routine, and periodic reports from hospital administrators measuring the cost-effectiveness of one's activities. "Many [practitioners became] so alienated and angered by the relentless pricing of their day that they [wound] up having no desire to do more than the minimum required for the financial bottom line," according to one report in the *New England Journal of Medicine*.[18] Accentuated by ever-decreasing reimbursements for work carried out, this mindset remains a problem that few governmental or commercial interests have put into their health-delivery equations.

One of the gravest omissions doctors can make, as drilled into us as medical students and residents, is to miss something on physical examination. Our teachers stressed that a rectal examination and determination of the presence of blood in the stool were integral parts of *every* workup. A few years ago, I witnessed a horrifying example of such an exclusion. I occasionally chatted with a security guard at one of the medical school buildings. One day he mentioned that he was passing occasional flecks of red blood with his stools and was to be checked through his health plan. Sometime later he told me that during the hurried visit the screening nurse attributed the bleeding to hemorrhoids and assured him that it would stop with local care. After some months we met again. He said that the bleeding had worsened and that he had returned to the clinic on several occasions for help and advice. Each time the nurse practitioner and the physician implicated the hemorrhoids. Although I told him he should demand a detailed examination, nothing was done. I did not see him again for some time but one day walked past and noticed that he had lost weight. I eventually found out that he had extensive tumor spread in his liver from an undiscovered cancer of the rectum that could easily have been felt by a simple examination. Inexcusably, no one had ever done one. He died a year later. I still remain shocked by this progression of events that began with the exclusion of a basic practice and ended in an unnecessary death. Significantly, recent data confirmed my anecdotal impression, finding that cancers are diagnosed later in individuals like the security guard who are covered by low-cost insurance than among those with more comprehensive plans.[19] Even more discouraging are analyses showing that lack of health coverage results in 45,000 deaths each year, a fatality rate 40 percent higher than for those who are insured.[20] At the same time the Institute of Medicine, an organization of experts providing advice to the nation on matters of health, reported that 20,000 people die in the United States each year because of lack of coverage.[21] Regardless of whose numbers are correct, all seem unacceptable, although probably not dissimilar to numbers of deaths from automobile accidents, trauma, and criminal behavior.

It seems clear that the traditional, market-driven structure of health-care delivery is developing serious cracks, despite good treatment delivered to many people. A recent survey updating the 2000 World Health Organization ranking rated the U.S. health-care system thirty-seventh in the world, even though it spent more per capita than any other developed country.[22] Their reasons may have included the inconstant distribution of quality care throughout a citizenry of broad ethnicity and striking financial disparity. Life expectancy in the United States also remains near the bottom. In 2006 the mortality rate for males ranked 42nd, females 43rd, and infants 36th.[23] Although international comparison may not be fully useful because of unique features of this country, these figures have gained attention among lawmakers. An even more threatening specter is that the present generation of young people may be the first to survive for a shorter time than their parents, possibly a result of the obesity epidemic and the high incidence of diabetes.

The continuing monetary advantages attained by health plans in the face of unremitting costs and sometimes problematic service fuel the low opinion the public holds about the availability and expense of coverage for themselves and their families; those with pre-existing conditions seeking new or additional insurance have been at particular risk. The salaries that private HMOs and even nonprofit plans award their executives, the exemption of the companies from antitrust laws, and the economic gains expected by their investors have compounded public and professional disquiet, particularly as the cost of coverage increases.[24] Anthem Blue Cross, California's largest private health insurer, announced a rise in premiums of 39 percent for their enrollees who purchased individual coverage within the past two years, noting that expenses had increased because many of their healthy subscribers were dropping their policies in the recession, leaving sicker patients with more insurance needs in the pool. At the same time their huge parent company, WellPoint, announced a yearly profit of $2.7 billion in the last quarter of 2009, and the salary of the chief executive officer was raised to over $13 million, a 51 percent increase that is still dwarfed by the salaries of some executives in the pharmaceutical industry.[25]

In some instances, such gains have arisen from blatant financial inconsistencies.[26] The Hospital Corporation of America (HCA), the largest of the HMOs, has approximately 200 hospitals under its umbrella. Yet fees for given procedures vary markedly depending upon the insurance status of the patient. At one of their hospitals in Oklahoma, for instance, the charge for a brain operation was $14,600 when billed to Blue Cross and $13,900 when billed to Medicare. But if the patient was *uninsured*, the total became $85,400. A hospital in Florida charged Medicare patients $6,200 for an appendectomy, individuals commercially insured $7,000, but $35,200 for those without coverage. Although HCA accumulated nearly $22 billion in revenue in 2003, it overcharged the uninsured the year before by over $2 billion and defrauded federal programs by $63 million. Penalties for these activities came to $1.7 billion. About the same time government agencies forced Tenet, the second largest HMO, to pay nearly $380 million in civil damages and criminal fines for comparable irregularities. Other major companies have been similarly penalized for reimbursement fraud. One can only marvel at the societal benefits of our laissez-faire system as these and similar figures emerge.

Changing social dynamics during the past quarter-century in the United States have challenged the long-established responsibilities of academic medical institutions. Usually located in the larger cities, teaching hospitals bear the brunt of social problems of the urban poor, budgetary constraints, public apathy, lack of political will, or obstruction by vested interests. Low-income housing, sex education, gun control, and alcohol and drug use are inadequately addressed or controlled. The surgeons often find themselves the final arbitrators of the end products of these shortcomings as they try to save the lives of the victims of poverty, street crime, domestic violence, substance abuse, and self-indulgence. At the same time the pressures from the business side of medicine have influenced surgical practices in private institutions and in teaching hospitals alike. Over 20 million elective operations are performed each year, an astonishing figure that contrasts dramatically with the relative handful carried out a century before.[27] This evolution has broadened much of the long-established character, goals, and careers of those in the field. It has altered the types of approaches, the procedures, ancillary technologies, and the spectrum of surgically treated disease in almost unrecognizable ways.

In response to these and other dynamics, university-affiliated clinical departments have grown in size and activity, shifting from their traditional focus of care for all into business models driven by commercial pressures. Increasingly they resemble for-profit hospitals, with the number of "patient contacts" and "physical interventions" becoming the prime measures of "productivity." As one official in the American Association of Medical Colleges put it: "The rules are changing. We're going to make it explicit that you [faculties of teaching hospitals] should be generating money."[28] Those in academic medicine have become increasingly discouraged about the progressive industrialization of their profession, institutional emphasis on increased practice revenues, cost containment, and growing financial constraints for ongoing clinical programs. With pressures on the faculties to see more patients in less time and the individuals cared for generally sicker than those in community hospitals, the need for close relationships and supervision of trainees is greater than ever. One crucial result is that time spent previously on education, mentoring, research, and other intellectual pursuits has too often declined to unsupportable levels. Indeed, it has become clear to medical school deans, curriculum committees, program directors, and to the residents and students themselves that teaching is taking second place to clinical demands.

The volunteer clinical instructor, so long the mainstay of training institutions, has become increasingly burdened by the pressures of the marketplace, administrative impositions, and not always subtle insistence by department heads and hospital administrators to keep the coffers filled.[29] Directives to shorten hospital stays, increase numbers of office visits, and carry out more invasive procedures have frustrated the abilities of dedicated teachers to find the time to act as mentors or role models. Conscientious educators are also raising concerns that the corporate control of health care is inhibiting the professional maturation of their charges and instilling values at odds with the enduring tenets of the profession. One warned particularly against emphasizing the business of medicine in a university-based setting. "I think the student who learns medicine in an environment where the bottom line involves cash flow will become a different kind of person than someone educated in an atmosphere where we at least hold out that the bottom line is the satisfaction of the patient's needs."[30] Despite strenuous efforts to make ethics and concern for the patient paramount in medical education, this situation remains unsolved and a continuing subject of concern.

The pursuit of research in the life sciences has been a further victim of the corporate emphasis on income-generating, patient-based activities.

Numbers of medical students and residents seeking careers as clinical investigators in academic settings have declined, at least in part due to financial pressures from educational debts, the prospect of relatively low career salaries, and difficulties in acquiring consistent laboratory funding. In contrast to the 1960s, when half the grant applications to the National Institutes of Health were accepted, only about 12 percent have been successful since the mid-1990s. In 2007 the NIH budget fell for the fifth consecutive year, a decline in size and duration never before experienced.[31] Similarly, in areas of the country where managed care has become the most prevalent and available clinical income is used to finance nonfederally supported studies, ongoing investigations have decreased and sometimes ceased.[32] Established researchers are well aware of this trend. First-time applicants are even more aware as they experience particularly low acceptance rates for their proposals. In response, voices in the academic community are expressing ever-louder alarm that one or more generations of scientists will be lost—both basic scientists and clinical researchers committed to applied biology and trained to translate laboratory findings into the practical treatment of human disease.

We are beginning to see the results of diminished research funding in practical form. Despite unprecedented advances in biology, clinical medicine, and drug discovery, it is now considerably more usual to interview medical students and train residents who wish to obtain an additional degree in business administration, public health, or health-care policy than those aspiring toward translational investigations. It is also interesting that a small but growing proportion of graduating seniors interested in the basic sciences are choosing positions in biotechnology industries. As part of the American Recovery and Reinvestment Act of 2009, the NIH received $200 million in monies to stimulate research in science and health. These Challenge Grants were meant to provide two years of advances in funding for biomedical and behavioral research in high-priority subjects. The recent government "stimulus plan" forwarded in 2010 has also improved funding for science. But with the current swing in political sentiment against government spending, it may take some time for the research enterprise to recover or even stabilize at existing levels of funding.

I do not mean to imply that the existing multifaceted system of medical care is ineffectual, or that the mission of academic institutions is faltering. Overall, medical advances continue to produce some of the best results of diagnosis and treatment anywhere for a large proportion of the population. Positive changes in health-care policies are evolving at the same time. Massachusetts, for instance, has mandated coverage for all their citizens, with penalties attached for those who forgo health insurance. Although the debate continues, all but a small percentage of the public are now covered. On a federal level, considerable energy has been expended toward enhancing public health measures such as the campaign against smoking (despite the continuing chicaneries of the tobacco companies), control of hypertension, identification and treatment of diabetes, and appreciation of the epidemic of obesity. The gradual introduction of computerized patient records in hospitals is streamlining diagnosis, focusing care plans, and improving communication and collaborations among specialists treating individuals with complex conditions. The electronic referencing of an array of pharmaceuticals that address virtually any condition is increasing efficacy and reducing duplication.

However, ensuring equity of access and uniform quality of distribution and delivery remains the compelling problem. A multitier system remains firmly in place; those who subscribe to the best insurance programs are served well, whereas those with less effective or absent coverage may not be. It is considered anathema to mention and those in power deny it, but rationing is a fact of life for many people.[33] Third-party payers already restrict care through excessive fees and co-payments, denying recompense to many with potentially expensive pre-existing conditions, reducing hospital stays, and abbreviating physician interactions.[34] Reimbursement to providers is often limited and extra charges to patients high. Encouraged by lobbyists and contributions from vested interests, the federal government relies on the free market to regulate drug costs, yet blocks importation of the same drugs from other countries at reduced rates. Many patients, particularly the elderly on fixed incomes and on expensive medications, simply cannot afford the monthly drain on their resources.

The marketplace may not be an appropriate venue for the social mission of medicine. The increase in investor-owned specialty hospitals or clinics, and the concentration on profit by third-party payers and associated industries have accelerated expenses. One result is that more and more physicians are forced to become entrepreneurs to survive, sometimes limiting their practices to patients with the highest incomes and best insurance, or over-testing to increase revenue. To add to the confusion, a recent analysis examined economic differences between cohorts of for-profit and not-for-profit hospitals. Over three-quarters of the not-for-profit institutions performed more effectively in regard to both expenses and efficiency.[35] Indeed, the author of a recent book has pointed out that mortality rates are 6 percent higher in investor-owned hospitals than in nonprofit institutions, yet treatment costs 3–13 percent more.[36]

Some medical communities have organized themselves effectively to reduce costs. The lesson from Grand Junction, Colorado, seems particularly relevant. Its average per capita Medicare spending in 2007 was 24 percent below the national average and as much as 60 percent lower than the most expensive regions in the United States.[37] Among changes made by the medical establishment there, leadership by family physicians appeared to be the most important factor. Equalization of all payment for all patients, regardless of coverage, was another. Incentives for control and transparency of costs for every doctor became part of the medical culture; with yearly reviews of the practices and cost profiles of all involved, payment was withheld from specialists performing excessive procedures who were then educated about working within the norms of the community. Low-cost care at the end of life, with much interaction with elderly patients about advance directives, was emphasized. Why other parts of the country have not applied these approaches is unclear.

Medical professionals facing the inequitable distribution of health care on a daily basis are caught in the middle. Their primary responsibility is helping individual patients regardless of financial constraints. On the one hand, the existing private system works well for many subscribers. On the other, at least some safety net for the large numbers with insufficient coverage has obvious appeal. Many fear, however, that the expenses of such a universal scheme might reduce the best we expect to a lower level of care, with less use of beneficial but costly technical advances. They fear we may face limitations on our choices of doctor and treatment strategies.

Many in the medical establishment too have an aversion to changing the existing system. As useful and financially appealing as these advances are, they seem to have driven the system from what the practitioner may do *for* the patient to what he or she may do *to* the patient. It may be that if increased attention is given to the maintenance of healthy lifestyles and public health measures that keep chronic conditions at bay, the eventual costs for a more completely insured public may decline.

All other industrialized and many developing countries have initiated strategies for universal health care. The United States, almost alone, remains wedded to the influence of market forces, even though the government pays about half the direct and indirect costs in the present hybrid of private and public insurance plans; in the latter category, Medicare, Medicaid, and the Children's Health Insurance Program cover about 100 million people.[38] The annual health expenditure of $2.2 trillion is currently 16 percent of the gross domestic product, a figure projected to rise to 20 percent in the next seven years. This figure is about twice that of the relevant budget of virtually all other nations.[39] Despite this vast financial outlay and contrary to accepted opinion, many patients now wait to see their primary care providers for longer periods than patients in France, Canada, Holland, and other countries with single-payer schemes. Waiting times for specialized care in nationalized systems may be long and some of the current practices and technologies that we take for granted may not be immediately available. To avoid delay, for instance, a relatively few Canadians come across the border and pay out of pocket for diagnosis and treatment. Those who desire private insurance in the United Kingdom for prompt attention are free to purchase it.

Even with limitations that include older facilities and less general use of expensive technology, it is interesting to consider the benefits of universal health care, as exemplified particularly by the British system. Because everyone is covered if illness or accident strikes, the specter of financial ruin is obviated and concerns about cancellation of coverage for a pre-existing condition or job change precluded. Trainees enter primary care in adequate numbers because they do not have educational debt and will earn as much as specialists. These primary physicians follow accepted treatment protocols, and without threat of litigation, order relatively few unnecessary or expensive tests. They are paid commensurate with both patient load and quality of care. With all medical records computerized, the National Health Service can determine if the results of an individual practitioner meet established criteria, while annual peer review allows comprehensive and helpful discussion of problems. All citizens choose their primary doctor, who sends them to specialists as needed. Although hardly perfect and under constant economic constraints, this and other systems that many other countries have developed are relatively efficient and inexpensive, consistently popular, and greatly appreciated by the public. There is much here to consider.

Often with good reason, there remains in the United States a prevailing distrust of government and government interventions. Unfortunately, those in professional practice have as few solutions as those immersed in policy decisions, although emotionally many are convinced that some variety of national health service is the only answer. I have come to feel that there is little eventual alternative.

Despite ongoing dialogue and debate concerning universal health care, it appears that powerful and influential vested interests and lobbyists for the medical industry itself will continue their efforts to prevent a divided government from designing a system to accommodate as much of their equally divided constituency as possible. Some of my own long-held opinions about tempering at least some of the problems inherent in the existing system have begun to jell during the current political imbroglio. As one who continues to hold relatively idealistic views about the traditional aims of the medical profession, I offer several hardly original but possible suggestions to consider.

First, health-care reform measures would be easier to accept if they were carried out in a graded and sequential fashion over time. Assuming that general coverage would be mandated as currently occurs in Massachusetts, the eligibility age for those covered by a Medicare-like public option could be lowered by ten years at five-year intervals. Willing persons not yet in the system would keep their existing coverage as before.

The serious dearth of primary care doctors must be addressed. Perhaps some educational debt could be relieved for individuals committed to the field. In addition, as in Britain, the salaries of these persons could be raised to levels commensurate with those of specialists. Appropriately trained nurse practitioners and physician's assistants could carry out more routine activities, freeing up time for the physician to spend with fewer patients. More young graduates would then be attracted into a rewarding profession.[40]

The educational debt accrued by the majority of young doctors not only takes years to pay back but may influence their choice of specialty. Federal subsidization of medical education attached to a mandated period of service in the Indian Health Service, rural areas, clinics and hospitals in inner cities, and other underserved sites might be one solution. Indeed, such an infusion of educated manpower would markedly help the 96 million poor and high-risk people who live in rural and urban areas with inadequate health resources. Like older physicians who spent two or more years in the armed services, young graduates could donate equivalent time as general medical officers, while those with significant residency experience in their field could carry some of the burden of existing specialists, which might reduce their present attrition rate. Government agencies could give such individuals a reasonable stipend during their period of service, forgive their educational debts, and at the same time expunge existing for-profit lending agencies from the system. Some have also suggested tuition loan rebates for those who desire careers as physician-scientists in academic centers but whose earning potential is limited.

Although many politicians are lawyers and are unwilling to address the subject, tort reform would reduce unnecessary and damaging lawsuits that increase medical costs and limit access to doctors. Indeed, the Congressional Budget Office has estimated that appropriate reform of medical liability would subtract about $54 billion from federal expenses over the next decade.[41] To practice medicine without the continuing threats of potential lawsuits would decrease unneeded tests and reduce costs. Perhaps a mandated, uniform, and universal national screening system by professional experts, impervious to appeal, could block frivolous suits and let through only "deserving" ones for full litigation. The additional stipulation that "the loser pays all" would reduce further the existing litigatory feeding frenzy.

A cap on the profits of private insurers and the pharmaceutical industry would allow direction of excess funds back into the system to aid consumers who need help. Along with reasonable limitations of drug costs could be the increased application of well-tested generics. Restricting the top-heavy salaries of company executives to more reasonable levels would increase public good will.

As proffered in the recent legislation, tax credits could be introduced for persons who pay for individual policies or those obtained through state-managed health insurance exchanges. Medicare-like coverage of all for catastrophic medical care could be implemented. Routine insurance would continue through existing private or employer-based schemes.

One means to subsidize, at least in part, the expenses of the majority of patients unable to afford the most advanced (and expensive) treatments might be for third-party payers to increase the costs selectively for those able to pay for optimal care. Indeed, such a system is at least partially in place through differing rates of insurance coverage. Such a strategy might also temper the endless debate about tax breaks for the rich.

There have been successful models for volunteer surgical services for those without insurance. In one, for instance, volunteers in Los Angeles have spent a few hours a month caring for over 6,500 nonemergent patients in a fifteen-year period.[42] Surgical results were exemplary, complications were few, and follow-up was consistent. The program not only included medical professionals but hospital administrators, nurses, lawyers, and laymen. If initiated in increased numbers of inner cities, such local philanthropic support would relieve, in part at least, state and federal responsibilities.

Although expensive to implement, the replacement of the existing stacks of paper charts, lab reports, and other patient-associated information with electronic medical records will not only allow more effective communication between the primary care physician and specialist but substantially increase safety for the patient. These will allow more efficient use of services and diminish repetition of tests and drugs.

As has been evident from much of what I have said in this chapter, I am one of the many people who believe that health care is a right. Throughout human history, those more fortunate have had advantages over those less so in many aspects of life. The Protestant ethic on which the United States is built has further suggested that individuals who work hard will attain success in life, and that poverty is the fault of those who do not strive enough.[43] While many have thrived on that premise almost since its inception, the country currently faces marked social changes, with shifting demographics, a decline of the middle class, increasing separation between the rich and everyone else, diminishing productivity, and significant unemployment. Most accept that everyone in society needs an automobile or home insurance. Why should medical insurance be different? Federal intervention is hardly a panacea, but as far as medicine is concerned there seems little choice but to try to repair a system that is badly damaged. We must not deny the promise of the medical advances that have developed during the past century for individuals financially unable to take advantage of them.

However, this is a book about surgeons and surgery. Despite all the dialogue, arguments, and political recriminations, I am encouraged by those currently in the field and those entering it. Having spent a professional career in an academic center, I have seen much of the best that it can offer, have interacted with often selfless individuals involved in advancing patient care, have viewed and participated in relevant applied research, and have been stimulated by teaching the young. I believe that university-affiliated institutions, with a mission to treat all comers with the best evidence-based information available, regardless of insurance status, remain an important model for health care. It is difficult for me to imagine that any future system in the richest country in the world could not use effectively the lessons it provides.

Notes
Acknowledgments
Index

NOTES

Introduction

1. H. C. Polk, Jr., Quality, safety, and transparency, *Annals of Surgery* 242 (2005): 293.

1. Three Operations

1. J. Ochsner, The surgical knife, *Bulletin of the American College of Surgeons* 84 (1999): 27.
2. Sir H. Dale, *The Harveian Oration on "Some Epochs in Medical Research"* (London, H.K. Lewis, 1935), 9.
3. H. Dodd and F. B. Cockett, *The Pathology and Surgery of the Veins of the Lower Limbs* (Edinburgh: E. and S. Livingston, 1956), 3.
4. J. Homans, Operative treatment of varicose veins and ulcers, based on a classification of these lesions, *Surgery, Gynecology and Obstetrics* 22 (1916): 143.
5. D. McCord, *The Fabrick of Man: Fifty Years of the Peter Bent Brigham* (Portland, Maine: Anthoensen Press, 1963), 18.
6. C. B. Ernst, Current concepts: Abdominal aortic aneurysm, *New England Journal of Medicine* 328 (1993): 1167.
7. N. L. Tilney, G. L. Bailey, and A. P. Morgan, Sequential system failure after rupture of abdominal aortic aneurysms: An unsolved problem in post-operative care, *Annals of Surgery* 178 (1973): 117.
8. K. M. Flegal, M. D. Carroll, C. L. Ogden, and C. L. Johnson, Prevalence and trends in obesity among US adults 1999–2000, *Journal of the American Medical Association* 288 (2002): 1723.
9. J. Stevens, J. J. Cai, E. R. Pamuk, D. F. Williamson, M. J. Thum, and J. L. Wood, The effect of age in the association between body-mass index and mortality, *New England Journal of Medicine* 388 (1998): 1.
10. J. C. Hall, J. McK. Watts, P. E. O'Brien, et al., Gastric surgery for morbid obesity: The Adelaide Study, *Annals of Surgery* 211 (1990): 419.
11. C. Rosenthal, Europeans find extra options for staying slim, *New York Times*, Jan. 3, 2006, D7.
12. J. McGuire, C. Wright, and J. N. Leverment, Surgical staplers: A review, *Journal of the Royal College of Surgeons of Edinburgh* 42 (1997): 1.
13. N. T. Soper, M. L. Brunt, and K. Kerbl, Laparoscopic general surgery, *New England Journal of Medicine* 330 (1994): 409.

2. The Teaching Hospital

1. C. W. Walter, Finding a better way, *Journal of the American Medical Association* 263 (1990): 1676.

2. F. D. Moore, The Brigham in Emile Holman's day, *American Journal of Surgery* 80 (1955): 1094.

3. E. H. Thomson, *Harvey Cushing: Surgeon, Author, Artist* (New York: Neale Watson Academic Publications, 1981), 74.

4. H. K. Beecher and M. B. Altschule, *Medicine at Harvard: The First 300 Years* (Hanover, N.H.: University Press of New England, 1977), 487.

5. F. C. Shattuck, The dramatic story of the new Harvard Medical School, *Boston Medical and Surgical Journal* 193 (1920): 1059.

6. K. M. Ludmerer, *Learning to Heal: The Development of American Medical Education* (New York: Basic Books, 1985), 48.

7. N. N. Nercessian, Built to last, *Harvard Medical Alumni Bulletin* (Winter 2002): 47.

8. W. I. T. Brigham, *The History of the Brigham Family: A Record of Several Thousand Descendants of Thomas Brigham the Emigrant* (New York: Grafton Press, 1907), 128.

9. Beecher and Altschule, *Medicine at Harvard*, 320.

10. K. M. Ludmerer, *Time to Heal: American Medical Education from the Turn of the Century to the Era of Managed Care* (Oxford: Oxford University Press, 1999), 18.

11. Beecher and Altschule, *Medicine at Harvard*, 168.

12. L. F. Schnore and P. R. Knights, Residence and social structure: Boston in the antebellum period, in *Nineteenth Century Cities: Essays in the New Urban History*, ed. S. Thernstrom and R. Sennett (New Haven: Yale University Press, 1969), 249.

13. M. J. Vogel, *The Invention of the Modern Hospital: Boston 1870–1930* (Chicago: University of Chicago Press, 1980), 15.

14. Ibid., 12.

15. G. Williams, *The Age of Agony* (London: Constable, 1975), 89.

16. C. Woodham-Smith, *Florence Nightingale* (London: Constable, 1950), 157.

17. R. Jones, Thomas Wakley, plagiarism, libel and the founding of the *Lancet, Journal of the Royal Society of Medicine* 102 (2009): 404.

18. The pecuniary condition of the medical profession in the United States, *Boston Medical and Surgical Journal* 4 (1831): 9.

19. M. Kaufman, *American Medical Education: The Formative Years, 1765–1910* (Westport, Conn.: Greenwood Press, 1976), 155.

20. H. W. Felter, *History of the Eclectic Medical Institute* (Cincinnati: Published for the Alumni Association, 1902), 39.

21. P. Starr, *The Social Transformation of American Medicine* (New York: Basic Books, 1982), 93.

22. A. Flexner, *Medical Education in the United States and Canada: A Report to the Carnegie Foundation for the Advancement of Teaching* (New York: Carnegie Foundation for Higher Education, 1910).

23. R. Shryock, *American Medical Research, Past and Present* (New York: Commonwealth Fund, 1947), 49.

24. O. W. Holmes, Currents and counter-currents in medical science, in O. W. Holmes, *Medical Essays 1842–1882* (Boston: Houghton-Mifflin, 1883), 203.

3. Evolution of a Profession

1. G. Corner and W. Goodwin, Benjamin Franklin's bladder stone, *Journal of the History of Medicine and Allied Sciences* 8 (1953): 359.
2. Sir J. Bell, *Principles of Surgery* (London: Longman, Hurst, Rhes, Orme, 1808), 417.
3. R. Holmes, *The Age of Wonder: How the Romantic Generation Discovered the Beauty and Terror of Science* (New York: Pantheon Books, 2008), 306.
4. D'A. Power, Robert Liston (1794–1847), *Dictionary of National Biography*, 1909, 11:1236.
5. J. Duncan, Modern operating theaters, *British Medical Journal* 2 (1898): 299.
6. E. J. Browne, *Charles Darwin: A Biography, vol. 1: Voyaging* (New York: Alfred A. Knopf, 1995), 62.
7. C. Bell, On lithotomy, *Lancet* 12 (1827): 773.
8. E. Riches, The history of lithotomy and lithotrity, *Annals of the Royal College of Surgeons of England* 43 (1968): 185.
9. W. Moore, *The Knife Man* (New York: Broadway Books, 2005), 221.
10. Court of King's Bench, Cooper v. Whatley, *Lancet* 1 (1828): 353.
11. H. Ellis, *A History of Surgery* (London: Greenwich Medical Media, 2001), 25.
12. R. French, The anatomical tradition, in *Companion Encyclopedia of the History of Medicine*, ed. W. Bynum and R. Porter (London: Routledge, 1993), 81.
13. W. Osler, *Principles and Practice of Medicine* (New York: Appleton, 1912), 492.
14. E. Masson, *Elève des Sangues* (1854), cited in *The Rise of Surgery: From Empiric Craft to Scientific Discipline*, ed. O. H. Wangensteen and S. D. Wangensteen (Minneapolis: University of Minnesota Press, 1978), 250.
15. Ellis, *A History of Surgery*, 50.
16. F. H. Garrison, *An Introduction to the History of Medicine* (Philadelphia: W. B. Saunders, 1963), 220.
17. A. F. Guttmacher, Bootlegging bodies: A history of bodysnatching, *Bulletin of the Society of Medical History of Chicago* 4 (1935): 352.
18. J. H. Warner and J. M. Edmonson, *Dissection: Photographs of a Rite of Passage in American Medicine: 1880–1930* (New York: Blast Books, 2009), 17.
19. J. Walsh, *History of Medicine in New York: Three Centuries of Medical Progress* (New York: National Americana Society, 1919), 2:382.
20. Graveyard ghouls arrested with a cargo of corpses, *Philadelphia Press*, Dec. 5, 1882.
21. L. F. Edwards, The famous Harrison case and its repercussions, *Bulletin of the History of Medicine* 31 (1957): 162.
22. H. K. Beecher and M. B. Altschule, *Medicine at Harvard: The First 300 Years* (Hanover, N.H.: University Press of New England, 1977), 38.
23. B. W. Brown, Successful issue following the administration of 7 pounds of metallic mercury, *Association Medical Journal (London)* 1 (1853): 12.
24. G. M. Beard and A. D. Rockwell, *A Practical Treatise on the Medical and Surgical Uses of Electricity* (New York, 1878), 579.
25. F. Treves, Intestinal obstruction, its varieties, with their pathology, diagnosis and treatment, *The Jacksonian Prize Essay of the Royal College of Surgeons of England* (London, 1884), 476.
26. Ellis, *A History of Surgery*, 67.

27. O. H. Wangensteen and S. D. Wangensteen, *The Rise of Surgery: From Empiric Craft to Scientific Discipline* (Minneapolis: University of Minnesota Press, 1978), 227.

28. Ibid., 238.

29. J. Marion Sims, *The Story of My Life* (rpt.; New York: Da Capo Press, 1968), 116.

30. J. A. Shepherd, *Spencer Wells* (Edinburgh: E. and S. Livingstone, 1965), 97.

31. Fanny Burney, A mastectomy, Sept. 30, 1811, in *The Journals and Letters of Fanny Burney* (Madame d'Arblay), ed. J. Hemlow (Oxford: Oxford University Press, 1975), 6:596–616, cited in Holmes, *Age of Wonder*, 306.

32. L. D. Vandam, Anesthesia, in R. Warren, *Surgery* (Philadelphia: W. B. Saunders, 1963), 277.

33. Ellis, *A History of Surgery*, 89.

34. Ibid., 93.

35. F. D. Moore, Surgery, in *Advances in American Medicine: Essays at the Bicentennial*, ed. J. Z. Bowers and E. F. Purcell (New York: Josiah Macy, Jr., Foundation, 1976), 627.

36. S. D. Gross, A century of American surgery, in *A Century of American Medicine 1776–1876*, ed. E. H. Clark (rpt.; Brinklow, Md.: Old Hickory Bookshop, 1962).

37. R. J. Dubos, *Louis Pasteur, Free Lance of Science* (Boston: Little, Brown, 1950) 300.

38. T. D. Brock, *Robert Koch: A Life in Medicine and Bacteriology* (Washington, D.C.: ASM Press, 1999), 289.

4. Steps Forward and Steps Backward

1. E. C. Cutler, Harvey (Williams) Cushing, *Science* 90 (1939): 465.

2. S. J. Crowe, *Halsted of Johns Hopkins: The Man and His Men* (Springfield, Ill.: Charles C. Thomas, 1957), 66.

3. H. K. Beecher and M. B. Autschule, *Medicine at Harvard: The First 300 Years* (Hanover, N.H.: University Press of New England), 413.

4. H. Clapesattle, *The Doctors Mayo* (Minneapolis: University of Minnesota Press, 1941), 448.

5. Ibid., 407.

6. Sir Frederick Treves, *Plarr's Lives of Fellows of the Royal Society of England* (London: Royal College of Surgeons, 1930), 2:434.

7. F. Treves, The Cavendish Lecture on some phases of inflammation of the appendix, *British Medical Journal* 1 (1902): 1589.

8. F. D. Moore, Surgery, in *Advances in American Medicine: Essays at the Bicentennial*, ed. J. Z. Bowers and E. F. Purcell (New York: Josiah Macy, Jr., Foundation, 1976), 645.

9. *Vital Statistics of the United States for 1935, 1950, 1972, 1973* (Washington, D.C.: U.S. Government Printing Office, 1975).

10. Moore, Surgery, 639.

11. W. B. Cannon, The movements of the intestines studied by means of the Roentgen rays, *American Journal of Physiology* 6 (1902): 251.

12. Crowe, *Halsted of Johns Hopkins*, 21.

13. Ibid., 27.

14. W. A. Dale, The beginnings of vascular surgery, *Surgery* 76 (1974): 849.

15. G. Majno, *The Healing Hand: Man and Wound in the Ancient World* (Cambridge, Mass.: Harvard University Press, 1975), 403.

16. O. H. Wangensteen, J. Smith, and S. D. Wangensteen, Some highlights on the history of amputation reflecting lessons in wound healing, *Bulletin of the History of Medicine* 41 (1967): 97.

17. R. M. Goldwyn, Bovie: The man and the machine, *Annals of Plastic Surgery* 2 (1979): 135.

18. H. Cushing and W. T. Bovie, Electro-surgery as an aid to the removal of intracranial tumors, *Surgery, Gynecology and Obstetrics* 47 (1928): 751.

19. R. Stevens, *American Medicine and the Public Interest* (New Haven: Yale University Press, 1971), 244.

20. E. C. Cutler and R. Zollinger, *Atlas of Surgical Operations* (New York: MacMillan, 1939).

21. J. S. Edkins, The chemical mechanism of gastric secretion, *Journal of Physiology* 34 (1906): 135.

22. W. Beaumont, *Experiments and Observations on the Gastric Juice and the Physiology of Digestion* (Plattsburgh: F. P. Allen, 1833).

23. F. D. Moore, The gastrointestinal tract and the acute abdomen, in R. Warren, *Surgery* (Philadelphia: W. B. Saunders, 1963), 764.

24. F. D. Moore, The effect of definitive surgery on duodenal ulcer disease: A comparative study of surgical and non-surgical management in 997 cases, *Annals of Surgery* 132 (1950): 654.

25. A. Ochsner, P. R. Zehnder, and S. W. Trammell, The surgical treatment of peptic ulcer: A critical analysis of results from subtotal gastrectomy and from vagotomy plus partial gastrectomy, *Surgery* 67 (1970): 1017.

26. L. R. Dragstedt and F. M. Owens, Supra-diaphragmatic section of the vagus nerves in treatment of duodenal ulcer, *Proceedings of the Society for Experimental Biology and Medicine* 53 (1943): 152.

27. M. J. Blaser and J. C. Atherton, *Helicobacter pylori* persistence: Biology and disease, *Journal of Clinical Investigation* 113 (2004): 321.

28. R. P. H. Logan and M. M. Walker, ABC of the upper gastrointestinal tract: Epidemiology and diagnosis of *Helicobacter pylori* infection, *British Medical Journal* 323 (2001): 920.

5. War and Peace

1. F. D. Moore, Surgery, in *Advances in American Medicine: Essays at the Bicentennial*, ed. J. Z. Bowers and E. F. Purcell (New York: Josiah Macy, Jr., Foundation, 1976), 662.

2. O. H. Wangensteen, S. D. Wangensteen, and C. Klinger, Wound management of Ambroïse Paré and Dominique Larrey: Great French military surgeons of the sixteenth and nineteenth centuries, *Bulletin of the History of Medicine* 46 (1972): 218.

3. F. Nightingale, *Notes on Nursing for the Labouring Classes* (London: Harrison, 1861), 29.

4. G. H. B. Macleod, *Notes on the Surgery of the War in the Crimea* (Philadelphia: J. B. Lippincott, 1862), 328.

5. L. Strachey, Florence Nightingale, in *Eminent Victorians* (Harmondsworth: Penguin Books, 1971), 121.

6. J. S. Billings, Medical reminiscences of the Civil War, *Transactions and Studies of the College of Physicians of Philadelphia* 27 (1905): 115.

7. G. A. Otis and D. L. Huntington, *Medical and Surgical History of the War of the Rebellion, 1861–1865* (Washington, D.C.: United States War Department Surgeon General's Office, 1870), pt. 3, vol. 2, 877.

8. N. M. Rich and D. G. Burris, "Modern" military surgery: 19th century compared with 20th century, *Journal of the American College of Surgeons* 200 (2005): 321.

9. D. R. Welling, D. G. Burris, and N. M. Rich, Delayed recognition–Larrey and Les Invalides, *Journal of the American College of Surgeons* 202 (2006): 373.

10. H. B. Shumaker, Jr., Arterial aneurysms and arteriovenous fistulas: Sympathectomy as an adjunct measure in operative treatment, in *Vascular Surgery in World War II*, ed. D. C. Elkin and M. E. DeBakey (Washington, D.C.: Office of the Surgeon General, 1955), 318.

11. G. Majno, *The Healing Hand: Man and Wound in the Ancient World* (Cambridge, Mass.: Harvard University Press, 1975), 292.

12. J. P. Bennett, Aspects of the history of plastic surgery since the 16th century, *Journal of the Royal Society of Medicine* 76 (1983): 152.

13. H. D. Gillies, *Plastic Surgery of the Face* (London: Henry Frowde, 1920).

14. A. C. Valdrier and A. Lawson Whale, Report on oral and plastic surgery and on prosthesis appliances, *British Journal of Surgery* 5 (1918): 151.

15. J. M. Dubernard, B. Lengelé, E. Morelon, et al., Outcome 18 months after the first human partial face transplantation, *New England Journal of Medicine* 357 (2007): 2451.

16. O. Cope, Management of the Cocoanut Grove burns at the Massachusetts General Hospital, *Annals of Surgery* 117 (1943): 801.

17. G. W. Gay, Burns and scalds, *Boston Medical and Surgical Journal* 93 (1865): 349.

18. C. A. Moyer, H. W. Margraf, and W. W. Monafo, Jr., Burn shock and extravascular sodium deficiency: Treatment with Ringer's solution with lactate, *Archives of Surgery* 90 (1965): 799.

19. F. D. Moore, Metabolism in trauma: The meaning of definitive surgery–the wound, the endocrine glands and metabolism, *The Harvey Lectures, 1956–1957* (New York: Academic Press, 1958), 74.

20. F. D. Moore, *A Miracle and a Privilege: Recounting a Half Century of Surgical Advance* (Washington, D.C.: Joseph Henry Press, 1995), 110.

21. P. C. Oré, *Transfusion du Sang* (Paris: Ballière, 1886).

22. R. Lower, "Tractatus de corde," cited in A. R. Hall, Medicine and the Royal Society, in *Medicine in Seventeenth Century England*, ed. A. G. Debus (Berkeley: University of California Press, 1974), 439.

23. S. Pepys, *Diary and Correspondence of Samuel Pepys, Esq., FRS.*, Nov. 18, 1666 (London: Bickers and Son, 1877), 4:161.

24. J. J. Abel, L. C. Rowntree, and B. B. Turner, On the removal of diffusible substances from the circulating blood by means of dialysis, *Transactions of the Association of American Physicians* 28 (1913): 51.

25. J. R. Brooks, Carl W. Walter, MD: Surgeon, inventor, and industrialist, *American Journal of Surgery* 148 (1984): 555.

26. I. S. Ravdin and J. E. Rhoads, Certain problems illustrating the importance of knowledge of biochemistry by the surgeon, *Surgical Clinics of North America* 15 (1935): 85.

27. S. J. Dudrick, D. W. Wilmore, H. M. Vars, and J. E. Rhoads, Long-term parenteral nutrition with growth development and positive nitrogen, *Surgery* 64 (1968): 134.

28. R. U. Light, The contributions of Harvey Cushing to the techniques of neurosurgery, *Surgical Neurology* 55 (1991): 69.

29. T. I. Williams, *Howard Florey: Penicillin and After* (Oxford: Oxford University Press, 1984), 57.

30. G. Macfarlane, *Alexander Fleming: The Man and the Myth* (Cambridge, Mass.: Harvard University Press, 1984), 98.

31. L. Colebrook and Gerhard Domagk, *Biographical Memoires of Fellows of the Royal Society*, vol. 10 (1964).

32. A. Schatz, E. Bugie, and S. A. Waksman, Streptomycin, a substance exhibiting antibiotic activity against gram positive and gram negative bacteria, *Proceedings of the Society for Experimental Biology and Medicine* 55 (1944): 66.

6. The Promise of Surgical Research

1. J. C. Thompson, Gifts from surgical research. Contributions to patients and surgeons, *Journal of the American College of Surgeons* 190 (2000): 509.

2. F. D. Moore, The university and American surgery, *Surgery* 44 (1958): 1.

3. J. A. Buckwalter, C. Saltzman, and T. Brown, The impact of osteoarthritis: Implications for research, *Clinical Orthopaedics and Related Research* 427 suppl. (2004): S6.

4. J. Antoniou, P. A. Martinean, K. B. Fillon, et al., In-hospital cost of total hip arthroplasty, *Journal of Bone and Joint Surgery* 86 (2004): 2435.

5. J. Charnley, Anchorage of the femoral head prosthesis to the shaft of the femur, *Journal of Bone and Joint Surgery* 42 (1960): B28.

6. K. O'Shea, E. Bale, and P. Murray, Cost analysis of primary total hip replacement, *Irish Medical Journal* 95 (2002): 177.

7. F. H. Garrison, *An Introduction to the History of Medicine* (Philadelphia: W. B. Saunders, 1963), 347.

8. R. D. French, *Anti-Vivisection and Medical Science in Victorian Society* (Princeton: Princeton University Press, 1975).

9. C. Darwin, letter to E. Ray Lankester, cited in E. J. Browne, *Charles Darwin*, vol. 2: *The Power of Place* (New York: Alfred A. Knopf, 2002), 421.

10. Quoted in S. Benison, A. C. Barger, and E. L. Wolfe, *Walter B. Cannon: The Life and Times of a Young Scientist* (Cambridge, Mass.: Harvard University Press, 1987), 172.

11. Quoted in ibid., 281.

12. L. H. Weed, Studies on cerebro-spinal fluid: The theories of drainage of cerebrospinal fluid with an analysis of the methods of investigation, *Journal of Medical Research* 31 (1914): 21.

13. W. Osler, On sporadic cretinism in America, *American Journal of the Medical Sciences* 106 (1893): 5.

14. W. Osler, Sporadic cretinism in America, *American Journal of the Medical Sciences* 114 (1897): 337.

15. M. Bliss, *The Discovery of Insulin* (Chicago: University of Chicago Press, 1982), 20.

16. E. L. Opie, *Disease of the Pancreas* (Philadelphia: J. B. Lippincott, 1903).

17. S. Wild, G. Roglic, A. Greer, R. Sicree, and H. King, Global prevalence of diabetes: Estimates for 2000 and projection for 2030, *Dial Care* 27 (2004): 1047.

18. Current data available at http://www.cdc.gov/features/diabetesfactsheet/.

19. F. M. Allen and J. W. Sherrill, Clinical observations on treatment and progress in diabetes, *Journal of Metabolic Research* 2 (1922): 377.

20. F. M. Allen, E. Stillman, and R. Fitz, *Total Dietary Regulation in the Treatment of Diabetes* (New York: Rockefeller Institute for Medical Research, 1919), 184.

21. I. Murray, Paulesco and the isolation of insulin, *Journal of the History of Medicine and Allied Sciences* 26 (1971): 150.

22. M. Bliss, *Banting, A Biography* (Toronto: McClelland and Stewart, 1984).

23. J. Cheymol, Il y a cinquante ans Banting et Best "découvraient l'insuline," *Histoire des Sciences Médicales* 6 (1972): 133.

24. Bliss, *The Discovery of Insulin*, 112.

25. F. G. Banting, C. H. Best, J. B. Collip, W. R. Campbell, and A. A. Fletcher, Pancreatic extracts in the treatment of diabetes mellitus: Preliminary report, *Canadian Medical Association Journal* 2 (1922): 141.

26. F. G. Banting, C. H. Best, J. B. Collip, W. R. Campbell, A. A. Fletcher, J. J. R. MacLeod, and E. C. Noble, The effect produced on diabetes by extracts of pancreas, *Transactions of the Association of American Physicians* 37 (1922): 1.

27. Bliss, *The Discovery of Insulin*, 243.

28. Ibid., 211.

29. J. Hunter, Lectures on the principles of surgery (1786),in *The Works of John Hunter*, ed. James F. Palmer (London, Longman, Rees, Orme, Brown, Green, and Longman, 1837), 1:436.

30. J. W. White, The result of double castration in hypertrophy of the prostate, *Annals of Surgery* 22 (1895): 2.

31. P. Starr, *The Social Transformation of American Medicine* (New York: Basic Books, 1982), 343.

7. Operations on the Heart

1. G. Majno, *The Healing Hand: Man and Wound in the Ancient World* (Cambridge, Mass.: Harvard University Press, 1975), 401.

2. R. Warren, The heart, in R. Warren, *Surgery* (Philadelphia: W. B. Saunders, 1963), 650.

3. B. Cabrol, *Alphabeton Anatomikon* (Lyon: Pierre and Jacques Chouet, 1624), 99.

4. E. J. Trelawney, "Percy Bysshe Shelley (1792–1822)," in J. Sutherland, *The Oxford Book of Literary Anecdotes* (Oxford: Oxford University Press, 1975), 192.

5. T. Billroth, Krankheiten der Brust, in *Handbuch der Allgemeinin und Speziellen Chirurgie*, ed. M. Pitha and T. Billroth (Stuttgart: F. Ennke, 1882), 3:163.

6. S. Paget, *Surgery of the Chest* (1896), cited in H. B. Shumacker, Jr., *The Evolution of Cardiac Surgery* (Bloomington: Indiana University Press, 1992), 3.

7. Baron D. J. Larrey, *Clinique Chirurgicale, Exercée Particulièrment dans le Camps et les Hôpitaux Militaires depuis 1792 jusqu'en 1829* (Paris: Gabon, 1829), 2:284.

8. Shumacker, Jr., *The Evolution of Cardiac Surgery*, 8.

9. W. G. MacPherson, A. A. Bowlby, C. Wallace, and C. English, *History of the Great War–Medical Services Surgery of the War* (London: H. M. Stationary Office, 1922), 1:11–12.

10. D. E. Harken, Foreign bodies in and in relation to the thoracic blood vessels and heart, *Surgery, Gynecology and Obstetrics* 83 (1946): 117.

11. Cited in G. W. Miller, *King of Hearts: The True Story of the Maverick Who Pioneered Open Heart Surgery* (New York: Random House, 2000), 4.

12. W. S. Edwards and P. D. Edwards, *Alexis Carrel: Visionary Surgeon* (Springfield, Ill.: Charles C. Thomas, 1974), 8.

13. R. E. Gross and J. P. Hubbard, Surgical ligation of a patent ductus arteriosus: Report of first successful case, *Journal of the American Medical Association* 112 (1939): 729.

14. R. H. Bartlett, Surgery, science, and respiratory failure, *Journal of Pediatric Surgery* 12 (1997): 401.

15. Cited in W. H. Hendren, Robert E. Gross, 1905–1988. *Transactions of the American Surgical Association* 107 (1989): 327.

16. R. E. Gross, Complete surgical division of the patent ductus arteriosis: A report of 14 successful cases, *Surgery, Gynecology and Obstetrics* 78 (1944): 36.

17. R. E. Gross, Surgical correction for coarctation of the aorta, *Surgery* 18 (1945): 673.

18. C. Crafoord and G. Nylin, Congenital coarctation of the aorta and its surgical treatment, *Journal of Thoracic Surgery* 14 (1945): 347.

19. E. C. Pierce, R. E. Gross, A. H. Bill, Jr., and K. Merrill, Jr., Tissue culture evaluation of the viability of blood vessels stored by refrigeration, *Annals of Surgery* 129 (1949): 333.

20. R. E. Gross and C. A. Hufnagel, Coarctation of the aorta: Experimental studies regarding its surgical correction, *New England Journal of Medicine* 233 (1945): 287.

21. A. Blalock and E. A. Park, Surgical treatment of experimental coarctation (atresia) of aorta, *Annals of Surgery* 119 (1944): 445.

22. V. T. Thomas, *Pioneering Research in Surgical Shock and Cardiovascular Surgery: Vivien Thomas and His Work with Alfred Blalock* (Philadelphia: University of Pennsylvania Press, 1985), 58.

23. W. S. Stoney, Bill Longmire and the blue baby operation, *Journal of the American College of Surgeons* 198 (2004): 653.

24. A. Blalock and H. Taussig, Surgical treatment of malformations of the heart in which there is pulmonary stenosis or pulmonary atresia, *Journal of the American Medical Association* 128 (1945): 189.

25. T. Tuffier, La chirurgie du coeur, Cinquième Congres de la Societé Internationale de Chirurgie, Paris, July 19–23, 1920 (Brussels: L. Mayer, 1921), 5.

26. O. Becker, Uber die sichtbaewn Erscheinungen der Blutbewegen in der Netzhant, *Archives of Ophthalmology* 18 (1872): 206.

27. H. Cushing and J. R. B. Branch, Experimental and clinical notes on chronic valvular lesions in the dog and their possible relation to a future surgery of the cardiac valves, *Journal of Medical Research* 17 (1908): 471.

28. L. Brunton, Preliminary notes on the possibility of treating mitral stenosis by surgical method, *Lancet* 1 (1902): 352.

29. Letter from H. Souttar to D. E. Harken, cited in Shumacker, *The Evolution of Cardiac Surgery*, 40.

30. C. S. Beck and E. C. Cutler, A cardiovalvulotome, *Journal of Experimental Medicine* 40 (1924): 375.

31. E. C. Cutler, S. A. Levine, and C. S. Beck, The surgical treatment of mitral stenosis, *Archives of Surgery* 9 (1924): 689.

32. T. Treasure and A. Hollman, The surgery of mitral stenosis 1898–1948: Why it took 50 years to establish mitral valvuloplasty, *Annals of the Royal College of Surgeons of England* 77 (1995): 145.

33. J. J. Collins, Dwight Harken: The legacy of mitral valvuloplasty, *Journal of Cardiac Surgery* 9 (1994): 210.

34. D. E. Harken, L. B. Ellis, P. F. Ware, and L. R. Norman, The surgical treatment of mitral stenosis. I. Valvuloplasties, *New England Journal of Medicine* 239 (1948): 801.

35. L. B. Ellis and D. E. Harken, The clinical results of the first five hundred patients with mitral stenosis undergoing mitral valvuloplasty, *Circulation* 11 (1955): 4.

36. L. B. Ellis and D. E. Harken, Closed valvuloplasty for mitral stenosis: A twelve-year follow up on 1571 patients, *New England Journal of Medicine* 270 (1964): 643.

8. The Mechanical Heart

1. F. Trendelenburg, Zur Operation der Embolie der Lungenarterien, *Zentralblatt für Chirurgie* 35 (1908): 92.

2. E. C. Cutler, Pulmonary embolectomy, *New England Journal of Medicine* 209 (1933): 1265.

3. A. Ochsner, cited in R. W. Steenburg, R. Warren, R. E. Wilson, and L. E. Rudolf, A new look at pulmonary embolectomy, *Surgery, Gynecology and Obstetrics* 107 (1958): 214.

4. C. J. J. LeGallois, *Expériences sur le principe de la vie, notamment sur celui des mouvemens du coeur, et sur le siège de ce principe* (Paris: D'Hautel, 1812).

5. C. E. Brown-Sequard, Récherches expérimentales sur les propriétés physiologiques et les usages du sang rouge et du sang noir et leurs principaux élements gazeux, l'oxygène, et acide carbonique, *Journal de le Physiologie de l'Homme et des Animaux* 1 (1858): 95.

6. T. G. Brodie, The perfusion of surviving organs, *Journal of Physiology* 29 (1903): 266.

7. J. MacLean, The discovery of heparin, *Circulation* 19 (1959): 75.

8. C. A. Lindbergh, An apparatus for the culture of whole organs, *Journal of Experimental Medicine* 62 (1935): 409.

9. J. H. Gibbon, Jr., Development of the artificial heart and lung extracorporeal blood circuit, *Journal of the American Medical Association* 206 (1968): 1983.

10. J. H. Gibbon, Jr., The development of the heart-lung apparatus, *Review of Surgery* 27 (1970): 231.

11. F. D. Moore, *A Miracle and a Privilege: Recounting a Half Century of Surgical Advance* (Washington, D.C.: J. Henry Press), 224.

12. J. H. Gibbon, Jr., Application of a mechanical heart and lung apparatus to cardiac surgery, *Minnesota Medicine* 37 (1954): 171.

13. W. G. Bigelow, W. K. Lindsay, R. C. Harrison, R. A. Gordon, and W. F. Greenwood, Oxygen transport and utilization in dogs at low body temperatures, *American Journal of Physiology* 160 (1950): 125.

14. C. A. Hufnagel, Permanent intubation of the thoracic aorta, *Archives of Surgery* 54 (1947): 382.

15. C. A. Hufnagel, The use of rigid and flexible plastic prosthesis for arterial replacement, *Surgery* 37 (1955): 165.

16. C. A. Hufnagel, P. D. Vilkgas, and H. Nahas, Experience with new types of aortic valvular prosthesis, *Annals of Surgery* 147 (1958): 636.

17. A. Starr and M. L. Edwards, Total mitral replacement: Clinical experience with a ball valve prosthesis, *Annals of Surgery* 154 (1961): 726.

18. W. B. Fye, The delayed diagnosis of myocardial infarction: It took half a century, *Circulation* 72 (1980): 262.

19. World Health Organization, World Health Report 2004: *Changing History* (Geneva: World Health Organization, 2004), 120.

20. H. B. Shumacker, Jr., *The Evolution of Cardiac Surgery* (Bloomington: Indiana University Press, 1992), 231.

21. W. B. Cannon, Studies of the circulation of activity in endocrine glands. V. The isolated heart as an indicator of adrenal secretion induced by pain, asphyxia, and excitement, *American Journal of Physiology* 50 (1919): 399.

22. E. C. Cutler, Summary of experiences up-to-date in the surgical treatment of angina pectoris, *American Journal of the Medical Sciences* 173 (1927): 613.

23. C. S. Beck, The development of a new blood supply to the heart by operation, *Annals of Surgery* 102 (1935): 801.

24. A. M. Vineberg, Development of an anastomosis between the coronary vessels and a transplanted internal mammary artery, *Canadian Medical Association Journal* 45 (1941): 295.

25. A. Carrell, Aorto-coronary bypass: Address to the American Surgical Association, 1910, cited in Shumacker, *The Evolution of Cardiac Surgery*, 139.

26. R. G. Favaloro, Saphenous vein autograft replacement of severe segmental artery occlusion, *Annals of Thoracic Surgery* 5 (1968): 334.

27. R. C. Fox and J. P. Swazey, *The Courage to Fail* (Chicago: University of Chicago Press, 1974), 151.

28. H. H. Dale and E. A. Schuster, A double perfusion pump, *Journal of Physiology* 64 (1928): 356.

29. A. Carrel and C. A. Lindbergh, Culture of whole organs, *Science* 31 (1935): 621.

30. D. Liotta and D. A. Cooley, First implantation of cardiac prosthesis for staged total replacement of the heart, *Transactions of the American Society for Artificial Internal Organs* 15 (1969): 252.

31. M. E. DeBakey, C. W. Hall, et al., Orthotopic cardiac prosthesis: Preliminary experiments in animals with biventricular artificial hearts, *Cardiovascular Research Center Bulletin* 71 (1969): 127.

32. D. A. Cooley, D. Liotta, et al., Orthotopic cardiac prosthesis for two-staged cardiac replacement, *American Journal of Cardiology* 24 (1969): 723.

33. R. Bellah, Civil religion in America, in R. Bellah, *Beyond Belief: Essays in Religion in a Post-traditional World* (New York: Harper and Row, 1970), 168.

34. R. C. Fox and J. P. Swazey, *Spare Parts: Organ Replacement in American Society* (Oxford: Oxford University Press, 1982), 95.

35. J. Kolff, Artificial heart substitution: The total or auxiliary artificial heart, *Transplantation Proceedings* 16 (1984): 898.

36. W. C. DeVries, J. L. Anderson, L. D. Joyce, et al., Clinical use of the total artificial heart, *New England Journal of Medicine* 310 (1984): 273.

37. W. C. DeVries, The permanent artificial heart in four case reports, *Journal of the American Medical Association* 259 (1988): 849.

38. W. S. Pierce, Permanent heart substitutes: Better solutions lie ahead, *Journal of the American Medical Association* 259 (1988): 891.

39. F. D. Moore, *Transplant: The Give and Take of Tissue Transplantation* (New York: Simon and Schuster, 1972), 275.

40. L. W. Miller, F. G. Pagini, S. D. Russell, et al., for the Heartmate II Clinical Investigators, *New England Journal of Medicine* 357 (2007): 885.

41. J. G. Copeland, R. G. Smith, F. A. Arabia, et al. Cardiac replacement with a total artificial heart as a bridge to transplantation, *New England Journal of Medicine* 351 (2004): 859.

9. The Transfer of Organs

1. J. E. Murray, ed., Human kidney transplant conference, *Transplant* 2 (1964): 147.

2. R. Küss and P. Bourget, *An Illustrated History of Organ Transplantation* (Rueil-Malmaison, France: Laboratoires Sandoz, 1992), 8–23.

3. J. Dewhurst, Cosmas and Damian, patron saints of doctors, *Lancet* 2 (1988): 1479.

4. R. M. Goldwyn, Historical introduction, in G. Baronio, *Degli Innesti Animali [On the Grafting of Animals]* (1804; Boston: Boston Medical Library, 1975), 17.

5. Cited in D. Hamilton, *The Monkey Gland Affair* (London: Chatto and Windus, 1986), 12.

6. F. Lydston, Sex gland implantation: Additional cases and conclusions to date, *Journal of the American Medical Association* 66 (1916): 1540.

7. Cited in Hamilton, *The Monkey Gland Affair*, 28.

8. C. Moore, Physiologic effects of non-living testis grafts, *Journal of the American Medical Association* 94 (1930): 1912.

9. P. B. Medawar, The behavior and fate of skin autografts and skin homografts in rabbits, *Journal of Anatomy* 78 (1944): 176.

10. F. D. Moore, *Give and Take: The Development of Tissue Transplantation* (Philadelphia: W. B. Saunders, 1964), 14.

11. R. H. Lawler, J. W. West, P. H. McNulty, E. J. Clancey, and R. P. Murphy, Homotransplantation of the kidney in the human, *Journal of the American Medical Association* 144 (1950): 844.

12. C. Dubost, N. Oeconomos, J. Vaysse, et al., Note préliminaire sur l'étude des fonctions rénales greffes chez l'homme, *Bulletin et Mémoires de la Societe des Medicines et Hôpitalieres de Paris* 67 (1951): 105.

13. D. M. Hume, J. P. Merrill, et al., Experiences with renal transplantation in the human: Report of nine cases, *Journal of Clinical Investigation* 34 (1955): 327.

14. J. E. Murray, Reflections on the first successful kidney transplant, *World Journal of Surgery* 6 (1982): 372.

15. J. E. Murray, J. P. Merrill, G. J. Dammin, et al., Study on transplant immunity after total body irradiation: Clinical and experimental investigations, *Surgery* 48 (1960): 272.

16. J. Hamburger, J. Vaysse, J. Crosnier, et al., Transplantation d'un rein entre non-monozygotes après irradiation du recouver, *Presse Médicale* 67 (1959): 1771.

17. R. Schwartz and W. Dameshek, Drug induced immunological tolerance, *Nature* 183 (1959): 1682.

18. J. E. Murray, A. G. R. Sheil, R. Moseley, et al., Analysis of mechanisms of immunosuppressive drugs in renal homotransplantations, *Annals of Surgery* 160 (1964): 449.

19. J. E. Murray, Remembrances of the early days of renal transplantation, *Transplantation Proceedings* 13 (1981): 9.

20. J. E. Murray, J. P. Merrill, J. H. Harrison, R. E. Wilson, and G. J. Dammin, Prolonged survival of human-kidney homografts by immunosuppressive drug therapy, *New England Journal of Medicine* 268 (1963): 1315.

21. T. E. Starzl, T. L. Marchioro, and W. R. Waddell, The reversal of rejection in human renal homografts with subsequent development of "homograft tolerance," *Surgery, Gynecology and Obstetrics* 117 (1963): 385.

22. C. N. Barnard, Human heart transplantation: An evaluation of the first two operations performed at the Groote Schuur Hospital, Cape Town, *American Journal of Cardiology* 22 (1968): 811.

23. P. Mollaret and M. Goulon, Le coma dépassé et necroses nerveuses controles massives, *Revue Neurologique* 101 (1959): 116.

24. A definition of irreversible coma, Report of the Ad Hoc Committee of the Harvard Medical School to Examine the Definition of Brain Death, *Journal of the American Medical Association* 205 (1968): 337.

25. The thirteenth report of the human renal transplant registry, prepared by the Advisory Committee to the Renal Transplant Registry, *Transplantation Proceedings* 9 (1977): 9

26. I. Penn, The incidence of malignancies in transplant recipients, *Transplantation Proceedings* 7 (1975): 325.

27. R. R. Lower, E. Dong, Jr., and N. E. Shumway, Suppression of rejection crises in the cardiac homograft, *Annals of Thoracic Surgery* 1 (1965): 645.

28. Transplants: Guarded outlook, *Newsweek*, July 21, 1969, 109.

29. R. C. Powles, A. J. Barrett, H. M. Clink, et al., Cyclosporin A for the treatment of graft versus host disease in man, *Lancet* 2 (1978): 1327.

30. R. Y. Calne, D. J. G. White, S. Thiru, et al., Cyclosporin A in patients receiving renal allografts from cadaver donors, *Lancet* 2 (1978): 1323.

31. J. F. Borel, The history of Cyclosporin A and its significance, in *Cyclosporin A: Proceedings of an International Symposium on Cyclosporin A*, ed. D. J. G. White (Amsterdam: Elsevier, 1972), 5.

32. Canadian Multi-center Transplant Group, A randomized clinical trial of Cyclosporin in cadaveric renal transplantation, *New England Journal of Medicine* 309 (1983): 809.

33. European Multi-centre Trial, Cyclosporin in cadaveric renal transplantation: One year follow-up of a multi-center trial, *Lancet* 2 (1983): 986.

34. F. K. Port, R. M. Merion, E. C. Rays, and R. A. Wolfe, Trends in organ donation: Transplantation in the United States, 1997–2006, *American Journal of Transplantation* 8, pt. 2 (2008): 2911.

35. M. Simmerling, P. Angelos, J. Franklin, and M. Abecassis, The commercialization of human organs for transplantation: The current status of the ethics debate, *Current Opinion in Organ Transplantation* 11 (2006): 130.

36. C. Chelda, China's human-organ trade highlighted by US arrest of "salesman," *Lancet* 351 (1998): 735.

37. N. Scheper-Hughes, Neo-cannibalism: The global trade in human organs, *Hedgehog Review* 3 (Summer, 2001).

10. Making a Surgeon, Then and Now

1. P. Starr, *The Social Transformation of American Medicine* (New York: Basic Books, 1982), 224.

2. F. D. Moore, Surgery, in *Advances in American Medicine: Essays at the Bicentennial*, ed. J. Z. Bowers and E. F. Purcell (New York: Josiah Macy, Jr., Foundation, 1976), 630.

3. K. M. Ludmerer, *Time to Heal: American Medical Education from the Turn of the Century to the Era of Managed Care* (Oxford: Oxford University Press, 1999), 86.

4. Ibid., 181.

5. E. W. Fonkalsrud, Reassessment of surgical subspecialty training in the United States, *Archives of Surgery* 104 (1972): 760.

6. American College of Surgeons and American Surgical Association, Surgical manpower, in *Surgery in the United States: A Summary on the Study on Surgical Services for the United States* (New York, American College of Surgeons and American Surgical Association, 1975), ch. 4.

7. L. Sokoloff, The rise and decline of the Jewish quota in medical school admissions, *Bulletin of the New York Academy of Medicine* 68 (1992): 497.

8. F. D. Moore, *A Miracle and a Privilege: Recounting a Half Century of Surgical Advance* (Washington, D.C.: Joseph Henry Press, 1995), 55.

9. M. Bliss, *William Osler: A Life in Medicine* (Oxford: Oxford University Press, 1999), 962.

10. J. K. Inglehart, The American health care system: Teaching hospitals, *New England Journal of Medicine* 329 (1993): 1054.

11. D. A. Asch and R. M. Parker, The Libby Zion case: One step forward or two steps backward? *New England Journal of Medicine* 318 (1988): 771.

12. M. L. Wallach and L. Chao, Resident work hours: The evolution of a revolution, *Archives of Surgery* 136 (2001): 1426.

13. T. R. Russell, From my perspective, *Bulletin of the American College of Surgeons* 85 (2000): 4.

14. A. C. Powell, J. S. Nelson, N. N. Massarweh, L. P. Brewster, and H. P. Santry, The modern surgical lifestyle, *Bulletin of the American College of Surgeons* 94 (2009): 31.

15. J. E. Fischer, Continuity of care: A casualty of the 80 hour work week, *Academic Medicine* 79 (2004): 381.

16. S. M. Zaré, J. Galanko, K. E. Behrns, et al., Psychological well-being of surgery residents before the 80-hour work week: A multi-institutional study, *Journal of the American College of Surgeons* 198 (2004): 633.

17. T. F. Dodson and A. L. B. Webb, Why do residents leave general surgery? The hidden problem in today's programs, *Current Surgery* 62 (2005): 128.

18. T. J. Leibrandt, C. M. Pezzi, S. A. Fassler, E. E. Reilly, and J. B. Morris, Has the 80 hour work week had an impact on voluntary attrition in general surgery residency programs? *Journal of the American College of Surgeons* 202 (2006): 340.

19. E. J. Thomas, D. M. Studdert, H. R. Burstin, et al., Incidence and types of adverse events and negligent care in 1992 in Utah and Colorado, *Medical Care* 38 (2000): 261.

20. L. T. Kohn, J. M. Corrigon, and M. S. Donaldson (eds.), *To Err Is Human: Building a Safer Health System* (Washington, D.C.: National Academic Press, 2000).

21. L. L. Leape, Error in medicine, *Journal of the American Medical Association* 272 (1994): 1851.

22. R. L. Pincus, Mistakes as a social construct: An historical approach, *Kennedy Institute of Ethics Journal* 11 (2001): 117.

23. L. B. Andrew, Physician suicide, available at http://emedicine.medscape.com/article/806779-overview (accessed March 4, 2011).

24. F. D. Moore, *Metabolic Care of the Surgical Patient* (Philadelphia: W. B. Saunders, 1959), vii.

11. Shifting Foundations

1. K. B. Stitzenberg and G. F. Sheldon, Progressive specialization within general surgery: Adding to the complexity of workforce planning, *Journal of the American College of Surgeons* 201 (2005): 925.

2. American Medical Association, Freida Online, General surgery training statistics, 2009. Available at https://freida.ama-assn.org/ama/pub/education-careers/graduate-medical-education/freida-online.shtml (accessed March 4, 2011).

3. Association of American Medical Colleges, Record number of U.S. medical school seniors apply to residency programs. Match participation by international medical graduates continues to rise. Available at http://www.aamc.org/newsroom/news-releases/2007/87960/070315.html (accessed March 23, 2011).

4. National Resident Matching Program (NRMP) 2006, www.nrmp.org (accessed March 23, 2011).

5. W. H. Hendron, Robert Edward Gross, 1905–1988. *Transactions of the American Surgical Association* 107 (1989): 327.

6. B. A. Davies, A review of robotics in surgery, *Proceedings of the Institution of Mechanical Engineers* 214 (1999): 129.

7. Healthcare Cost and Utilization Project (HCUP), Nationwide Inpatient Sample (NIS) 2000–2008. Available at http://hcup-us.ahrq.gov/db/nation/nis/nisrelatedreports.jsp (accessed March 23, 2011).

8. N. T. Berlinger, Robotic surgery: Squeezing into tight places, *New England Journal of Medicine* 354 (2006): 20.

9. J. May, Endovascular repair of abdominal aortic aneurysms, *Australian and New Zealand Journal of Surgery* 72 (2002): 908.

10. D. Sanghavi, Baby steps, *Boston Globe Magazine*, May 29, 2005, 19.

11. G. I. Barbash and S. A. Glied, New technology and health care costs: The case of robot-assisted surgery, *New England Journal of Medicine* 363 (2010): 701.

12. J. C. Ho, X. Gu, S. R. Lipsitz, et al., Comparative effectiveness of minimally invasive vs. open radical prostatectomy, *Journal of the American Medical Association* 302 (2009): 1557.

13. R. A. Cooper, The coming era of too few physicians, *Bulletin of the American College of Surgeons* 93 (2008): 11.

14. R. A. Cooper, It's time to address the problem of physician shortages: Graduate medical education is the key, *Annals of Surgery* 246 (2007): 527.

15. H. T. Debas, Surgery: A noble profession in a changing world, *Annals of Surgery* 236 (2002): 263.

16. K. Bland and G. Isaacs, Contemporary trends in student selection of medical specialties, *Archives of Surgery* 137 (2002): 259.

17. G. Miller, The problem of burnout in surgery, *General Surgery News* 36 (2009): 20.

18. J. E. Fisher, The impending disappearance of the general surgeon, *Journal of the American Medical Association* 298 (2007): 2191.

19. S. M. Cohn, M. A. Prince, and C. L. Villareal, Trauma and critical care workforce in the United States: A severe surgeon shortage appears imminent, *Journal of the American College of Surgeons* 209 (2009): 446.

20. B. Jancin, Programs aim to bolster ranks of cardiac surgeons, *American College of Surgeons: Surgery News* 4 (2008): 11.

21. A. Grover, K. Gorman, T. M. Dall, et al., Shortage of cardiothoracic surgeons is likely by 2020, *Circulation* 1120 (2009): 488.

22. National Ambulatory Medical Care Survey: 2007 Summary (20 November 2010), CDC/National Center for Health Statistics. Center for Disease Control and Prevention. Available at: http://www.cdc.gov/nchs/data/nhsr027.pdf (accessed March 23, 2011).

23. D. D. Trunkey, A growing crisis in patient access to emergency care: A different interpretation and alternate solutions, *Bulletin of the American College of Surgeons* 91 (2006): 14.

24. C. W. Burt, L. F. McCaig, R. H. Valverda, Analysis of ambulance transports and diversions among U.S. emergency departments, *Annals of Emergency Medicine* 47 (2006): 317.

25. L. F. McCaig et al., National Hospital Ambulatory Medical Care Survey: 2003 Emergency Department Summary (Hyattsville, MD: National Center for Health Statistics, Centers for Disease Control and Prevention). Available at: http://www.cdc.gov/nchs/data/ad/ad358.pdf.

26. F. M. Pieracci, S. R. Eachempari, P. S. Barie, and M. A. Callahan, Insurance status, but not race, predicts perforation in adult patients with acute appendicitis, *Journal of the American College of Surgeons* 205 (2007): 445.

27. H. R. Burstin, W. G. Johnson, S. R. Lipsitz, and T. A. Brennan, Do the poor sue? A case-control study of malpractice claims and socioeconomic status, *Journal of the American Medical Association* 154 (1994): 1365.

28. D. G. Nathan and J. D. Wilson, Clinical research at the NIH: A report card, *New England Journal of Medicine* 349 (2003): 1860.

29. A. Zugar, Dissatisfaction with medical practice, *New England Journal of Medicine* 350 (2004): 69.

30. L. E. Rosenberg, Physician-scientists: Endangered and essential, *Science* 283 (1999): 331.

31. S. A. Wells, Jr., The surgical scientist, *Annals of Surgery* 224 (1996): 239.

32. A. B. Haynes, T. G. Weiser, W. R. Berry, et al. (Safe Surgery Saves Lives Study Group), A surgical safety checklist to reduce morbidity and mortality in a global population, *New England Journal of Medicine* 360 (2009): 491.

33. D. C. Ring, J. H. Herndon, and G. S. Meyer, Case 34–2010: A 65-year-old woman with an incorrect operation on the left hand, *New England Journal of Medicine* 363 (2010): 1950.

34. W. W. Souba, The new leader: New demands in a turbulent, changing environment, *Journal of the American College of Surgeons* 197 (2003): 79.

12. Unsolved Challenges

1. I. Redlener and R. Grant, America's safety net and health care reform: What lies ahead? *New England Journal of Medicine* 36 (2009): 123.

2. Cited by G. Annas, Organ transplants: Are we treating the modern miracle fairly? in *Human Organ Transplantation: Societal, Medical-legal, Regulatory and Reimbursement Issues*, ed. D. Cowan, J. Kantonovitz, et al. (Ann Arbor, Mich.: Health Administration Press, 1987), 166.

3. Treatment methods for kidney failure, National Institute of Diabetes and Digestive and Kidney Disease, National Institutes of Health. Available at: http://kidney.niddk.nih.gov/kudiseases/pubs/kidneyfailure/index.htm (accessed March 23, 2011).

4. S. Woolhandler, T. Campbell, and D. U. Himmelstein, Cost of healthcare administration in the United States and Canada, *New England Journal of Medicine* 349 (2003): 768.

5. *Focus* (News from Harvard Medical, Dental, and Public Health Schools), Feb. 5, 2010.

6. E. S. Fisher, J. P. Bynum, and J. S. Skinner, Slowing the growth of health care costs: Lessons from regional variation, *New England Journal of Medicine* 360 (2009): 849.

7. E. S. Fisher, D. Goodman, and A. Chandra, Disparities in health and health care among Medicare beneficiaries: A brief report of the Dartmouth Atlas Project, Robert Wood Johnson Foundation, June 5, 2008. Available at http://www.rwjf.org/pr/product.jsp?id=31251 (accessed March 7, 2011).

8. S. Saul, Need a knee replaced? Check your ZIP code, *New York Times*, June 11, 2007, H6.

9. R. A. Deyo, Back surgery: Who needs it? *New England Journal of Medicine* 356 (2007): 2239.

10. E. S. Fisher, cited in Saul, Need a knee replaced?

11. T. Bodenheimer, K. Grumbach, and R. A. Berenson, A lifeline for primary care, *New England Journal of Medicine* 360 (2009): 26.

12. M. B. Rosenthal, Nonpayment for performance? Medicare's new reimbursement rule, *New England Journal of Medicine* 357 (2007): 16.

13. R. M. Wachter, The "dis-location" of U.S. medicine: The implications of medical outsourcing, *New England Journal of Medicine* 354 (2006): 661.

14. R. M. Kirkner, Medical tourism up, posing ethical dilemmas for US docs, *General Surgery News* 36 (2009): 10.

15. J. Greenwald, The outsourced patient, *Proto* (Winter 2008), 10. Available at http://protomag.com/assets/the-outsourced-patient (accessed March 7, 2011).

16. www.planethospital.com, October, 2005.

17. www.vivcaxxine.com, October, 2005.

18. P. Hartzband and J. Groopman, Money and the changing culture of medicine, *New England Journal of Medicine* 360 (2009): 101.

19. K. Sack, Study links diagnosis of cancer to insurance, *New York Times*, Feb. 18, 2008, A10.

20. A. P. Wilper, S. W. Woolhandler, K. E. Lasser, et al., Health insurance and mortality in U.S. adults, *American Journal of Public Health* 99 (2009): 2289.

21. Institute of Medicine, *Care without Coverage: Too Little, Too Late* (Washington, D.C.: National Academy Press, 2002).

22. C. J. L. Murray and J. Frenk, Ranking 37th: Measuring the performance of the U.S. health care system, *New England Journal of Medicine* 362 (2010): 98.

23. World Health Organization, World Health Report 2000: *Health systems: Improving performance* (Geneva: World Health Organization, 2000).

24. R. B. Reich, Bust the health care trusts, *New York Times*, Feb. 24, 2010, A21.

25. K. Q. Seelya, Raising rates and eyebrows, *New York Times*, Feb. 10, 2010, A9.

26. D. D. Trunkey, A growing crisis in patient access to emergency care: A different interpretation and alternative solutions, *Bulletin of the American College of Surgeons* 91 (2006): 14.

27. H. C. Polk, Jr., Quality, safety, and transparency, *Annals of Surgery* 242 (2005): 1.

28. Cited in K. M. Ludmerer, *Time to Heal: American Medical Education from the Turn of the Century to the Era of Managed Care* (Oxford: Oxford University Press, 1999), 374.

29. R. H. Murray and V. L. Bonham, Jr., The threatened role of volunteer faculty members, *Academic Medicine* 66 (1991): 445.

30. J. R. Krevans, Medicine's dying angels, *Johns Hopkins Magazine* (Aug. 1989), 40.

31. S. J. Heinig, J. Y. Krakower, H. B. Dickler, and D. Korn, Sustaining the engine of U.S. biomedical discovery, *New England Journal of Medicine* 357 (2007): 1042.

32. E. G. Campbell, J. S. Weissman, and D. Blumenthal, Relationship between market competition and the activities and attitudes of medical school faculty, *Journal of the American Medical Association* 278 (1997): 222.

33. S. L. Isaacs and S. A. Schroeder, California dreamin': State health care reform and the prospect for national change, *New England Journal of Medicine* 358 (2008): 1537.

34. R. Kuttner, Market-based failure: A second opinion on U.S. health care costs, *New England Journal of Medicine* 358 (2008): 549.

35. P. V. Rosenau and S. H. Linder, Two decades of research comparing for profit versus non-profit performance in the U.S., *Social Science Quarterly* 84 (2003): 2.

36. J. Geyman, *The Corrosion of Medicine: Can the Profession Reclaim Its Moral Legacy?* (Monroe, Maine: Common Courage Press, 2008).

37. T. Bodenheimer and D. West, Low cost lessons from Grand Junction, Colorado, *New England Journal of Medicine* 363 (2010): 15.

38. Centers for Medicare and Medicaid Services, National Health Expenditure Fact Sheet. Available at http://www.cms.hhs.gov/NationalHealthExpendData/25_ NHE_Fact_Sheet.asp (accessed March 23, 2011).

39. S. Rosenbaum, Medicaid and national health care reform, *New England Journal of Medicine* 361 (2009): 21.

40. B. Woo, Primary care: The best job in medicine? *New England Journal of Medicine* 355 (2006): 846.

41. Senator Chuck Grassley, Health care reform: A Republican view, *New England Journal of Medicine* 361 (2009): :25.

42. S. R. Matula, J. Beers, J. Errante, et al., Operation Access: A proven model for providing volunteer surgical services to the uninsured in the United States, *Journal of the American College of Surgeons* 209 (2009): 769.

43. M. Weber, *The Protestant Ethic and the Spirit of Capitalism* (New York: Charles Scribner and Sons, 1959).

ACKNOWLEDGMENTS

Many people helped in this book's evolution. My teachers and mentors were of enduring importance, particularly as their wisdom and encouragement from so many years ago percolated subliminally to the surface as I wrote. The debt all surgeons owe to such individuals who molded their own careers is incalculable. I am especially indebted for the practical advice of colleagues and friends who kindly reviewed parts of the emerging text, particularly David Brooks, Bridget Craig, Robert Gray, Nicholas O'Connor, Robert Sells, and Howard Snyder. Their suggestions, criticism, and advice were most welcome. Brian Bator cheerfully aided with the illustrations. My conversations with Caprice Greenberg and Damanpreet Bedi, newly minted surgical residents, about the changes in the academic curriculum and in their own training during the past few years were most enlightening. Christine Royse in the Admissions Department of the Brigham and Women's Hospital and social worker Paul Faircloth spent much time describing the problems they face in ensuring adequate coverage for the patients. I am particularly grateful to Michael Zinner, Surgeon-in-Chief of the Brigham and Women's Hospital, for generously providing me with an office and secretarial help during the years the project took to emerge. He has guided the Department of Surgery through an unprecedented and unrelenting period of social, financial, professional, and educational turbulence. Donald Cutler, my accomplished and experienced literary agent, suggested sensible and sometimes ingenious means of organizing and embellishing the developing manuscript. It would not have achieved completion without his gentle goading and wise advice. The encouragement and editing of Michael Fisher and Kate Brick of Harvard University Press have improved the book immeasurably. I am most appreciative of their substantial efforts. My daughters, Rebecca, Louise, Victoria, and Frances, have put up with the vagaries of a surgical father during most of their lives, yet have escaped to become talented and productive members of society. Most especially, my wife, Mary, has consistently provided me with an aura of calm and productivity. I owe her more than I can ever express.

INDEX

Abbott, Edward, 69
Abbott Laboratories, 125
Abraham, E. P., 124
academic medicine, 291, 314
Accreditation Council for Graduate
  Education, 286
Addison, Joseph, 136
Addison, Thomas, 77
adrenal glands, 257
African Americans, 62, 173–176, 244
Agatha, Saint, 220
Allen, Frederick, 143–144
Allgemeines Krankenhaus, 70
ambulance personnel, responsibilities
  of, 154
ambulances, 36, 101, 290
American Association of Medical
  Colleges, 287, 314
American Board of Surgery, 86, 87, 88
American Cancer Society, 150
American Civil War, 10, 67, 100, 101
American College of Surgeons, 86, 87,
  117, 260, 263
American Cyanamid Company, 125
American Medical Association, 47
American Recovery and Reinvestment
  Act, 315
American Society for the Prevention of
  Cruelty to Animals, 137
amputations, 53, 98, 99
anatomy, understanding of, 60–63, 133
anatomy schools, 61
André, Brother, 158
anesthesia: cocaine used as, 83;
  introduction of, 68–69; local, 83;
  and obesity surgery, 27–28, 33;
  pharmacological advances in, 23,
  33; resistance to, 70; risks of, 75–76.
  See also chloroform anesthesia; ether
  anesthesia; spinal anesthesia
anesthesiology, 11, 76
aneurysms, aortic, 17–25, 133,
  275–276

Angel of Bethesda, The (Mather), 45
angina pectoris, 195–199
animal experimentation: advances from,
  139; antivivisectionist movement,
  136–138; in art and fiction, 136;
  in cancer research, 148; in diabetes
  research, 144–148; for heart disease,
  197; in heart surgery research, 164,
  168, 170, 172, 174, 177, 189, 192; for
  mechanical hearts, 204–205, 207–208;
  in organ transplantation, 220, 223–
  224, 227–228; physiology understood
  through, 133–134; pre-anesthesia, 133;
  standards and regulations, 138
Anthem Blue Cross, 312
Anthony of Padua, Saint, 220
anthrax, 73
antibacterials, 120–121
antibiosis, 121
antibiotics: bacteria-resistant, 117, 124;
  introduction of, 116–117. See also
  specific antibiotics
anticoagulants, 111–112; heparin, 111,
  188
antimicrobials, 124
antisepsis, 72, 97, 99
antiseptics, 101
antivivisectionist movement, 136–138
aorta, 19
aortic coarctation, 170–172, 193
aortic stenosis, 192–194
appendicitis/appendectomy, 77–80
Arataeus, 141
Aristotle, 158
arteriograms, 19–20
arteriosclerosis, 16–17, 18, 196, 276
artificial heart, 202–212
asepsis: advances in sterilization,
  81–82, 112; early uses and
  improvements, 9, 71–75, 77, 84;
  effects of, 67, 97, 116; present day
  techniques, 131; resistance to, 57; use
  in wartime, 101

Atlas of Surgical Operations (Cutler and Zollinger), 89
atomic bomb, 227
autopsy, 133–134

bacteria: antibiotic-resistant, 117–118, 124; role in peptic ulcer disease, 95–96
bacteriology, 120
Bailey, Charles, 183–184, 185
Banting, Frederick, 144–148
bariatric surgery, 25–30, 32–34, 96. *See also* gastric bypass surgery
Barnard, Christiaan, 229, 233
Barnes Hospital, 41
Baronio, Giuseppe, 221, 223
Battle of Crécy, 98
Bavolek, Cecelia, 191
Baylor College of Medicine, 204–206
Beaulieu, Jacques de, 54
Beaumont, William, 89–90
Beck, Claude, 198
Bedi, Damanpreet, 281–283
Bell, John, 65
Bellah, Robert, 206–207
Berman, Elliott, 94–95
Bernard, Claude, 133
Best, Charles, 145–148
Bigelow, Wilfred, 192
Billroth, Theodor, 91–92, 160
biomedical innovation, funding, 204, 205–206, 208, 210
biotechnology industry, 315
bladder stones, 52–54
Blalock, Alfred, 172–177, 192, 279
bleeding, control of, 84–85, 90, 94, 98
blood banks, 111, 113
blood groups, 111
bloodletting, 55–57, 109–110, 143, 152
blood pressure cuff, 11
blood transfusions, 82–83, 101, 109–111, 188
blue babies, 173–176, 192, 279
Blundell, James, 110
bodies, trafficking in, 62, 238–239
bodysnatching, 61–63

bone grafts, 105
bone marrow transplantation, 233
Boothby, Walter, 11, 76
Borel, Jean, 234
Boston City Hospital, 37, 42
Botox, 118
Bovie, William, 85
brain death, 159, 229–230
breast cancer, 148–149, 254, 256–258
Brigham, Peter Bent, 15–16, 38–39, 42, 43
Brigham, Uriah, 38
Brigham and Women's Hospital, 2, 39, 258–259. *See also* Peter Bent Brigham Hospital; Robert Breck Brigham Hospital
Brinkley, J. R., 222
British Medical Research Council, 122
Brock, Russell, 184
Brunton, Lauder, 180, 181, 184
Budd-Chiari syndrome, 213, 215
Burcham, Jack, 209
Burke, William, 62
Burney, Fanny, 68
burn management, 106–108
Burrows, Mary, 306
Bush, Vannevar, 149–150

Cabral, Barthelemy, 158
Caligula, 221
Calne, Roy, 227, 233, 235
Campbell, Bruce, 218–219
cancer, 230–231; research and treatment, 148–149. *See also specific types*
cardiac catheterization, 182–183, 191
cardiac surgeons, 288
cardiology, 161
cardiopulmonary bypass, 184, 189–191, 194–195, 201
cardio-thoracic surgeons, 289
Carnegie, Andrew, 149
Carnegie Corporation, 48
Carnot, Sadi, 166–167
Caroline of Ansbach, 64
Carrel, Alexis: antiseptic solution introduced, 101; antivivisectionist's protest, 137; continuing influence of,

167; heart research, 171, 188, 199, 204; suturing technique, 167, 170, 223; transplantation research, 223
Caserio, Santo, 166
cataract surgery, 3–5
cathode ray, 81
Catholic hospitals, 244
CAT scans, 79
cautery, 84–85
Celsus, 53–54, 98, 109
cephalosporins, 124
Chain, Ernst, 122–124
Charnley, John, 131
Cheever, David, 8–11, 13–15, 254, 285
chest wounds, 153–157, 164
childbirth, 69–71, 110–111, 116
Children's Health Insurance Program, 318
Children's Hospital (Boston), 37, 42, 278
China, 113, 238, 309
chloroform anesthesia, 69, 100
cholera, 73
circulatory system, 11–12, 56, 110, 161–162
Clark, Barney, 208–209
clostridium, 118–119
Clowes, George, 146, 147
Cocoanut Grove nightclub fire, 106–107
Code of King Hammurabi of Mesopotamia, 265
Cold War, 112–113
Collins, Wilkie, 136
Collip, J. B., 146–148
colostomy, 64
Columbia University School of Medicine, 41
commoditization of the human body, 62, 238–239, 308–309
common bile duct, 214
Company of Barber Surgeons, 61
compound fracture, 71–72
Cooley, Denton, 202–203, 205–206
Cooper, Astley, 13, 221
coronary bypass surgery, 200–201, 308

corticosteroids, 126
Cosmas, Saint, 220
Costello, Joseph, 16, 18–20, 22–25, 34, 246, 258, 262, 264, 276
Council of Tours, 58
Cournand, André, 183
Crafoord, Clarence, 171
Crawford, Jane, 65–66
cretinism, 140–141
Crile Clinic, 80
Crimean War, 99, 101
criminals, bodies of executed, 61–62
Cross, David, 269–270
Cruikshank, Thomas, 58
Curley, James Michael, 40
Cushing, Harvey: career satisfaction, 75, 76; characteristics of, 253; expectations of, 242; on faculty system, 49; and heart research, 177, 180; on injuries of war, 100–101; and operative hygiene, 9, 117; reputation of, 14; staff of, 9; surgical advances, adoption of, 11, 83, 85; teaching responsibilities of, 134–135
Cutler, Elliott, 88–89, 181–182, 183, 187, 197
Cyclosporin A, 234, 235
cyclotron, 109

Dakin, Henry, 101
Damian, Saint, 220
Darwin, Charles, 53, 137
Darwinian theory of evolution, 135, 136
Daumier, Honoré, 58
Davy, Humphry, 68
death: beliefs about, 158–159; in children, 45; delaying through technology, 159–160, 202–203, 212; and end-of-life criteria, 159, 160, 229–230; organ donation and, 219, 229–230. *See also* brain death
death committees, 299
DeBakey, Michael, 204–205
De Curtorum Chirugia per Insitionem (Tagliacozzi), 104
de Gaulle, Charles, 21

Denis, Jean, 110
dentistry, 220
DeVries, William, 207–210
diabetes mellitus, 141–148, 316
diagnostic medicine, 134
diagnostic procedures, advances in,
    81–82. *See also* technological advances
dialysis, 94, 102, 118–119, 218,
    299–300
dialysis machine, 207, 210
diathermy (electrocautery), 85
digitalis, 161
disease, moral doctrine of, 44
diverticulosis, 254
doctor-patient relationship, 264
Doctor's Riot, 62
Domagk, Gerhard, 121
Doyle, Arthur Conan, 136
ductus arteriosis, 167–170, 279
Dunant, J. H., 99–100

Eakins, Thomas, 72
Edward VII, 77–78
Ehrlich, Paul, 119–120, 122
Eli Lilly and Company, 146, 147
Eliot, Charles William, 37, 47, 137
embolectomy catheter, 179
embolus, arterial, 178–180
emergency rooms, 153–157, 250–251,
    289–290
endocrine system, 126, 139–149,
    197–198
endoscopy, 275–277
Esperanza, Carmen, 213–217
ether anesthesia, 11, 14, 68–69, 75–76,
    83
experimentation on animals. *See* animal
    experimentation
experimentation on humans, questions
    of, 210–211, 265

face masks, 9
face transplants, 105–106
facial reconstruction, 103–106
Faraday, Michael, 68
Favaloro, René, 200
Félix, Charles François, 59–60

fetal surgery, 277–278
fistula-in-ano (anal fistula), 59–60
Fitz, Reginald, 77
Fleming, Alexander, 101, 120–124
flexible image transmission camera
    systems, 31
Flexner, Abraham, 48
Florey, Howard, 121–124
Fogarty, Thomas, 179
Foley embolectomy catheter, 179
Food and Drug Administration (FDA),
    207, 208, 209, 210, 212
Forssmann, Werner, 182–183
Franco-Prussian War, 73, 98, 143
Franklin, Benjamin, 52
French Imperial Academy of Medicine,
    67
Freud, Sigmund, 83

Galen, 56, 60, 84, 132, 158
gallbladder functions, 214, 254–255
gallbladder surgery, 31, 32, 83, 86, 277
gallstones, 254–255
gangrene, 71, 79, 99, 100, 118–119
gas gangrene, 118–119
gastric bypass surgery, 25–30, 32–34,
    67, 277
gastric physiology, 89–90, 92–93
gastritis (peptic disease), 94–95
gastroenterostomy, 92–93
general practitioners, 241, 243, 251
genomic therapy, 297
George II, 64
germ theory of disease, 73
Gibbon, John, Jr., 184, 186, 188–191
Gibbon, Mary, 189
Gillette, King, 10
Gillies, Harold, 104–105
Gilman, Daniel Coit, 40
gland grafting, 221–223
goiters, 125, 140
Gothergill, John, 195
grafts, future of, 296. *See also specific types*
Grand Junction, Colorado, 317
Greenberg, Caprice, 283–284, 290
Gross, Robert, 168–172, 176–177, 271,
    278

Gross, Samuel, 72
gunshot wounds, 98–99, 100, 153–157, 163–164
Gutenberg, Johannes, 60

Halsted, William Stewart: contributions of, 82–84, 86, 134–135, 139; influence of, 88, 135; mastectomy popularization, 256; and resident training, 242–243; on standardized education, 87; surgical technique of, 76–77, 86, 164
Hare, William, 62
Harken, Dwight, 164–165, 183–184, 204
Harrison, William Henry, 62
Harvard Medical School: anesthesiology department, 76; beginnings, 36–37; the Brigham and, 2, 15, 39–40, 42, 135, 139; Eliot's reforms of, 37, 47; and faculty salaries, 49; 1900 expansion, 37–38
Harvey, William, 11–12, 56, 110
Haydon, Murray, 209
health care: changes, 258–260; community involvement in, 317; cost-effective priorities, 262–263; equity of access to, 316, 318–319, 322; legislating, 299–300; outsourcing, 287, 307–309; urban and rural, 290, 320. *See also* socioeconomics of medical care
health care litigation, 260, 265, 290, 318, 320
health care reform, 287, 299, 316, 318–322
health care system: bureaucracy in, 301–302; market-driven structure of, 290, 300–303, 311–316, 318
health insurance. *See* insurance, health
health maintenance organizations (HMOs), 300, 305–307, 312
heart: anatomy and role in circulation, 161–162; early understanding of, 11–12; mechanical, 202–212; as symbol, 158, 160
heart attacks, 17, 196–197

heart-lung machine, 184, 189–191, 194–195, 201
heart surgery, 184; for adult abnormalities, 178–185, 192–194; advances in, 125, 164–166, 184, 189–192, 194–195, 200–202, 275–276; for angina relief, 198; for congenital anomalies, 167–172, 173–176, 191–193; coronary bypass, 200–201; early instances, 160–161, 163–164, 180–181; emergency, 165–166; opposition to, 169, 181, 187; valve replacement in adults, 192–194, 275
heart transplantation, 202–203, 206, 212, 229, 233
Heberden, William, 195
Henry VIII, 61
heparin, 111, 188
hernia repair, 63–65, 86
Herrick, Richard, 225–226
Herrick, Ronald, 225–226
Hippocrates, 56, 141, 158
hip replacement surgery, 130–131
hirudin, 111
Hogarth, William, 136
Holmes, Oliver Wendell, 50, 70
Homans, John, 13
hormone replacement therapy, 199
Hospital Corporation of America (HCA), 312–313
hospitals: history of, 43–46; investor-owned specialty, 316–317; for-profit vs. not-for-profit, 316–317; operative hygiene in, 71–75; public distrust of, 8, 43, 45; reforms in, 50, 99; sanitary conditions, 45; university-affiliated, 2, 48–49, 258–259, 291–292, 313–315. *See also* military hospitals; *specific hospitals*
Howard University College of Medicine, 244
HR1, 299–300
Hufnagel, Charles, 170–172, 193–194
Huggins, Charles, 148–149, 257
Humana Corporation, 209
human body, commoditization of, 62, 238–239, 308–309

Hume, David, 224–225, 271
Hunter, John, 61, 89, 132, 220
Hunter, William, 61
hydrocephalus treatment, 139
hysterectomy, 86

I. G. Farben Company, 121
imaging technology, 19–20, 31, 79,
    182–183. *See also* X-rays
immune system function, 231–232
immunization in wartime, 101, 118
immunologic tolerance, 236
immunosuppression, 227–228, 230
immunosuppressive drugs, 234–236
indigent, treatment of, 16, 38, 39–40,
    42, 45
Industrial Revolution, 44–45
infection, understanding, 72–74
infection control: in Chinese hospitals,
    113; early methods of, 70–71,
    98; immunization for, 101; with
    antibiotics, 116–124; in war wounds,
    98–101
Innocent VIII, 110
Institute of Medicine, 311
insulin, 141–148
insurance, health, 6, 316, 318, 321. *See
    also* insurance companies; Medicaid;
    Medicare; uninsured patients
insurance companies: cost control
    strategies, 27, 80, 298–299, 302–303,
    305, 310; executive salaries in,
    312, 321; legislative protections,
    312; medication coverage by, 304;
    profits, 312–313; public respect for,
    312; reforms proposed, 321–322;
    reimbursement fraud by, 312–313. *See
    also* third-party payers
internal medicine. *See* general
    practitioners
intestinal obstruction, treatment for,
    63–65
intravenous fluids and nutrition,
    114–116
intravenous tubing, 112–114
investor-owned specialty hospitals,
    316–317

iodine, 125, 140–141
iron lung, 160

Jacobson, Conrad, 14, 262
Jarvik, Robert, 207–210
Johns Hopkins Hospital, 40, 48,
    82–83, 242
Johns Hopkins Medical School, 23,
    40–41, 48–49
Johns Hopkins University, 134
Johnson, Samuel, 136
Joint Commission International, 308
Joyce, James, 89

Karp, Haskell, 202–206
Kelly, John, 21
kidney transplantation: abroad,
    308–309; advances in, 228–229,
    235; early efforts, 218, 223,
    224–226; legislating coverage for,
    299–300; monitoring prior to, 215;
    morbidity and mortality, 230–231,
    235; research, 128–130, 223–229;
    results of, 219, 226; statistics, 236
Knox, Robert, 62
Koch, Robert, 72, 73, 119, 136
Kolff, Willem, 207–208, 210
Koller, Carl, 83
Korean War, 98, 102, 172

Laennec, René-Théophile-Hyacinthe,
    159
Lahey Clinic, 80
Lancet, 55
Landseer, Edwin, 136
Landsteiner, Karl, 111
Langerhans, Ernst, 141–142
laparoscopy, 30–32, 274
Larrey, Baron Dominique Jean, 53, 68,
    101, 163
Lasker, Mary, 150
Lasker Foundation, 150
Lautz, David, 25–26, 33–34
Laverne, Shirley, 25–29, 96, 259, 262,
    274
Lavoisier, Antoine, 188
leeches, 57, 111

Leeuwenhoek, Anthony van, 72
Leo I, 220
Leonardo da Vinci, 60
leprosy, 105
liability insurance, 290–291
Lindbergh, Charles, 188, 204
Liotta, Domingo, 204–206
Lister, Joseph, 71–72, 75, 78, 132, 256
Lister, Joseph Jackson, 73
lithotomy, 52–54
liver, 213–214
liver transplantation, 214–217
Long, Crawford, 69
Louis XIV, 59–60, 110
Lower, Richard, 110, 187–188
lungs, artificially supported, 159
lymphocytes/lymph nodes, 232, 234
lysozyme, 121–122

MacLean, Jay, 188
Macleod, J. J. R., 145, 146, 148
Magendie, Françoise, 133
Malpighi, Marcello, 12
malpractice insurance, 289
managed care, 300. *See also* health
  maintenance organizations (HMOs)
marginal ulcer, 92
Mark, Saint, 220
market-driven health care, 290,
  300–303, 311–316, 318
Marshall, Barry, 96
Marston, Jonathan, 308–309
MASH units (mobile army surgical
  hospitals), 102, 103
Massachusetts General Hospital: the
  Brigham and, 2, 15, 41–42; faculty
  and staff, 37, 244; first successful
  operation under anesthesia, 17;
  medical training opportunities, 46;
  private practice plans, 49; relations
  with Harvard Medical School, 40;
  surgery statistics, 63; wealthy patrons
  of, 42
mastectomy, 68, 86, 256–258
Mather, Cotton, 45
Mayo, Charles, 76, 80, 117
Mayo, William, 76, 77, 80, 117

Mayo Clinic, 80, 126
McDowell, Ephraim, 65–66, 67
mechanical heart, 202–212
mechanical respiration, 159–160
Medawar, Peter, 223–224, 225, 236
Medicaid, 300, 303–304, 318
medical bureaucracy, 301–302
medical care, nonsurgical advances
  in, 125; nutritional, 114–116;
  pharmaceutical, 111–112; resistance
  to, 71
Medical College of Ohio, 62–63
medical education: changes, 258–261;
  cost controls and reductions in,
  314; costs, 48, 285–286, 318, 320;
  history of, 37, 40–42, 44–47, 61–63;
  postgraduate, 76, 80–81; reforms,
  40–42, 49–50. *See also* residency
  programs
medical profession: limitations, 50–51;
  after World War II, 127, 243–244;
  professional standards of, 46–47;
  respect for, 46, 49, 58
medical records, electronic, 316, 321
medical schools: acceptance
  demographics, 244; admission
  process, 269–271; admission
  standards, 37, 47; applicant
  demographics, 271–272; application
  statistics, 268; competency of
  graduates, 37; curricular changes in,
  84, 272–273; funding of, 48; for-
  profit, 47, 49; reforms, 37, 47. *See also*
  specific medical schools
medical tourism, 308–309
Medicare, 299–300, 303–305, 307,
  312–313, 317–318
medicine, future of, 296–302
Meharry Medical College, 244
meningitis, 137
menopause, 199
Merck Company, 123, 124, 126
microbiology, 73
microscope, invention of, 73
midwives, 70–71
military hospitals: MASH units, 102,
  103; Nightingale's reforms in, 99

mitral stenosis, 178–185
molecular biology, 152
Molière, 58
Moore, Francis, 130, 190, 211, 246, 266; contributions to medicine, 107, 109, 184
Morbidity/Mortality Conference, 249–250, 262
morbid obesity, 25–30, 96. *See also* bariatric surgery
Morgan, J. P., 149
Morton, William, 69, 70
Mount Sinai Hospital, 244
MRI visualization, 79
Mullins, Giles, 52–55, 57, 63, 67, 265
Murray, Joseph, 218, 219, 225, 227–228, 231
myxedema, 140

Napoleon Bonaparte, 52, 89, 101
Napoleonic Wars, 53, 101
Napoleon III, 52
National Health Service (U.K.), 318–319
National Heart Institute, 204, 205, 206, 208
National Institutes of Health, 138, 150, 151–152, 315
national transplant list, 215–216
needles, 81–82, 111
New York Hospital, 46
New York State Commissioner of Health, 260
Nightingale, Florence, 45–46, 99–100
nitrous oxide, 68
Notes on Hospitals (Nightingale), 100
Novartis, 234
nurses, 99–100, 249
nursing reforms, 45–46
nutrition, parenteral, 114–116

obesity: in children, 26; epidemic of, 26, 143, 316. *See also* morbid obesity
Ochsner Clinic, 80
Opie, Eugene, 142
organ donation: cadavers for, 224–225, 238; death and, 219, 229–230;

moral and ethical questions about, 215, 229; national transplant list for, 215–216; need for, 236; and surgical techniques, 277
organ transplantation: challenges of, 237–239; future of, 236–237; historical, 219–221; outside the United States, 238, 308–309; pharmaceutical research and, 234–236; rejection in, 224, 228, 232; for sexual vitality, 221–223; socioeconomics of, 237–239; symbol of, 220. *See also specific organs*
O'Rourke, Tommy, 157, 161, 174
orthopedics, 131
Osler, William, 23, 50, 56–57, 116, 140, 196
outcomes research, 292
ovarian cyst removal, 65–66, 67
ovaries, removal of, 257
Ovid, 109

Paget, Stephen, 160
Palazola, Joe, 230–231
pancreas, 141–148
pancreatic tumors, 254
Paré, Ambroïse, 98, 132, 158
parenteral nutrition, 114–116
Paris Faculty of Medicine, 60
Pasteur, Louis, 72, 73, 136
pathologists, 251
patient records, computerized, 316, 321
patients: admission process, 18–19, 247, 262; advocates for, 302–303; care for, 258–259; expectations, 264, 280; and relationship with doctor, 264–265; and rights, 264; and safety protocols, 262
Patient's Bill of Rights, 264
Paulesco, Nicolas, 144, 145
pedical grafts, 198
pedical tube grafts, 104, 105
peer review, early forms of, 79
penicillin, 122–124
Pennsylvania Hospital, 46, 48
peptic ulcer disease, 89–93, 95–96, 254

Pepys, Samuel, 52, 110
pericarditis, 163, 198
Peter, Saint, 220
Peter Bent Brigham Hospital:
  advancement of medical reforms,
  50; ambulances, 36; application and
  admission statistics, 269; association
  with Harvard Medical School, 2, 15,
  39–40, 42, 135, 139; beginnings,
  17–19, 38–39; described, 8–9, 17–18,
  35–36; endowment, 2, 15–16, 38,
  39; first surgical patient, 2, 7–15,
  35–36; indigent care, 16; operative
  hygiene, 9–11; opposition to, 41–42;
  private practice plans, 49; residency
  application process, 240–241; surgical
  advances, 16, 18, 22–25; surgical
  costs, 24–25
Pfizer, 123
pharmaceutical advances, 111–112,
  116, 125, 234–236
pharmaceutical industry: academic
  laboratory collaborations, 125, 126,
  147; after World War II, 97, 123,
  125–126; executive salaries in, 312,
  321; growth of, 126; legislative
  protections of, 316; patents by, 147;
  reforms proposed, 321. *See also specific
  companies*
pharmacology, experimental, 119–120
Philip VI, 98
physicians: declining numbers of,
  286–287; educational debt, 318, 320;
  history of, 43–44, 50, 58; income
  of, 318–319, 320; leadership in
  health care reform, 317. *See also specific
  specialties*
physician scientists, 291
physiology, understanding, 132–134,
  139. *See also* animal experimentation
pituitary gland, 126, 257
plastic and reconstructive surgery,
  103–106
polio, 125, 160
polio vaccine, 150
Pope, Alexander, 136
Presbyterian Hospital (New York), 41

Priestley, Joseph, 68
Principles and Practice of Medicine, The
  (Osler), 56–57
prisoners: executed, body parts from,
  222, 225, 238, 309; experimentation
  on, 222
prisoners of war, 103–104
prostate cancer, 148, 254, 274–275
prosthetics, 296
psychiatrists, 251
public health, 43, 45, 49, 125, 149, 316
puerperal fever, 70–71
pulmonary embolectomy, 17, 186–189
pyloric obstruction, 92

Queen Mary's Hospital, 104–105

radiation, 227–228
radiologists, 251, 307–308
radiology departments, 81
Red Cross, 100
research, university-based: beginnings,
  134–135, 139; challenges faced,
  291–294; funding, 149–152, 291,
  315; future of, 291; pharmaceutical
  industry collaborations, 125, 126,
  147. *See also* animal experimentation
residency programs, 84, 88, 127, 242;
  admissions, 268–272; application
  process, 240–242, 244–246; attrition
  rate, 243; changes in, 253–254,
  273–274; legislation, 260–262;
  length of, 242–243, 267; nurses' role
  in, 249; structure of, 246–253
residents: demographics, 263, 267,
  268–269, 288; educational debt,
  284–286; emergency rotations, 153,
  290; goodbye ceremony, 267–268;
  income, 130, 253, 285
respirators, 159–160
resurrectionists, 61–63
rheumatic heart disease, 177–185
Richards, Dickinson, Jr., 183
Robert Breck Brigham Hospital, 39
robotics, 274–275, 279–280
Rockefeller, John D., 149
Rockefeller Foundation, 48–49, 122

Roentgen, Wilhelm, 81, 164
Roosevelt, Franklin D., 149
Royal College of Surgeons, 134
Royal Infirmary of Edinburgh, 53
Royal Navy, 68
Rush, Benjamin, 56
Russians, 150
Rutgers University, 124

Salvarsan, 120, 121
Sandoz, 234
Sauerbruch, Ferdinand, 183
scalpels, 1, 10–11
Schroeder, William, 209
Science: The Endless Frontier (Bush), 150
sedatives, 65, 67–68
Sells, Robert, 113
Semb, Bjarne, 209
Semmelweis, Ignaz Philipp, 70–71
sepsis, 70
septal defect, 190–192
Servetus, Michael, 60–61
Shakespeare, William, 89
Shelley, Percy Bysshe, 158
shock wave treatment, 54
Shumway, Norman, 233
Sims, Marion, 65–67
Sir William Dunn School of Pathology,
    121–124
skin grafts, 105, 108, 221, 223–224,
    226, 296
sleep apnea, 25, 27
smallpox, 101
socioeconomics of medical care, 62,
    238–239, 281, 304; and emergency
    rooms, 290; historical, 8, 38, 39–40,
    42–44, 45; in hospital, 244, 248–
    249; market-driven model, 300–303,
    311–317; percent of GDP, 318; at
    teaching hospitals, 48, 313–314;
    uninsured and, 311, 312–313. *See also*
    third-party payers
Souttar, Henry, 181, 184
specialization, growth in, 243, 288
spinal anesthesia, 83
Squibb, 123

standards of care, 86
stapling instruments, 29, 30–34
Starzl, Thomas, 228
St. Bartholomew's Hospital, 52–53
St. Elizabeth's Hospital, 244
stem cell therapy, 296–297
Stenberg, Leif, 209
sterilizers, development of, 112
steroids, 126, 228
stethoscope, 159
Stevenson, Robert Louis, 136
St. Luke's Hospital, 205
St. Martin, Alexis, 90
St. Mary's Hospital, 120–121
stomach cancer, 254
stomach removal, 95
streptomycin, 124, 125
sulfanilamide, 121, 125
surgeons: academic, 129–131,
    149, 291–294; battlefield, 100;
    certification requirements, 86–88,
    134; characteristics, 43–44, 251–253,
    263, 265–266; declining numbers,
    287–288, 294; dissatisfaction and
    disillusionment, 264; emergency calls
    and, 290–291; income, 286,
    288–289; insurance requirements
    for, 289, 290–291; in the Middle
    Ages, 58–59; of the nobility, 59–60;
    physicians vs., 58; respect for, 58,
    60, 65; suicide rates among, 264;
    volunteer care by, 321. *See also specific
    specialties*
surgery, 254–256; after World War
    I, 101; alternatives to, 63–65; in the
    ancient world, 57–58; and costs, 15,
    279–281; future of, 296–302; and
    morbidity and mortality, 54–55,
    64–65, 67, 70–72, 99, 116–117;
    in operating theaters, 9, 53; and
    operative hygiene, 9–10, 33, 54,
    70–74, 75, 81–82, 84; outpatient,
    262; patient preparation for, 55;
    religious objections to, 58; risks,
    117, 178–180, 263–264; ritualistic
    aspects, 14; time required for, 53,

55, 75, 77; in twenty-first century,
5–6, 292–293, 302–303; violence of,
53–55, 57, 68. *See also specific surgical
interventions*
surgical care: pharmacological adjuncts,
125; post-trauma supportive
measures, 108–111, 112–114,
114–116; sterilization, 112
surgical education: contributors to, 134;
costs, 284–285; twenty-first century,
281–286. *See also* residency programs
surgical profession: basic tenets,
266; challenges faced, 293–294;
foundations threatened, 280–281
Surgical Safety Checklist, 292
surgical scientists, 129–131
Sushruta, 103–104, 158
sutures, 24, 66–67, 167, 169
syphilis, 104, 120, 137
syringes, glass, 111

Tagliacozzi, Gasparo, 104
Taussig, Helen, 173–175, 192
teaching hospitals. *See* hospitals,
university-affiliated
technological advances: ball valve,
193–194; blood bag, 112; bypass
machine, 184, 189–191, 194–195,
201; computerized patient records,
316; delaying death through,
159–160, 202–203, 212;
electrocautery, 85–86; embedded
micro-apparatuses, 296; fiber-optics,
54; Foley embolectomy catheter, 179;
in imaging, 19–20, 31, 79, 81,
182–183; in needles, 111; plastic
tubing, 112–113; resistance to,
182–183; robotics, 274–275,
279–280; scalpels, 10; stapling
instruments, 29, 30–34; sterilization,
112; synthetic grafts, 172; syringes,
111; valvulotome, 181
teeth, transplantation of, 220
teleradiologists, 287, 307–308
testis, 221–223
tetanus toxoid vaccine, 118

tetralogy of Fallot, 173–176
Texas Heart Institute, 202–203
Textbook of Surgery (Homans), 13
third-party payers: cost-reduction
programs, 308–311; HMOs, 300,
305–307, 312; market-driven model,
303, 310; public respect for, 310,
312; reimbursement limitations, 316;
restriction of care methods, 305–307,
316. *See also* insurance companies
Thomas, Vivien, 172–176
Thompson, Leonard, 147
thyroid, 197–198
*Total Dietary Regulation in the Treatment of
Diabetes* (Allen), 143
transplantation biology, 224
transplant list. *See* national transplant
list
trauma care. *See* war, advances resulting
from
Trelawney, E. J., 158
Treves, Frederick, 64, 78
tuberculosis, 73, 119, 124, 125, 137,
207
Tufts University Medical School, 244
tumor removal, 64, 86
Turner, Mary Agnes, 7–15, 34, 35–36,
43, 157, 200, 246, 254, 258, 262,
264, 295
typhoid, 101

uninsured patients, 304, 311–313, 321
universal health care, 318–319, 322
university hospitals: expansion of,
258–259; market-driven structure,
313–315; private practice plans,
48–49; socioeconomics of health care,
48, 313–314; statistics, 2; surgical
careers, 291–292
University of Michigan Medical
School, 41, 48
University of Minnesota, 192
University of Oxford, 128–129
University of Pennsylvania, 48
University of Toronto, 147
University of Utah, 207–209

University of Wisconsin, 76
Upjohn, 126

vaccines: opposition to, 136; polio, 125, 150; rabies, 73, 136; smallpox, 101; tetanus, 118; typhoid, 101
valve replacement, 192–194, 275
valvulotome, 181
varicose veins, 7–15, 254
Varro, 72
vascular reconstruction of aortic aneurysms, 16–18, 22–25
vascular system function, 11–14
vein grafts, 200–201
Venables, James, 69
ventricular-assist devices, 212
Vesalius, Andreas, 60
vesico-vaginal fistula repair, 66–67
Victoria, Queen of England, 69
Vietnam War, 98, 102
Virgil, 220
vitamins, 125
vitriol (sulfuric acid), 84–85
Voltaire, 50
Voronoff, Serge, 222

Waksman, Selman, 124
war, advances resulting from: bone grafts to replace missing jaws, 105; gunshot wounds, treatment for, 98–99, 100; heart surgery, 163, 164–165; mass immunizations, 101; Nightingale's reforms, 99; overview, 96–98; pedical tube grafts, 105;

pharmacological, 126; plastic and reconstructive surgery, 103–106; transportation of the injured, 101–102; wound care, 101
war, devastation of, 98–101. *See also specific wars*
warfarin, 112
Warren, J. Collins, 17–18, 135
Warren, John Collins, 17, 69
Warren, Richard, 17, 18, 23–25, 187
Warren, Robin, 96
Washington University, 41
Washkansky, Louis, 229
Waters, Ralph, 76
Watska, Adolf, 9, 10
Watson, Thomas, 189
Weed, Louis, 139
WellPoint, 312
Wells, H. G., 136
Wells, Horace, 69, 70
Wells, Spencer, 67
Whatley, Thomas, 55
World War I, 9, 101, 104–105
World War II, 118, 122–123, 164–165, 227
wound care, 101, 296
wound healing, 125
Wren, Christopher, 110
Wright, Almroth, 101
wrong-site surgery, 292–293

X-rays, 19–20, 81, 164, 227–228

Zion, Libby, 260–261, 263